Locoregional Radionuclide Cancer Therapy

Franklin C. L. Wong
Editor

Locoregional Radionuclide Cancer Therapy

Clinical and Scientific Aspects

Springer

Editor
Franklin C. L. Wong
Department of Nuclear Medicine
University of Texas, M. D. Anderson Cancer Center
Houston, TX
USA

ISBN 978-3-030-56266-3 ISBN 978-3-030-56267-0 (eBook)
https://doi.org/10.1007/978-3-030-56267-0

This Springer imprint is published by the registered company Springer Nature Switzerland AG
The registered company address is: Gewerbestrasse 11, 6330 Cham, Switzerland

Preface

Radionuclide therapy by systemic administration is becoming mainstay of cancer therapy. It has developed from radio-iodide ablation to radionuclide palliative treatment of intractable cancer bone pain (Sr-89, Sm-153 EDTMP and Ra-223) and further to radioimmunotherapy (Lu-177 PSMA and other ligands) as well as treatment of osseous metastasis (Ra-223). Locoregional radionuclide therapy (LRCT) has great potential of harnessing pharmacokinetic advantages to expand therapeutic windows but is still in developing stages. Although LRCT shares locoregional characteristics of the widely accepted cancer therapy external beam radiotherapy, wide adoption of LRCT is limited by lack of understanding of its effects and radiation dosimetry to the target organs and to the rest of the organism.

Recent advances in instrumentation, imaging algorithm, and radiation dosimetry modeling have allowed accurate imaging of minute amounts of radioactivity in small volumes. Therefore, this is a prudent time to revisit the theoretical bases and practical issues of LRCT in the application to human cancer. The scope of human cancer, the current therapies, and locoregional radiotherapy of cancer are reviewed in the first three chapters. The current practices of radionuclide therapy and locoregional delivery by interventional schemes are covered in Chaps. 4 and 5. Simulated radiation dosimetry of target tissues and surrounding tissues from common geometric models of commercially available radionuclides is explored in Chap. 6 followed by detailed imaging schemes to derive empirical image-based dosimetry for correlation in Chap. 7. Experimental findings in animal models of LRCT are examined in Chap. 8 followed by available animal models for different tumor types in Chap. 9 to provide guidance for further animal trials. The practical, logistical, and regulatory aspects of performing LRCT clinical trials are described in Chap. 10 to guide practitioners in LRCT. Current clinical nuclear medicine studies are reviewed in Chap. 11 as introduction to possible future studies in LRCT.

The practice of LRCT is a multidisciplinary effort. The book is written with the intent to introduce LRCT to scientists, physicians, and potential LRCT practitioners in related disciplines with the hope to cover minimum requisites from each discipline. More efforts from more practitioners are certainly needed for LRCT to develop further into clinical trials.

Houston, TX, USA Franklin C. L. Wong

Acknowledgments

The editor gratefully acknowledges each author who contributed to the writing of this book with extraordinary efforts. The continuous support from Springer's Project Coordinator Abha Krishnan and Springer Editor Margaret Moore is sincerely appreciated.

Contents

1 **Human Cancer: Epidemiology, Hallmarks, and Defense Strategies** . 1
Brian S. Wong, Calvin W. Wong, and Franklin C. L. Wong

2 **Cancer Treatment Modalities Systemic and Locoregional Approaches: Challenges and Opportunities of Multidisciplinary Approaches** 17
Roberto Carmagnani Pestana and Nuhad K. Ibrahim

3 **Cancer Radiotherapy: General Considerations and Human Radiobiology** 39
Alison K. Yoder, Matthew S. Ning, Melissa M. Joyner, and Lilie L. Lin

4 **Radionuclide Cancer Therapy: Unsealed Alpha- and Beta-Emitters** 61
A. Cahid Civelek and Franklin C. L. Wong

5 **Locoregional Therapy: Cancer Interventions with and Without Radionuclides** 89
Steven Yevich and Armeen Mahvash

6 **Radiation Dosimetry Considerations of Locoregional Radionuclide Cancer Therapy** 111
Franklin C. L. Wong and Richard B. Sparks

7 **Voxel-Based Targeted Radionuclide Therapy Dosimetry** 133
Greta S. P. Mok

8 **Locoregional Unsealed Radionuclide Cancer Therapy: Experimental Findings** 159
Franklin C. L. Wong

9 Animal Cancer Therapy Models: Ready Translation to Humans . . . 189
V. Behrana Jensen and Suzanne L. Craig

10 An Overview of the Regulations of Radiopharmaceuticals 225
Dao Le

11 Locoregional Radionuclide Cancer Therapy (LRCT) Using Sealed and Unsealed Radionuclides 249
Franklin C. L. Wong

Index 263

Contributors

A. Cahid Civelek, MD Department of Radiology, Division of Nuclear Medicine and Molecular Imaging, Johns Hopkins Medicine, Baltimore, MD, USA

Suzanne L. Craig, DVM Medical University of South Carolina, Division of Laboratory Animal Resources, Charleston, SC, USA

Nuhad K. Ibrahim, MD Department of Breast Medical Oncology, The University of Texas MD Anderson Cancer Center, Houston, TX, USA

V. Behrana Jensen, DVM UT MD Anderson Cancer Center, Department of Veterinary Medicine and Surgery, Houston, TX, USA

Melissa M. Joyner, MD, MBA Department of Radiation Oncology, The University of Texas MD Anderson Cancer Center, Houston, TX, USA

Department of Radiation Oncology, The University of Texas Medical Branch, Galveston, TX, USA

Dao Le, PharmD The University of Texas, MD Anderson Cancer Center, Houston, TX, USA

Lilie L. Lin, MD Department of Radiation Oncology, The University of Texas MD Anderson Cancer Center, Houston, TX, USA

Armeen Mahvash, MD Department of Interventional Radiology, Division of Diagnostic Imaging, University of Texas MD Anderson Cancer Center, Houston, TX, USA

Greta S. P. Mok, PhD Biomedical Imaging Laboratory, Department of Electrical and Computer Engineering, Faculty of Science and Technology, University of Macau, Macau SAR, China

Matthew S. Ning, MD, MPH Department of Radiation Oncology, The University of Texas MD Anderson Cancer Center, Houston, TX, USA

Roberto Carmagnani Pestana, MD Division of Cancer Medicine, The University of Texas MD Anderson Cancer Center, Houston, TX, USA

Richard B. Sparks, PhD CDE Dosimetry Services, Inc., Knoxville, TN, USA

Brian S. Wong, MD, MPH Department of Radiology, University of Texas Medical Branch, Galveston, TX, USA

Calvin W. Wong, BA Department of Biological Sciences, Rice University, Houston, TX, USA

Franklin C. L. Wong, MD, PhD, JD Department of Nuclear Medicine, University of Texas, M. D. Anderson Cancer Center, Houston, TX, USA

Steven Yevich, MD, MPH Department of Interventional Radiology, Division of Diagnostic Imaging, University of Texas MD Anderson Cancer Center, Houston, TX, USA

Alison K. Yoder, MD Department of Radiation Oncology, The University of Texas MD Anderson Cancer Center, Houston, TX, USA

Chapter 1
Human Cancer: Epidemiology, Hallmarks, and Defense Strategies

Brian S. Wong, Calvin W. Wong, and Franklin C. L. Wong

Introduction

Cancer Epidemiology: The Human Costs in 2018

Cancer is a group of noncommunicable diseases (NCDs) that is characterized by malignant tumor cells that grow and spread abnormally. Currently, there are at least 100 types of cancer known to affect humans. Malignant tumor cells have the ability to grow locally, spread to adjacent tissue, and invade distant sites through a variety of mechanisms. The dysregulated growth is understood to result due to changes on a genetic level through causes including environmental factors, infectious agents, and genetic mutations. The clinical presentation of cancer is directly related to the location and type of tissue that the cancer cell arises from.

The incidence of cancer is expected to increase in the future, and it is projected to become the leading cause of death in the twenty-first century [1]. In 2018, an estimated 18.1 million cases of cancer were diagnosed worldwide, with 1.7 million cases in the USA [1, 2]. An estimated 199.8 cases of cancer per 100,000 people were diagnosed worldwide in 2018 [1]. From 2011 to 2015, 439.2 cases of cancer were diagnosed per 100,000 people every year in the USA [3]. Differences in incidence rate can be attributed to factors including differences in population age,

B. S. Wong (✉)
Department of Radiology, University of Texas Medical Branch, Galveston, TX, USA
e-mail: bswong@utmb.edu

C. W. Wong
Department of Biological Sciences, Rice University, Houston, TX, USA
e-mail: cwong@rice.edu

F. C. L. Wong
Department of Nuclear Medicine, University of Texas, M. D. Anderson Cancer Center, Houston, TX, USA
e-mail: fwong@mdanderson.org

F. C. L. Wong (ed.), *Locoregional Radionuclide Cancer Therapy*,
https://doi.org/10.1007/978-3-030-56267-0_1

growth, and access to screening. The rate of new cancer diagnoses in the USA has been decreasing by an average of 1.8% per year for men over the past decade and has remained unchanged for women [2].

Malignant neoplasms trailed behind cardiovascular disease as the second leading cause of death in the USA in 2016, with approximately 600,000 deaths [4]. Worldwide, mortality rates for cancer in 2018 were estimated to be 218.6 per 100,000 for men and 182.6 per 100,000 for women [1]. The mortality rate for cancer in the USA was 196.7 per 100,000 for men and 139.5 per 100,000 for women per year from 2011 to 2015 [2]. Mortality rate differences can be attributed to differences in population demographics and access to healthcare. The mortality rate of cancer in the USA has been decreasing by an average of 1.8% per year for men and 1.4% per year for women between 1999 and 2015 [3]. The mortality rate decreased continuously from 1991 to 2015 by a total of 26% [2].

While decrease in mortality rate may be correlated with advances in modern medicine, cancer has caused significant social and financial burden worldwide. In 2015, cancer caused 208.3 million years of disability-adjusted life years (DALY) globally with the majority of years (96%) attributable to years of life lost (YLL) due to premature death [5]. Cancer disproportionately affected individuals belonging to a higher sociodemographic index (SDI). Men in the highest SDI quintile were three times more likely to develop cancer compared to men in the lowest SDI quintile. For women, this effect was less significant, with women in the highest SDI quintile having a 60% increased chance of developing cancer compared to women in the lowest SDI quintile. In addition to morbidity and mortality, economic burden is a significant concern to societies with large populations of cancer survivors. In the USA, the national economic burden of cancer care in 2017 was estimated to be 147.3 billion USD [6]. This estimate is projected to rise as cancer prevalence increases and novel treatments become the standard of care.

Solid tumors are the most common cancers both worldwide and in the USA. The most common types of cancer diagnosed worldwide and in the USA in 2018 are estimated to be lung cancer (11.6%), female breast cancer (11.6%), prostate cancer (7.1%), and colorectal cancer (6.1%) [1] and female breast cancer (15.3%), lung and bronchus cancer (13.5%), prostate cancer (9.5%), colorectal cancer (8.1%), and melanoma (5.3%) [2], respectively. Other forms of solid cancer known to affect significant numbers in the USA include gynecologic (6.3%), thyroid (3.1%), kidney (3.8%), bladder (4.7%), and head and neck cancers (3.7%). Liquid tumors also cause significant morbidity in the USA and include leukemia (3.5%), lymphoma (4.8%), and myeloma (1.8%) [2]. Selected solid cancers of concern are discussed below.

Breast Cancer Breast cancer refers to malignant tumors that arise from breast tissue and includes subtypes such as infiltrating ductal carcinoma (70–80%), infiltrating lobular carcinoma (8%), and mixed ductal and lobular carcinomas (7%). They are further differentiated by molecular subtypes based on expression of genes such as human epidermal growth factor 2 (HER2) which determine prognosis and guide therapy. Breast cancer is the most common type of cancer in the USA with an estimated 266,120 diagnoses and 41,400 estimated deaths in 2018 [2]. Worldwide, 2,088,849 new cases of breast cancer were diagnosed in 2018 and 626,679 number of deaths, placing breast cancer as the second most common cancer worldwide behind lung cancer [1]. From 1999 to 2004, incidence rates of breast cancer decreased 2.3 percent per year in the USA. Studies have shown that this could be explained by a discontinuation of hormone replacement therapy and less likely a decline in screening mammography. More recent data from 2005 to 2014 shows that the incidence of breast cancer has risen by an average of 0.4% per year in the USA, but this is likely due to earlier detection from increased screening [2]. Breast cancer mortality rates have steadily declined since the 1970s. Data from 2011 to 2015 shows that the mortality rate has decreased by an average of 1.8% per year in the USA [2]. The decrease in mortality is attributable to improved breast cancer screening and adjuvant therapy. The 5-year survival rate for Stage 1 breast cancer was 100% in the USA from 2007 to 2013. From 2008 to 2014, the 5-year survival rate for all stages of breast cancer was 81.1% [3].

Lung/Bronchogenic Cancer Lung cancers arise from lung tissue and are divided into small-cell lung carcinoma (10%), non-small-cell lung carcinoma (85%), and other subtypes (5%). Non-small-cell carcinomas are further divided into squamous cell carcinoma, adenocarcinoma, and large-cell carcinoma. In the USA, lung cancer was the second most common type of cancer with an estimated 234,030 new cases and 154,050 deaths in 2018 [2]. Globally, lung cancer was the most common cancer type with 2,093,876 new diagnoses and 1,761,007 deaths [1]. Between 2008 and 2014, the 5-year survival rate was 16.2% [3]. Between 2005 and 2014, the incidence of lung cancer has decreased for males by 2.5% and for females by 1.2%. Between 2011 and 2015, the mortality rate decreased for males by 3.8% and by 2.3% for females [2]. In 2015, lung and bronchogenic cancers were the leading cause of cancer death for men, with 36.4 million DALYs [5].

Prostate Cancer Prostate cancer affects the gland responsible for production of seminal fluid in men. In 2018, the US incidence was 164,690 projected new cases and 29,430 deaths [2]. Globally in 2018, there were 1,276,106 cases and 358,989 deaths [1]. In the USA, incidence rates decreased by 5.6% between 2005 and 2014, and mortality rates decreased by 2.9% between 2006 and 2015 [2]. Between 2008 and 2014, the 5-year survival rate was 95.9% [3]. Globally, prostate cancer is one of the most common cancers for men, causing 6.3 million DALYs in 2015 [5].

Colorectal/Pancreatic/Stomach and Liver Cancer Colorectal cancer begins in the large intestine and usually arises from polyps that form on the inside of the colon. In 2018, there were 140,250 new cases and 50,630 deaths in the USA. Globally, there were 1,096,601 new cases and 861,662 deaths for 2018. Between 1998 and 2014, incidence of colorectal cancer decreased by 2.9% for males (?). For females, there was a 4.1% decrease based on delay-adjusted incidence rates between 2008 and 2012. The mortality rate decreased between 2011 and 2015 by 2.5% for males and 1.8% for females. The 5-year survival rate between 2008 and 2014 was 57.8% [3]. For 2015, colorectal cancers caused 17 million DALYs [5].

Pancreatic cancers are characterized by difficult early detection and aggressive growth. In the USA, there were 55,440 new cases of pancreatic cancer and 44,330 deaths in 2018. Globally, there were 458,918 new cases and 432,242 deaths. Between 2010 and 2014, incidence rates increased by 0.9% for males and 1.0% for females. Mortality rate for males (increased/decreased) by 0.3% between 2011 and 2015. For the same time period, there was no statistically significant change in mortality rate for females. Between 2008 and 2014, the 5-year survival rate was 8.6% [3].

Most stomach cancers arise from the gastric mucosa, and their development is correlated with consumption of smoked and salty foods. As refrigeration of food has become more widespread instead of smoking and salting, stomach cancer incidence rates have generally declined. The incidence of stomach cancer in the USA was 26,240, and the mortality was 10,800 in 2018. Worldwide, the incidence was 1,033,701, and the mortality was 782,685 for 2018. The 5-year survival rate from 2008 to 2014 was 31.1% [3]. 11.7 DALYs were attributed to stomach cancer in 2015 [5].

Liver cancers arise when the liver has already been affected either by hepatitis, alcohol abuse, or hemochromatosis. For 2018, there were 42,220 new cases and 30,200 liver cancer-related deaths. Globally, 841,080 new cases and 781,631 deaths were observed for 2018. Based on data from 2005 to 2014, incidence rates have increased on average by 2.7% for males. For females, the average incidence rate has increased by 2.8% between 2010 and 2014. The mortality rate, however, increased for females by 2.7% and for males by only 1.6% based on data from 2011 to 2015. Prognosis for liver cancer remains relatively poor, with a 5-year survival rate of 14% between 2008 and 2014 [3]. In 2015, 20 million DALYs were attributable to liver cancer [7].

Melanoma Though sometimes inherited, melanoma often develops from excessive UV exposure and is common in populations with lighter skin types. Data collected from the USA indicated that there were 91,270 new cases and 9320 deaths, while globally there were 287,723 new cases and 60,712 deaths. Incidence rates have increased for males by 1.8% (adjusted for delay) based on data collected between 2005 and 2014, while more recent data from 2010 to 2014 also show an increase of 1.8% for males. For females, there was a 2.3% increase when adjusted for delay; the average annual percent change was similar. Mortality rate has generally decreased between 2011 and 2015, with males' mortality rate decreasing by 3% and females' by 0.7%. From 2008 to 2014, the 5-year survival rate was 65.2% [3].

Cervical and Uterine Cancers Cervical cancer is commonly associated with human papilloma virus (HPV) infection, as well as use of oral contraceptives over the long term. In the USA, 13,240 new cases and 4170 deaths were reported for 2018, while globally, there were 569,847 new cases and 311,365 cervical cancer-related deaths. The 5-year survival rate between 2008 and 2014 was 55.5% [3]. Cervical cancer caused seven million DALYs in 2015.

Cancer of the uterine corpus more likely occurs in postmenopausal women, with 63,230 new cases and 11,350 deaths in the USA in 2018. Meanwhile, there were 382,069 new cases and 89,929 deaths worldwide in 2018. On average, incidence rates for uterine corpus cancer have increased between 2005 and 2014 by about 1.2%, and mortality rates have increased by 1.9% between 2011 and 2015. The 5-year survival rate between 2008 and 2014 was 64% [3].

Bladder Cancer/Renal Cell Carcinoma Renal cell carcinoma and bladder cancer are often detected by blood in the urine. Among the US population, there were 81,190 new cases and 17,240 deaths in 2018. Globally, there were 549,393 new cases and 199,922 deaths from bladder cancer/renal cell carcinoma in 2018. The 5-year survival rate from 2008 to 2014 was 63.0% [3]. Bladder cancer caused 3.4 million DALYs in 2015 [5]. It also was more common in men than in women, with an odds ratio of 1 in 59 versus 1 in 239.

Differentiated Thyroid Cancer Differentiated thyroid cancer arises from follicular cells and is associated with swelling or nodules in the neck. For 2018, the USA had 53,990 new cases and 2060 deaths, while globally, there were 567,223 new cases and 41,071 differentiated thyroid cancer-related deaths. Incidence rates have increased by 3.9% for both males and females between 2005 and 2014. Changes in mortality rate are not reported, but mortality rate is low, at 0.9 deaths per 100,000 cases. Based on data from 2008 to 2014, there is a 97.2% 5-year survival rate [3].

Head/Neck Cancer Cancers of the head and neck are associated with smoking and HPV, and symptoms may be felt in the mouth, sinuses, throat, or nose. In 2018, there were 64,690 new cases and 13,740 deaths in the USA, while there were 479,996 incidences and 253,747 deaths globally. The 5-year survival rate for cancer of the oral cavity and pharynx was 48.1%, while that of cancer of the larynx was 52% [3].

Lymphoma Lymphomas can be classified as Hodgkin's lymphoma and non-Hodgkin's lymphoma and are characterized by enlarged lymph nodes and fatigue. The US population had 83,180 new cases and 20,960 deaths in 2018, while there were 589,580 new cases and 274,891 deaths worldwide. Between 2008 and 2014, the 5-year survival rate was 69.7% for Hodgkin's lymphoma and 66.2% for non-Hodgkin's lymphoma [3]. Non-Hodgkin's lymphoma caused 6.3 million DALYs in 2015 [5].

Myeloma and Leukemia Myeloma forms in plasma cells and is characterized by weakened bones and anemia, with 30,770 new cases and 12,770 deaths reported in the USA for 2018. Globally, however, there were 159,985 new cases and 106,105 deaths in 2018. The 5-year survival rate between 2008 and 2014 was 52.1% [3]. Leukemia refers to cancer of blood-forming tissues and may be characterized by swollen lymph nodes, frequent infections, and fatigue. Further, it may be classified into acute lymphoid leukemia, chronic lymphoid leukemia, acute myeloid leukemia, and chronic myeloid leukemia. In 2018, there were 60,300 new cases and 24,370 deaths in the US population. The 5-year survival rate varies according to type, with an overall survival rate of 55.4%, 64.6% for *ALL*, 73.1% for *CLL*, 28.8% for *AML*, and 70.0% for *CML* [3]. Leukemia caused 12 million DALYs in 2015 [5].

Biology of Human Cancers: Hallmarks and Vulnerabilities

Uncontrolled cell growth is the key concept to understand human cancer. Host interaction and subsequent growth and progression of cancer were categorized by six classical hallmarks of human cancer proposed by Hanahan in 2000 and 2011, describing cellular and subcellular events of cancer initiation and progression [8, 9]. Additional important events have been added for better understanding of both cancer biology and vulnerability, as outlined in the Table 1.1.

An understanding of these mechanisms has provided multiple biomarkers to screen for and monitor cancer initiation and development. While conventional chemotherapeutics suppress cancer growth by interfering with their duplicating and cell division phases, novel therapeutics have been designed to target specific vulnerabilities with less toxicity and tested in clinical trials.

Primary Cancer Hallmarks

Evasion of Growth Suppressors Without the ability to evade growth suppressors that trigger senescence, cancerous cells do not proliferate very much or for very long. The simplest way for the cancerous cell to evade growth suppressors is for there to be a loss of function of the growth suppressor. This is typically caused by

Table 1.1 Both classical and emerging hallmarks of cancer have formed novel paradigms for studying and understanding interactions of cancer biology. Understanding of cancer hallmarks has enabled efficient therapeutic targeting of cellular processes critical for therapy development

Cancer hallmark/events	Example of vulnerability
Evading growth suppressors	Cyclin-dependent kinase inhibitor
Avoiding immune destruction	Immune checkpoint inhibitor
Enabling replicating immortality	Telomerase inhibitor
Tumor promoting inflammation	Anti-inflammatory drug
Activating invasion and metastasis	Inhibitor of HGF/c-Met
Inducing angiogenesis	Inhibitor of VEGF signaling
Genome instability and mutation	PARP inhibitor
Resisting cell death	Proapoptotic BH3 mimetics
Deregulating cellular energetics	Aerobic glycolysis inhibitor
Sustaining proliferative signaling	EGFR inhibitor

mutation in the tumor suppressor gene (TSG) encoding a protein for negative regulation of cell growth and proliferation, as well as apoptosis. There are numerous TSGs, and among the more well-known human TSGs are TP53 and BRCA1. The prototypical TSG is usually involved in a larger cellular signaling pathway that controls whether the cell enters apoptotic, senescence, or proliferative pathways. Thus, without the protective mechanisms in place to cause a damaged or stressed cell to enter senescence, a cancerous cell is increasingly able to avoid growth suppressors as it accumulates more mutations that cause loss of function of TSGs. The importance of TP53 is perhaps illustrated by the finding that mice without the gene encoding it develop leukemias and sarcomas at a markedly elevated rate compared with wild-type mice [10].

Resisting Cell Death Should a cell evade senescence, apoptotic signaling pathways are in place to induce programmed cell death [11, 12]. Typically, these apoptotic pathways are triggered by indicators of increased cell stress or damage. More specifically, signs of inappropriate cell proliferation, such as energetically inefficient mitochondria, DNA damage, and increased oncogene signaling, contribute to activation of apoptotic mechanisms. The apoptotic mechanism is divided into two routes: the extrinsic and the intrinsic. The extrinsic route is dependent on the Fas receptor, while the intrinsic route incorporates a variety of intracellular indicators of cell health, DNA damage, and energetic efficiency. The extrinsic route activates caspase 8, and the intrinsic route activates caspase 9, both of which trigger cellular proteolysis, disassembly, and consumption by phagocytic cells. Though defects may occur at different stages in the apoptotic pathways, cancer cells most commonly evade apoptosis by mutations that trigger the signaling cascade. Mutations in TP53, for example, commonly eliminate an initiating signal from the intrinsic route. While apoptosis can be thought of as a "built-in" barrier to cancer, the cells that do become cancerous commonly acquire mutations in genes encoding apoptotic signaling or execution.

Enabling Replicative Immortality Another closely related hallmark is the replicative immortality of cancer cells: the ability to proliferate ad infinitum to reach macroscopic proportions. This ability is mediated by the functional presence of telomerase in immortalized cells [13]. Healthy cells lack functionally active telomerase and consequently exhibit progressive erosion of their telomeres as they divide. In fact, the number of divisions a cell can undergo may be described as a function of the length of the telomeres. As telomeres erode away, cells begin to undergo senescence or apoptosis [13]. Thus, the active telomerase in immortalized cells regenerates the sequences lost in mitosis, preventing the initiation of senescence and apoptosis in cells that have otherwise exceeded their replicative capacity.

Sustaining Proliferative Signaling So far, the ability of cancerous cells to evade senescence or apoptosis has primarily been discussed. The remaining discussion of the primary hallmarks of cancer will focus primarily on proliferation. Cancer cells must not only evade or resist destruction but also be able to sustain proliferative signaling. In contrast, healthy cells have highly regulated cell cycle signaling pathways for careful control of mitosis. Typically, the mitogenic signaling pathway requires a paracrine or endocrine growth factor to bind receptor tyrosine kinases on the surface of the cell [14, 15]. Cancer cells may constitutively produce the ligand for the growth factor receptors, resulting in autocrine mitogenic activity. Alternatively, cancer cells may synthesize and secrete factors that trigger paracrine mitogenic signaling [16]. The ability of the cancer cell to sustain proliferative signaling may also involve hyperproduction of the receptor protein, which leads to hypersensitivity to growth factor. Last, mutations in the gene encoding a receptor protein may render the protein active in the absence of ligand, or a mutation in a signaling component downstream of the receptor may result in growth factor-independent mitogenic signaling.

Activating Invasion and Metastasis As a cancerous cell becomes increasingly capable of sustaining proliferative signaling, it will also gain the ability to invade new tissues and metastasize, as exemplified by cases of epithelial-mesenchymal transition. While alterations to the shape and extracellular matrix of a cancerous cell are expected, a more common characteristic of carcinoma cells is the functional loss of E-cadherin, which is responsible for the formation of adherens junctions between adjacent epithelial cells. Without E-cadherin, a cancerous cell is free to migrate away from its neighboring epithelial cells, while reducing the mutation of genes necessary for E-cadherin function seems to suppress the migratory capability of a cancerous cell [17, 18]. Not all adhesion proteins, however, are downregulated in cases of invasive cancer. N-cadherin, for example, is upregulated in many cases of invasive carcinoma. This is consistent with the understanding that N-cadherin is normally expressed during organogenesis in migrating cells.

Invasion and metastasis of cancer is generally thought of as a stepwise progression with clearly defined stages. The process begins with local tissue invasion, entry into lymphatic and blood vessels, transport, and exit from the lumina of the vessels [19]. Then, development of nodular growths, called micrometastases, occurs, followed by colonization, resulting in macroscopic tumors. Invasiveness of epithelial tumor type is most well documented, although some neuroectodermal tumors and sarcomas have been documented undergoing processes analogous to epithelial-mesenchymal transition.

Inducing Angiogenesis The metabolic demands of such rapid cell division, growth, and migration necessitate sufficient oxygen supply. Thus, even relatively early on in development, cancer cells exhibit the ability to induce angiogenesis, the outgrowth of neovasculature from existing vessels. Angiogenesis occurs occasionally in adults only during wound healing and the follicular phase of menstruation in females. In contrast, angiogenesis is continuously activated around actively growing tumors to provide the oxygen and nutrients necessary to sustain tumor development [20]. Angiogenic processes are controlled by cell-surface receptors of endothelial cells. While there are both extracellular inducers and inhibitors of angiogenesis, the archetypal inducers implicated in tumor-related neovascularization are vascular endothelial growth factor-A and the fibroblast growth factor family. Tumor neovasculature can be distinguished from healthy vasculature by increased convolution, branching, leakiness, as well as erratic flow.

The induction of angiogenesis, however, is counteracted by endogenous proteins, such as thrombospondin-1, plasmin, and endostatin [21, 22]. This is evidenced by experiments in a murine model indicating that overexpression of these inhibitors slow tumor development [21, 23]. The findings suggest that these proteins, aside from serving to control temporary angiogenesis during would healing, may function as barriers to tumor formation.

Secondary/Emerging Hallmarks

Avoiding Immune Destruction Another hallmark of cancer development is the ability to evade immune destruction. Though the finer mechanisms remain relatively obscure, it is known that the immune system plays a critical role in monitoring and eradicating neoplasia and that tumors that reach macroscopic proportions must develop a way to avoid immune detection and destruction. This is consistent with the finding that, in experimental models, immunodeficient mice showed more susceptibility to cancer development than immunocompetent mice did [24, 25]. Further, there is evidence that certain types of epithelial tumors infiltrated with cytotoxic T lymphocytes and natural killer cells have better prognoses than do those that lack immune cell infiltration [26, 27].

Cancer cells develop the ability to evade immune activation or destruction by several mechanisms. The simplest way to avoid destruction is for the cells to directly synthesize and secrete immunosuppressive factors, such as transforming growth factor-β [28, 29]. There are, however, alternative methods, such as recruitment of immunosuppressive, inflammatory cells, such as myeloid-derived suppressor cells and regulatory T cells [30, 31]. Cancer cells are also able to thrive in an acidic microenvironment, which is known to be detrimental to certain immune cell processes.

Tumor-Promoting Inflammation Tumor development is also promoted by inflammation. While this seems paradoxical, because inflammation is typically a by-product of the immune system being activated, inflammation aids tumor development because it supplies cancerous cells with an influx of nutrients and growth factors that promote cell survival and proliferation [32–35]. Additionally, inflammatory cells may release reactive oxygen species, which accelerate the evolution of cancer cells to develop cancer hallmarks. Cancer cells are also able to recruit proinflammatory cells, which lead to favorable tumor microenvironment conditions.

Deregulating Cellular Energetics Associated with the deregulation of cellular proliferation and cell cycle processes in cancer cells is the deregulation of cellular energetics and metabolism. One well-known example of altered energetics in cancer is the finding that cancer cells depend disproportionately on glycolysis for their energy, even in the presence of oxygen. Because glycolysis produces much less adenosine triphosphate (ATP) than do the reactions in the mitochondria, it may be apparent that reliance on glycolysis is to the cancer's disadvantage. However, cancer cells compensate for this by upregulating the amount of glucose transporter, and, consequently, transport into the cell [36]. Additionally, it has been proposed that the relative ATP cost of relying on glycolysis is at least partially offset by the ability of increased glycolytic flux to generate more amino acids and nucleosides.

Under hypoxic conditions, electron carriers must be regenerated to continue glycolysis in the cytosol. The product of glycolysis, pyruvate, may be converted to lactate, to oxidize nicotinamide adenine dinucleotide to be available for more use in glycolytic flux. There are two types of cancer cells, in which lactate may meet markedly distinct fates. Some cells secrete the lactate they make, while others preferentially import lactate for use as their main energy source. Both types of cells may be present in a single tumor, and their use of lactate is synergistic.

Genome Instability and Mutation Thus far, many of the hallmarks and features of cancer have been discussed. However, since various mechanisms are in place to prevent their development, genomic instability and mutation are required for these hallmarks to arise. That is, cells often increase mutation rates to acquire enough loss or gain of function for tumorigenesis. This increase may be a result of increased sensitivity to mutagens or a defect in caretaker genes, which serve vital roles in preserving genomic integrity and stability [37]. Relatively recent advances in DNA sequencing technology have allowed for cancer genomes to be efficiently and thoroughly sequenced, thus providing insight into what patterns of mutation are more common in certain tumor types. Additionally, DNA sequencing has provided further evidence for increased variation in nucleotide sequence and gene copy number in cancer.

The understanding of the various hallmarks of cancer has numerous and far-reaching implications for routes of cancer treatment. Chemotherapeutics target the function or signal transmission of proteins related to each of the hallmarks of cancer. For example, the ability to evade growth suppressors in the cell may be counteracted by drugs that inhibit cyclin-dependent kinases, which govern progress of a cell through the cell cycle. The capacity for replicative immortality may be greatly reduced by drugs that target the activity of telomerase. Cancers that produce and are sustained by inflammation may be targeted by use of anti-inflammatory agents. The ability to induce angiogenesis can be crippled by inhibitors of angiogenesis signaling receptors, such as a VEGF receptor inhibitor. Additionally, drugs that interfere with the ability of cancer cells to resist apoptosis, such as BH3 mimetics, can kill cancer cells selectively. Because cancer cells are so heavily dependent on glycolysis for meeting their metabolic needs, inhibitors of glycolysis prove especially damaging to the cancer cell. The proliferation of cancer cells can also be curbed by inhibitors of growth signaling receptors like the epithelial growth factor receptor. Evasion of immune destruction can be countered by use of immune checkpoint inhibitors, which essentially block the recognition or production of molecules that prevent the immune system from either recognizing or attacking cancer cells. Cancer treatment can thus be tailored for the characteristics of the neoplasm.

Cancer Detection, Diagnosis, and Monitoring

Cancer detection could be by patient self-report or screening by serum tumor markers or imaging. About half of breast cancer patients undergoing surgery in MDACC report that the initial detection is by mammography, while the other half report self-examination. Voluntary colon cancer screening is another means of early cancer detection. Other screening tools include serum markers and specific gene or biomarkers on patients with high tumor risk. Cost is certainly a concern as illustrated by the unfavorable recommendation on lung cancer screening using chest CT.

Upon detection of suspected cancer, the definitive cancer diagnosis is by histopathology. Staging and restaging require noninvasive anatomic imaging (ultrasound, CT, and MRI) and functional imaging (bone scans, sestamibi parathyroid SPECT-CT, and PET-CT using F-18 FDG, F-18 Fluciclovine, and Ga-68 DOTATATE) because of high sensitivity and specificity.

During the course of cancer treatment, imaging tools are important in the monitoring of disease by differentiating tumor recurrence from post-treatment inflammation. After an oncologic patient completes treatment and achieves remission, imaging and serum marker remain reliable and sensitive objective means of long-term cancer monitoring (further detailed in Chap. 2).

Defenses and Defense Strategies Against Human Cancers: Differential Toxicity

The understanding of the scope of deleterious human costs of cancers demands effective cancer defenses (Chap. 1). Biologic insights of cancer hallmarks have indeed provided opportunities of defenses and defense strategies. For oncologic patients, defenses against cancer include targeted therapeutics at the cellular level, cytoreduction by surgery, and locoregional irradiation at the organ level as well as chemotherapy, immunotherapy, and combinations at the systemic level. Defenses at the population level include cancer screening, early cancer detection, cancer monitoring, and cancer prevention by vaccination, healthy environment, and education of healthy lifestyle.

Surgical debulking of tumor mass has the obvious advantages of tumor relief and has remained an effective means of definitive cancer treatment. Many difficulty tumor debulking procedures are performed under image-guidance before or during surgery. Major limitations are proximity to adjacent organs, uncertain tumor margins, and micro-metastatic tumor deposits.

Conventional chemotherapeutics suppress metabolically active fast-growing tumors but may have intolerable adverse effects on fast growing human cells in the lungs, bowels, heart, eyes, or ears. Targeted therapeutics are specific to selected pivotal metabolic pathways unique to specific cancer cells to harness the differential toxicity to the tumor. Similarly, immunotherapy using checkpoint release therapeutics enhance the recognition and recruitment of host immune mechanisms against recognized tumor, delivering differential toxicity to tumors but (presumably and arguably) no harm to normal organs (Chap. 2).

Conventional and image-guide radiotherapy locoregionally deliver high radiation doses to the target tumor but lower doses to surrounding tissues (Chap. 3). Because of precision of radiation beam and dose tolerance by neighboring organs, differential toxicity to the tumor is still limited to modest tumor dose to 2–5 Gy/session and up to 10 Gy/day. External beam radiation is typically delivered in discontinuous fractions because of practical consideration of optimal use of equipment to treat more patients. Radionuclide therapy by systemic administration of radiopharmaceuticals makes use of prolonged continuous radiation exposure over hours to days to deliver radiation-absorbed doses in both high dose rate initially and low dose rates. It has been proven very efficacious such as in thyroid cancer ablation but nevertheless expose other organs to radiation (Chap. 4). Implantation of radioactive particles linked on needles is another approach (brachytherapy) to treat prostate cancer using I-125 seeds. For better tumor-to-background irradiation to avoid systemic toxicity, locoregionally radionuclide therapies deliver radioactive (Y-90) microspheres to tumors in the liver via hepatic arteries (Chap. 5) or implant balloon filled with I-125 Iotrex into postsurgical cavity to treat brain tumor bed. In an ongoing MDACC clinical trial, P-32 labeled particles are injected intratumorally under endoscopic ultrasound guidance into unrespectable pancreatic cancers to study their safety and efficacy.

Radiation therapy results in fractions of nonspecific ablation of tumor and normal tissues at the location of irradiation, with specific tissue responses being the immediate concern. Ongoing studies are underway to harness tumor vulnerabilities. One example is the detection of tumor genome instability and mutation and use of PARP inhibitor to enhance efficacy of radiation therapy. Another example is the detection of tumor hypoxia and ancillary medication such as metformin as radiation sensitizers. Furthermore, trials are underway to further explore serum immune responses and abscopal effects that were reported with melanoma patients treated under radiotherapy. Other than continuous irradiation of tumor and tissues under varying dose rates, radionuclide therapy is like radiation therapy but may result in different biomarker changes and different efficacies. The interaction and results between radionuclide therapy, cancer hallmarks, and cancer vulnerabilities remain to be further studied.

Each of the above therapeutic modalities has made great strides in different pace in reducing mortality, morbidity, and human suffering. Nevertheless, cancer recurrence over protracted periods indeed occurs often. The goals of effective cancer treatment include eradication of initial tumor burden and elimination of tumor recurrence. With advances in chemotherapy, radiotherapy, radionuclide therapy, and surgery, combinations of any or all therapeutic modalities upon initial cancer presentation and upon recurrence are important treatment options that need to be validated by clinical trials. The premises are to harness the synergy of combinations and sequences and to decrease toxicity from each therapeutic component below tolerable limits. For instance, a trial of combination of immune checkpoint release medication and radiation therapy of lung cancer to observe abscopal effects is underway in MDACC. The development of combinations and sequences of using therapeutic modalities are regulated in clinical trials. There are additional sets of regulation on the use of radiation and radionuclides for cancer therapy.

The central theme of most cancer therapeutic measures is to have high differential toxicity to the tumor to assure efficacy while maintaining low organ and systemic toxicities to assure of patient safety. Patient safety and therapeutic efficacy are the explicit goals of each modality or each combination under public supervision in Phase I, II, and III clinical trials.

The deployment of locoregional radionuclide cancer therapy (LRCT) requires understanding of the radiation dosimetry from radionuclides deposited in the body (Chap. 6), the methodology of deriving dosimetry from noninvasive imaging of the patient (Chap. 7), and biodistribution of radiopharmaceuticals after initial deposition that may be observed in small and large animals (Chap. 8). A review of animal tumor models using radionuclides (Chap. 9) provides invaluable insight of in vivo biodistribution of known radiopharmaceuticals to inspire further translation to humans. The regulatory, logistic, and practical aspects of using radiopharmaceuticals in the clinical setting (Chap. 10) should certainly be observed to allow seamless transition of benchtop research from the laboratory to the clinics. Practical issues of human use of LRCT are discussed in Chap. 11, and contrast of the use of sealed and unsealed radionuclides for LRCT is addressed. These knowledge bases will allow better design of LRCT strategies to serve as important components of human cancer therapy.

References

1. Bray F, Ferlay J, Soerjomataram I, Siegel RL, Torre LA, Jemal A. Global cancer statistics 2018: GLOBOCAN estimates of incidence and mortality worldwide for 36 cancers in 185 countries. CA Cancer J Clin. 2018;68(6):394–424.
2. Siegel RL, Miller KD, Jemal A. Cancer statistics, 2018. CA Cancer J Clin. 2018;68(1):7–30.
3. Cancer Statistics Review, 1975–2015 – Previous Version – SEER Cancer Statistics Review [Internet]. SEER. [cited 2019 Sep 15]. Available from: https://seer.cancer.gov/archive/csr/1975_2015/index.html
4. National Vital Statistics Reports Volume 67, Number 5 July 26, 2018, Deaths: Final Data for 2016. 76.
5. Global Burden of Disease Cancer Collaboration, Fitzmaurice C, Allen C, Barber RM, Barregard L, Bhutta ZA, et al. Global, regional, and national cancer incidence, mortality, years of life lost, years lived with disability, and disability-adjusted life-years for 32 cancer groups,

1990 to 2015: a systematic analysis for the global burden of disease study. JAMA Oncol. 2017;3(4):524–48.
6. Financial Burden of Cancer Care | Cancer Trends Progress Report [Internet]. [cited 2019 Sep 15]. Available from: https://progressreport.cancer.gov/after/economic_burden
7. Global Burden of Disease Liver Cancer Collaboration, Akinyemiju T, Abera S, Ahmed M, Alam N, Alemayohu MA, et al. The burden of primary liver cancer and underlying etiologies from 1990 to 2015 at the global, regional, and national level: results from the global burden of disease study 2015. JAMA Oncol. 2017;3(12):1683–91.
8. Hanahan D, Weinberg RA. Hallmarks of cancer: the next generation. Cell. 2011;144(5):646–74.
9. Hanahan D, Weinberg RA. The hallmarks of cancer. Cell. 2000;100(1):57–70.
10. Ghebranious N, Donehower LA. Mouse models in tumor suppression. Oncogene. 1998;17(25):3385–400.
11. Adams JM, Cory S. The Bcl-2 apoptotic switch in cancer development and therapy. Oncogene. 2007;26(9):1324–37.
12. Intrinsic tumour suppression | Nature [Internet]. [cited 2019 Sep 11]. Available from: https://www.nature.com/articles/nature03098
13. Blasco MA. Telomeres and human disease: ageing, cancer and beyond. Nat Rev Genet. 2005;6(8):611–22.
14. Witsch E, Sela M, Yarden Y. Roles for growth factors in cancer progression. Physiology. 2010;25(2):85–101.
15. Perona R. Cell signalling: growth factors and tyrosine kinase receptors. Clin Transl Oncol. 2006;8(2):77–82.
16. Cheng N, Chytil A, Shyr Y, Joly A, Moses HL. Transforming growth factor-β signaling–deficient fibroblasts enhance hepatocyte growth factor signaling in mammary carcinoma cells to promote scattering and invasion. Mol Cancer Res. 2008;6(10):1521–33.
17. Berx G, van Roy F. Involvement of members of the cadherin superfamily in cancer. Cold Spring Harb Perspect Biol. 2009;1(6):a003129.
18. Cavallaro U, Christofori G. Cell adhesion and signalling by cadherins and Ig-CAMs in cancer. Nat Rev Cancer. 2004;4(2):118–32.
19. Fidler IJ. The pathogenesis of cancer metastasis: the "seed and soil" hypothesis revisited. Nat Rev Cancer. 2003;3(6):453–8.
20. Hanahan D, Folkman J. Patterns and emerging mechanisms of the angiogenic switch during tumorigenesis. Cell. 1996;86(3):353–64.
21. Ribatti D. Endogenous inhibitors of angiogenesis: a historical review. Leuk Res. 2009;33(5):638–44.
22. Kazerounian S, Yee KO, Lawler J. Thrombospondins: from structure to therapeutics. Cell Mol Life Sci. 2008;65(5):700.
23. Nyberg P, Xie L, Kalluri R. Endogenous inhibitors of angiogenesis. Cancer Res. 2005;65(10):3967–79.
24. Immune-mediated dormancy: an equilibrium with cancer – Teng – 2008 – Journal of Leukocyte Biology – Wiley Online Library [Internet]. [cited 2019 Sep 11]. Available from: https://jlb.onlinelibrary.wiley.com/doi/full/10.1189/jlb.1107774.
25. Cancer immunoediting from immune surveillance to immune escape – Kim – 2007 – Immunology – Wiley Online Library [Internet]. [cited 2019 Sep 11]. Available from: https://onlinelibrary.wiley.com/doi/full/10.1111/j.1365-2567.2007.02587.x.
26. The impact of T-cell immunity on ovarian cancer outcomes – Nelson – 2008 – Immunological Reviews – Wiley Online Library [Internet]. [cited 2019 Sep 11]. Available from: https://onlinelibrary.wiley.com/doi/abs/10.1111/j.1600-065X.2008.00614.x.
27. Immune infiltration in human tumors: a prognostic factor that should not be ignored | Oncogene [Internet]. [cited 2019 Sep 11]. Available from: https://www.nature.com/articles/onc2009416
28. Yang L, Pang Y, Moses HL. TGF-β and immune cells: an important regulatory axis in the tumor microenvironment and progression. Trends Immunol. 2010;31(6):220–7.

29. Induction of Lymphoidlike Stroma and Immune Escape by Tumors That Express the Chemokine CCL21 | Science [Internet]. [cited 2019 Sep 11]. Available from: https://science.sciencemag.org/content/328/5979/749.
30. Mougiakakos D, Choudhury A, Lladser A, Kiessling R, Johansson CC. Chapter 3 – Regulatory T cells in cancer. In: Vande Woude GF, Klein G, editors. Advances in cancer research [Internet]. Academic Press; 2010 [cited 2019 Sep 11]. pp. 57–117. Available from: http://www.sciencedirect.com/science/article/pii/S0065230X1007003X.
31. Ostrand-Rosenberg S, Sinha P. Myeloid-derived suppressor cells: linking inflammation and cancer. J Immunol. 2009;182(8):4499–506.
32. DeNardo DG, Andreu P, Coussens LM. Interactions between lymphocytes and myeloid cells regulate pro- versus anti-tumor immunity. Cancer Metastasis Rev. 2010;29(2):309–16.
33. Grivennikov SI, Greten FR, Karin M. Immunity, inflammation, and cancer. Cell. 2010;140(6):883–99.
34. Qian B-Z, Pollard JW. Macrophage diversity enhances tumor progression and metastasis. Cell. 2010;141(1):39–51.
35. Cancer-related inflammation, the seventh hallmark of cancer: links to genetic instability | Carcinogenesis | Oxford Academic [Internet]. [cited 2019 Sep 11]. Available from: https://academic.oup.com/carcin/article/30/7/1073/2477107.
36. Tumor suppressors and cell metabolism: a recipe for cancer growth [Internet]. [cited 2019 Sep 11]. Available from: http://genesdev.cshlp.org/content/23/5/537
37. Negrini S, Gorgoulis VG, Halazonetis TD. Genomic instability — an evolving hallmark of cancer. Nat Rev Mol Cell Biol. 2010;11(3):220–8.

Chapter 2
Cancer Treatment Modalities Systemic and Locoregional Approaches: Challenges and Opportunities of Multidisciplinary Approaches

Roberto Carmagnani Pestana and Nuhad K. Ibrahim

Introduction

The past few decades have witnessed considerable progress toward the understanding of the molecular and immune hallmarks of cancer, which translated to significant advancements in cancer treatment. In addition to the wider implementation of multidisciplinary management approaches, advances in diagnostic (imaging and molecular) techniques, prevention, and early diagnosis resulted in improvement in the natural history of many cancers and allowed patients to enjoy prolonged cancer-free survival.

Given the multifaceted pathophysiology and heterogeneous presentation of cancer, a multimodal approach to its management has been proposed [1] (Fig. 2.1). One successful model is the multidisciplinary approach that requires upfront consultations with related disciplines or subspecialties of medicine to allow optimal integration of care [2, 3]. In fact, multidisciplinary tumor boards have developed into a vital component of clinical practice, as tools for the improvement and standardization of therapeutic decision-making. For illustration, in an international survey of practice including 148 centers from 39 countries, 95% of respondents reported having multidisciplinary team structures, and, furthermore, in 63% of

R. C. Pestana
Division of Cancer Medicine, The University of Texas MD Anderson Cancer Center, Houston, TX, USA
e-mail: RCarmagnani@mdanderson.org

N. K. Ibrahim (✉)
Department of Breast Medical Oncology, The University of Texas MD Anderson Cancer Center, Houston, TX, USA
e-mail: nibrahim@mdanderson.org

F. C. L. Wong (ed.), *Locoregional Radionuclide Cancer Therapy*,
https://doi.org/10.1007/978-3-030-56267-0_2

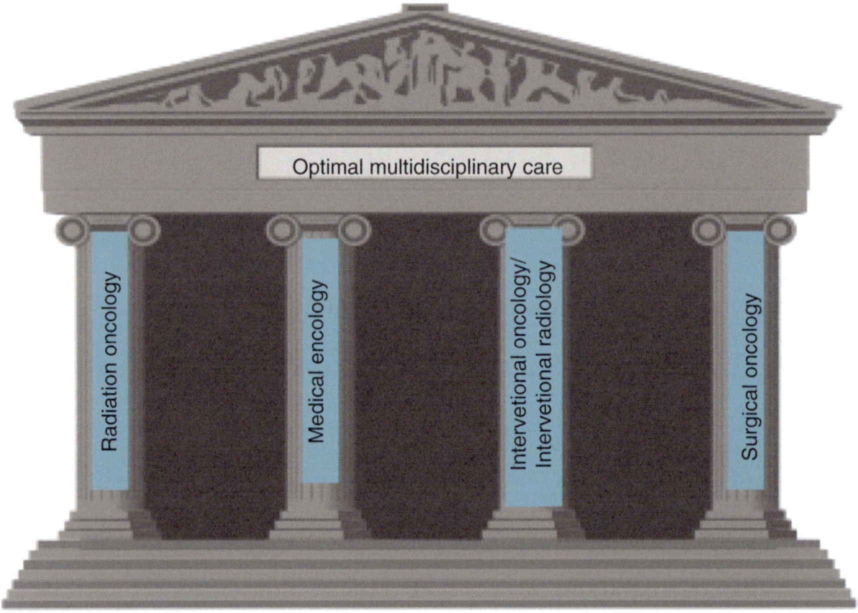

Fig. 2.1 The importance of all four principal oncology specialties is depicted. (Reprinted by permission from Springer Nature: Tree et al. [1])

Western European institutions, the multidisciplinary-team decision-making was a mandatory part of breast cancer care [4]. A notable study demonstrated the impact of such integration in oncologic outcomes – the introduction of multidisciplinary care for breast cancer patients in one Scottish region was associated with an 11% decrease in breast cancer-related mortality when compared with a region in which this was not implemented [5]. In the present chapter, we will explore the principles of locoregional and systemic cancer treatment modalities, with special focus on solid tumors.

Locoregional Cancer Therapy Modalities

Surgery

Surgery continues to be a mainstay in the "curative intent" management for most patients with localized solid malignancies and in some instances of oligometastases. Its role is vital in the continuum of cancer care, ranging from prevention to diagnosis and palliation.

The role of surgery in the treatment of cancer has seen remarkable changes over the past decades, and outcomes have improved substantially. Using colorectal cancer as a model, improvement of surgical techniques, and pre- and post-supportive care, the postoperative mortality after elective colorectal cancer resection dropped to 1%, in comparison to 17% in the 1960s [6].

During the late nineteenth and the early twentieth centuries, cancer surgery was dominated by rather mutilating radical dissection, being influenced by the principles of Dr. Williams Halsted, in breast cancer [7, 8] as an example; same can be said about sarcoma (amputation vs limb salvage) and many other solid tumors, as well. At that time, the established concept was that lymph nodes were the only destination of lymph-borne cancer cells and that tumor spread occurred in an orderly fashion, based on chronological and physical factors. Halsted postulated that cancer was a locoregional disease and that cure would increase with a more aggressive interpretation of what constituted the "region." Therefore, in Halsted's view, the cancer cells could be eradicated through the development of more advanced surgical techniques with en bloc dissection [9]. This foundation led Halsted to pioneer a radical procedure for breast cancer, introduced in 1882, involving the removal of all breast tissue, axillary lymph nodes, and both pectoralis muscles [10]. In the following decades, these principles were applied more broadly with the description of major operations for several cancers.

Challenges to the Halstedian theory of tumor spread evolved during the latter half of the twentieth century with the emergence of better understanding of the biology of cancer and metastasis. In contrast to Halstedian principles, tumor spread does not necessarily develop in an orderly fashion [11]. Rather, patterns of tumor spread are dictated by anatomic factors, as well as intrinsic characteristics of tumor cells and the normal tissue/microenvironment it reaches [11]. Breast cancer is viewed, instead, based on Fisher's hypothesis, as a systemic disease [7]. Therefore, more aggressive locoregional therapy would not necessarily lead to improved disease control [12]. This hypothesis was evaluated in randomized clinical trials, and the results provided, for the first time, an evidence basis for surgical oncologic treatments [7]. The landmark NSABP-B04 trial, initiated in 1971, randomized 1665 women with the aim of comparing the outcomes in three different groups: the first group was assigned to Halsted's radical mastectomy, while patients in the additional two underwent less radical surgeries, with or without postoperative radiation to the breast [13]. Remarkably, after 25 years of follow-up, survival outcomes were equivalent between groups [13]. The results supported Fisher's thesis and initiated a new era in surgical oncology aimed at decreased dissection but with more favorable outcomes.

The incorporation of (neo)adjuvant treatments, together with the ability to detect progressively smaller cancers through better imaging exams, has also contributed to further precluding the need for "radical" surgeries that may otherwise perceived to be "curable" however, mutilating. In breast cancer, patients who receive neoadjuvant systemic therapy are more likely to undergo breast-conserving surgery than those who opted for primary resection [14]. Further less invasive techniques that had impressive impact on patient care include the use of lymphatic mapping and sentinel node biopsy in early-stage melanoma and breast cancer [15, 16]. Another illustrative example is that of locally advanced rectal cancer, in which preoperative chemoradiotherapy, followed by surgery and subsequent adjuvant chemotherapy, was shown to provide better locoregional disease control while allowing more sphincter preservation [17]. In fact, preoperative chemoradiotherapy achieves pathologic complete response (pCR) in 12–38% of rectal cancer patients and might obviate the need for surgery, altogether [18, 19]. Published data of 1009 rectal cancer patients that underwent a "watch-and-wait" strategy rather than surgery after achieving clinical complete response reinforced the safety of this approach [18]. The 2-year local recurrence was 25.2% and local unsalvageable disease was rare. Moreover, 5-year disease-specific survival was 94% [18]. The same principles are under evaluation in breast cancer, in which studies have demonstrated that fine-needle aspiration and vacuum-assisted core biopsy are accurate in identifying patients with pCR [20–22]. A single-center phase II trial is underway accruing patients with triple-negative or HER2-positive breast cancer that achieve a pCR after neoadjuvant chemotherapy aim at the omission of breast surgery [23]. In some instances, however, more extensive surgery continues to be the preferred approach, henceforth the need to understand the tumor biology of different tumor types. One illustration is the use of total hepatectomy and orthotopic liver transplantation in selected early-stage hepatocellular carcinoma, which achieves local control of the cancer while, in addition, replacing the cirrhotic liver that remains at risk for the development of new malignant lesions [24].

Biomedical engineering resulted in the development of new surgical and less invasive techniques (Fig. 2.2). Laparoscopic surgery with high-resolution optics led to significant advances in cancer surgery, resulting in less morbid procedures with decreased patient discomfort, decreased hospital stay, and faster return to full activity while achieving comparable long-term results [25, 26]. Additionally, robotic technologies are changing traditional surgical approaches. Robotic-assisted surgeries allow the surgeon to manipulate the console while comfortably seated and enable high freedom of motion, avoiding the challenges with inflexible standard surgical instruments [27]. High cost is among the disadvantages of these new methods and is a challenge for widespread implementation [28].

Improvements in preoperative care of chronic comorbid diseases reduced surgical risks, and advancements in perioperative critical care allowed increasingly complex surgical procedures to be safer and with better outcomes [29]. In addition, advances in anesthesia have contributed to improved survival and decreased morbidity. For example, expanded use of regional blocks, for large visceral resections, has reduced the incidence of pulmonary atelectasis, infectious complications, pulmonary embolism and deep vein thrombosis, pain, and mortality [30].

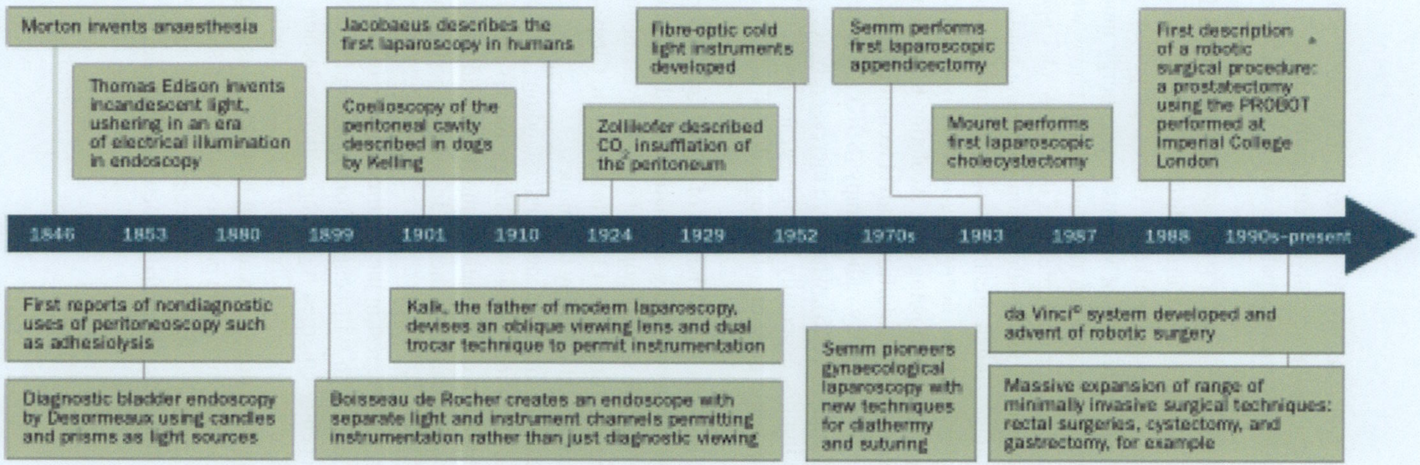

Fig. 2.2 Timeline of landmark developments in minimally invasive surgery. Minimally invasive surgery was first described over 150 years ago with the development of cystoscopy. The modern era of minimally invasive surgery was heralded by the gynecologists Steptoe and Semm in the 1960s and 1970s and was finally adopted by general surgeons in the late 1980s after publication of the first description of laparoscopic cholecystectomy by Mouret. Since then the range of minimally invasive techniques has proliferated massively across most surgical disciplines and for many procedures is now regarded as the "gold standard." (Reprinted by permission from Springer Nature: Wyld et al. [8])

Radiation Therapy

Radiation therapy is an integral modality for cancer management. It is estimated that 40% of cancer patients treated with curative intent receive radiation during their treatment, and around 50% of all oncologic patients will require radiation as part of their management [31, 32].

The era of radiation therapy started with Roentgen's report on the discovery of x-rays, in 1895, and with Pierre and Marie Curie's discovery of radium, 3 years later [33, 34]. Since, the field has witnessed marked advances, propelled by advances in technology, including the introduction of various beam energy modalities and more precise delivery of the external beam radiation to the tumor while sparing adjacent normal structures [32]. For example, less than 2 decades ago, radiation therapy was delivered as simple "fields," with minimal imaging guidance. In contrast, presently, targeted image-guided treatment with intensity modulated RT (IMRT) has been increasingly adopted, decreasing normal tissue radiation exposure, therefore reducing toxicity and allowing dose escalation to malignant tissues, to maximize antitumoral activity [35]. Additional novel techniques are stereotactic radiosurgery (SRS) and stereotactic body radiotherapy (SBRT), also referred to as stereotactic ablative radiotherapy (SARS), which are increasingly accepted for the radiation therapy of certain tumors, especially brain, lung, and prostate [36]. SARS denotes the delivery of one single dose or a few large dose fractions of 8–30 Gy per fraction [36].

Moreover, ongoing research has led to the use of novel radiation particles for cancer therapy. Proton therapy is a promising alternative with the potential to allow escalation of antitumor doses while sparing adjacent organs, given the unique depth dose properties of the proton radiation beam [32]. Please refer to Chap. 4 for a comprehensive discussion on cancer radiotherapy techniques.

Furthermore, an increasingly more refined understanding of the molecular mechanisms involved in radiation-induced tissue damage has resulted in expanded opportunities for multidisciplinary collaborations and the development of rational strategies investigating the use of radiation therapy in combination with novel drug agents (Fig. 2.3).

Finally, an increasing area of interest in the multimodal care of cancer is that of biomarkers to identify patients who will benefit from a particular treatment, and interesting findings have recently emerged regarding patient selection for postoperative radiation therapy. The combined analysis of two cohort studies, including 3213 patients, identified the detection of circulating tumor cells as a potential biomarker for the benefit of radiation therapy in patients with early-stage breast cancer [37]. Although this preliminary and hypothesis-generating data still require prospective validation, it highlights the potential of new technologies in optimizing management algorithms.

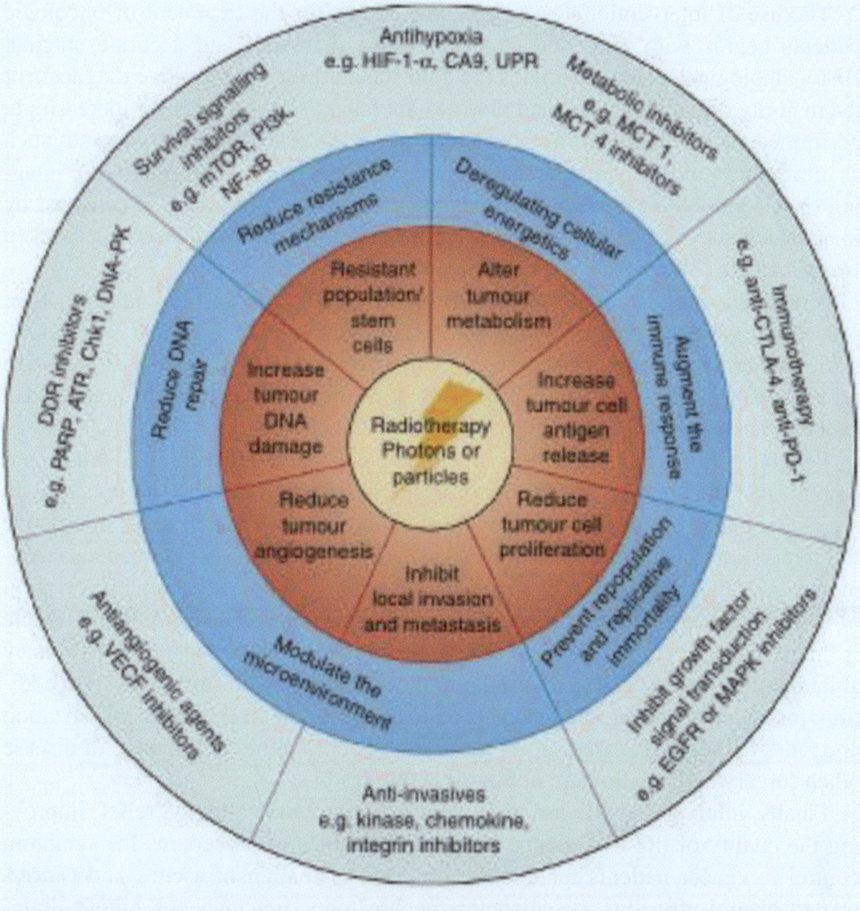

Fig. 2.3 RT has great potential to be combined with multiple classes of novel drugs. (Reprinted with permission from: Thompson et al. [32]. No changes were made from original pictue. License available under http://creativecommons.org/licenses/by/4.0/)

Interventional Radiology Procedures for the Cancer Patient

Interventional radiology is a fast-growing field that provides minimally invasive image-guided procedures for the diagnosis and treatment of cancer. The performance of the first angioplasty by Charles Dotter in 1964 initiated the era of minimally invasive procedures, and, today, interventional radiology is an important diagnostic and therapeutic modality in the management of various entities of solid tumors [38].

The use of interventional radiology procedures for the treatment of oncologic patients begins with procedures to establish a diagnosis and accurate staging. Histopathological analysis remains the gold standard for the definitive diagnosis of the majority of malignancies, and biopsies to obtain tissue samples are increasingly performed using minimally invasive techniques by interventional radiologists, such as ultrasound-guided, computed-tomography-guided, or magnetic resonance imaging (MRI)-guided core needle biopsies [39]. The direct visualization achieved by image guidance during biopsy improves efficacy and minimizes intervention related complications [39].

Moreover, interventional radiologists' role now extends to minimally invasive procedures with the goal of providing locoregional control of primary and metastatic cancer, frequently in combination with other modalities, as well as palliative procedures with the goal of managing complications of malignancy and control cancer-related symptoms [40].

Potentially curative interventional radiological methods, such as ablation and embolization techniques, are now part of the therapeutic arsenal against cancer. In selected clinical scenarios, these novel techniques provide an attractive alternative to surgery. For illustration, ablation of small kidney tumors using percutaneous techniques can obviate the need for surgery, with minimal morbidity, high preservation of kidney function, and satisfactory long-term local control [41]. Another example is that of hepatocellular carcinoma, in which, for selected patients, radiofrequency ablation achieves survival rates similar to those obtained with surgery [42]. In addition, for patients with primary or metastatic cancer in the liver, chemoembolization and radio-embolization are useful procedures to achieve the stabilization of disease when surgery and ablation are not feasible options [43, 44].

Finally, interventional radiology methods can provide palliation relief, improving the quality of life of patients. Common examples of procedures for symptom control in cancer patients include the drainage of malignant ascites and cancer-related pleural effusions, percutaneous nephrostomy, percutaneous biliary drainage, as well as stenting of the genitourinary, gastrointestinal, and respiratory tracts [45–48].

Systemic Cancer Therapies

Therapeutic modalities discussed above (surgery, radiation, and interventional radiology procedures) may be limited by the proximity of tumors to normal/vital structures that must be preserved or hampered by the presence of macro- or microscopic distant metastasis, limiting its efficacy. Consequently, systemic treatments are central to the management of cancer patients. The emphasis of drug development has shifted from cytotoxic antineoplastic therapies (in the form of single agents or combinations of agents) toward (1) molecules that target a specific "molecular targets" and (2) agents that stimulate or modulate the immune response against the cancer cells. In addition, substantial efforts are underway to explore strategies of combing such agents with cytotoxic or hormonal agents. These classes of drugs are referred to, respectively, as targeted cancer therapy and immunotherapy.

In the following sessions, we will review the different classes of systemic oncologic treatment modalities.

Cytotoxic Chemotherapy

Systemic therapy has been applied in the treatment of solid tumors since the 1950s and relative successes and impressive improvement of the natural history of numerous types of malignant tumors. In fact, chemotherapy allows for effective, safe, and curative treatment for the majority of patients with choriocarcinoma, germ-cell tumors, Hodgkin's lymphoma, high-grade non-Hodgkin's lymphoma, and pediatric acute lymphoblastic leukemia, to mention a few. However, it is important to recognize that many other tumors remain far from prolonged control of their disease or improvement in their survival.

The term "chemotherapy" was first used by German chemist Paul Ehrlich in the early 1900s, to designate chemicals used to treat human diseases. Cancer chemotherapy agents act as intracellular toxins, disrupting essential fundamental processes or pathways such as inducing lesions in DNA, inhibiting activity of cytoskeleton, or blocking essential metabolic reactions. These biochemical alterations ultimately lead to induction of apoptotic cell death. The main classes of cytotoxic chemotherapy treatments are (1) alkylating agents, (2) platinum salts, (3) antimetabolites, (4) tubulin-binding agents, and (5) camptothecins. Detailed description of the mechanism of action for specific cytotoxic agents is beyond the scope of this chapter. Different tumors may respond to different classes of drugs and to various degrees of efficacy; on the other hand, they may display primary or acquired resistance.

The era of modern chemotherapy started with the discovery of nitrogen mustard as an effective anticancer therapy. Substantial research on vesicant gases for military purposes was performed during World War 2 (WWII), notwithstanding the fact that gases were not used in combat in that era. The observation of significant bone marrow depletion in soldiers exposed to nitrogen mustard during an accidental spill led to a careful examination of the potential therapeutic effects of these chemicals. After promising preclinical data with nitrogen mustard, thoracic surgeon Gustaf Lindskog was pioneer in administering nitrogen mustard to a patient with upper airway obstruction due to advanced non-Hodgkin's lymphoma. Significant tumor response was observed, with encouraging initial results published in 1946 [49]. At that time, folate deficiency was found to be responsible for bone marrow failure mimicking the effects of nitrogen mustard; moreover, with Sidney Farber's observation that folic acid supplementation accelerated leukemia growth, research focused on the development of folate antagonists [50]. These compounds included aminopterin and amethopterin, currently called methotrexate, which were subsequently tested by Farber in children with leukemia achieving unequivocal remissions [50]. Advances in cytotoxic treatment for non-hematologic malignancies followed, and in the mid-1950s researchers identified greater uptake and use of uracil as a unique metabolic feature of rat hepatoma cells, which resulted in the synthesis of pyrimidine analog 5-fluorouracil (5-FU).

The development of additional active cytotoxic agents allowed for the next major breakthrough through the development of combination chemotherapy regimens: the VAMP regimen, combining amethopterin, vincristine, 6-mercaptopurine, and prednisone, for illustration, improved the rate and duration of remission for acute leukemia, achieving for, the first time, long-term remissions compatible with cure. The MOPP regimen, another successful example, allowed for complete remission rates near 80%, for patients with advanced Hodgkin's lymphoma. Since that time, significant advances have been made in the use of cytotoxic chemotherapy for various cancers, including lung, breast, prostate, colon, and stomach, among others. In metastatic colon cancer, for illustration, median survival has increased from 11 to 12 months with single agent 5-FU to 25–30 months with modern regimens [51, 52].

The concept that chemotherapy could achieve cure had a rolling effect on its application in earlier stages of malignancy, allowing for the development of adjuvant systemic therapies, based on the concept that many solid tumors are, in fact, systemic diseases and that adjuvant therapy helps control microscopic metastasis. Given substantial observations regarding high risk of systemic recurrence following surgery for localized breast cancer, two studies were initiated investigating the role of adjuvant chemotherapy [53]. The positive results of both studies provided proof of principle for this approach and allowed for the development of additional studies in breast cancer and in other tumor types, including colorectal, gastric, urothelial, and bone cancers, resulting in substantial improvement of the natural history of such cancers [54–57].

Hormonal Therapy

The relevance of hormones in the treatment of cancer was recognized early in the development of systemic oncologic treatments. In fact, Charles Huggins was awarded a Nobel Prize in 1966 for his research on hormonal strategies for the treatment of prostate adenocarcinoma. Hormonal therapy for the treatment of cancer has the objective to manipulate the endocrine milieu by interfering with either hormonal production, blockage of its receptors and thereby its downstream signaling activity, or degradation of the estrogen receptors on the malignant cells expressing such receptors to preclude the growth of hormone-sensitive malignancies. Like chemotherapy, hormonal therapy has broad applications in the treatment of malignancies, including the neoadjuvant, adjuvant, and metastatic settings. Further, its combination with CDK4/CDK6 inhibitors or mTOR inhibitors, in metastatic breast cancer setting, proved to be a very successful strategy in prolonging time-to-disease progression.

The most important examples of hormone-sensitive solid tumors are breast, prostate, and endometrial cancers. The role of hormonal signaling for other malignancies, however, remains unclear. Recent data has suggested that hormone receptor expression have prognostic implication across multiple tumor types, and hormone receptor is a candidate for drug development in low-grade glioma, gastric, squamous cell lung cancer, and pancreatic cancer; however, these findings still require further validation.

Targeted Therapy

With increasing knowledge of the genomic, molecular, and biochemical changes that take place during the processes of cancer development, progression, and distant metastasis, oncology drug development has shifted toward treatments that act on specific molecular targets considered drivers of tumor growth, inaugurating the era of *Precision Oncology* [58]. A dramatic development occurred in 2006, when a historical article by Druker et al. demonstrated the efficacy of imatinib, a drug that targets the unique molecular target abnormality that characterizes chronic myeloid leukemia, the BCR-ABL fusion protein [59, 60]. These landmark results provided proof of principle for the feasibility and efficacy of targeting specific molecular alterations. Results were also remarkable in determining that molecularly targeted treatment had the potential to convert malignancies into manageable chronic illnesses. Since then, the search for drugs to inhibit specific molecular targets has dominated cancer literature, and significant progress has been achieved. A recent interesting analysis by Marquart et al. estimated the percentage in the USA who benefit from genome-driven oncology, analyzing data from 2006 to 2018 [61]. Overall, considering all trials, the median response rate for molecularly targeted drugs was 54%, with a median duration of response achieving 29.5 months [61]. It is important to note, however, that based on treatments available at this time, the majority of patients will not benefit from molecularly targeted agents. For instance, this analysis suggests that less than 16% of cancer patients are eligible for and less than 7% benefit from these drugs [61].

Many molecular targets with effective targeted therapies were identified as well in solid tumors. While the list grows with time, we may mention a few, such as *BRAF* V600 mutations in melanoma, *ERBB2/HER2*- in breast cancer, cKIT in gastrointestinal stromal tumors (GIST), and the *BCR-ABL* fusion gene in chronic myeloid leukemia (CML) and epidermal growth factor receptor (EGFR)-mutant non-small cell lung cancer (NSCLC) [59–64]. For instance, EGFR is a receptor-tyrosine kinase that regulates cancer growth and proliferation. A mutation of this receptor is detected in 15% of lung adenocarcinomas in the USA and can lead to overexpression of the tyrosine kinase domain in the cell membrane, resulting in unregulated cell growth and proliferation. Tyrosine kinase inhibitors (TKIs) of EGFR are able to block these tumor-promoting properties in EGFR-mutated NSCLC, and first-generation TKIs achieve tumor control for a median of 11 months [65, 66]. However, resistance mechanisms can develop with loss of tumor control. A specific mutation within the EGFR exon 20 (T790M) was later identified as an acquired mechanism of resistance in approximately 50% of the cases [67]. This led to the development of third-generation TKIs with the ability to inhibit EGFR mutations that confer resistance. Osimertinib is a third-generation anti-EGFR TKI that specifically targets the T790M mutation. This compound showed significant activity in the second-line setting after frontline TKIs, with an objective response rate (ORR) of 67% and progression-free survival of 9.6 months. Osimertinib was later shown to be superior to first-generation TKIs in the frontline setting, with a median progression-free survival of 17 months [68].

Moreover, advances in medicinal chemistry, immunology, and molecular biology have led to novel approaches to inhibiting these molecular targets. In addition to small-molecule kinase inhibitors and antibody therapy (monoclonal, polyclonal, and bispecific antibodies), one area of recent progress is in antibody-drug conjugates (ADC) [69]. This approach consists of recombinant monoclonal antibodies that are covalently bound to cytotoxic chemicals via synthetic linkers. Such conjugates combine the antitumor potency of highly cytotoxic small-molecule drugs with the high selectivity and favorable pharmacokinetic profile of mAbs [69]. One example is ado-trastuzumab emtansine (TDM-1), which links the toxic antitubulin emtansine to trastuzumab, an anti-HER2 mAb. In the phase III TH3RESA trial, TDM-1 led to improvement in progression-free and overall survival compared to clinician's choice of therapy, for women with unresectable or metastatic HER2 amplified breast cancer after progression on first-line HER2 directed therapy [69, 70].

The increasing understanding of the molecular basis of cancer has also allowed for a paradigm shift in drug development. The choice of cancer therapy has been traditionally based on histologic classification. However, it has become clear that specific molecular alterations are present across different tumor types, and the appropriate targeted therapy can have efficacy regardless of tissue of origin. This concept has led to a new era in drug development, with novel clinical trial design and new regulatory challenges. Basket trials, for instance, are designed to evaluate the efficacy of a given targeted therapy based on its underlying mode of action rather than on cancer tissue of origin – examples include the ongoing NCI-MATCH (National Cancer Institute-sponsored Molecular Analysis for Therapy Choice) Trial and the ASCO-TAPUR (Targeted Agent and Profiling Utilization Registry) Study. We believe that we are witnessing the birth of *Genomic Oncology* field, which may overtake the traditional approach of cytotoxic or anti-hormonal disease-specific approaches that continue to govern our thinking and approach of disease-specific doctrines of therapy, to treat tumors beyond the limitation of the traditional organ-specific or even histology-oriented thinking.

Immunotherapy

Interest in tumor immunology and in strategies to use the immune system for cancer treatment started as early as the late 1800s. In 1893, the surgeon William Coley, considered the father of immunotherapy for cancer, observed cases of tumor regression following bacterial infection. Based on these observations, Dr. Coley prepared a mixture of killed *Serratia marcescens* and *Streptococcus pyogenes*, known as "Coley's toxins," which were effective in curing some types of cancers, particularly sarcomas, therefore pioneering cancer immunotherapy [71]. Later, in the 1970s and 1980s, the use of nonspecific enhancers of the immune system, such as BCG, interleukin-2, and interferon, was observed to generate clinical responses in patients with melanoma, bladder, or kidney cancer [72]. In the past decade, a more refined understanding of the mechanisms through which malignant cells evade the immune system, along with the availability of methods to interfere with this evasion, has revolutionized cancer treatment – these include immune checkpoint inhibitors, oncologic vaccines, and chimeric-antigen receptor T (CART) cells [73].

Recent advances in understanding the mechanisms of immune tolerance of the host to tumor-specific antigens have led to the development of immune checkpoint proteins such as monoclonal antibodies against PD-1, PDL-1, and CTLA-4 [73]. These agents interact with molecules involved in the antitumor immune activation, to reverse cancer-induced immune tolerance. These drugs are now approved for the treatment of melanoma, non-small cell lung cancer, urothelial cancers, renal cell carcinoma, hepatocellular carcinoma, and Hodgkin's lymphoma, among others and are remarkable for their potential to achieve long-term disease control and their overall favorable toxicity profile [74–79].

A complex network of biological pathways dictates the interactions between the immune system and malignant cells (Fig. 2.4). To initiate proper anticancer immune activation, two signals are required from antigen-presenting cells. The first signal to evoke activation occurs through binding of T cell receptor (TCR) to a matching antigen presented with MHC proteins on APCs. This interaction, however, is not enough for complete T cell activation, and a secondary signal is needed. This two-signal requirement is critical to modulate T cell activation, ensuring immunologic homeostasis. Therefore, co-inhibitory immune checkpoints are central for the maintenance of immune tolerance in normal tissues [80]. The two most vigorously studied immune checkpoints in the context of tumor immunotherapy are CTLA-4 and PD-1 – in fact, the characterization of these immune checkpoints led to Nobel Prize in Physiology or Medicine award to Dr. James Patrick Allison and Dr. Tasuku Honjo in 2018. These molecules regulate the immune system activation at diverse

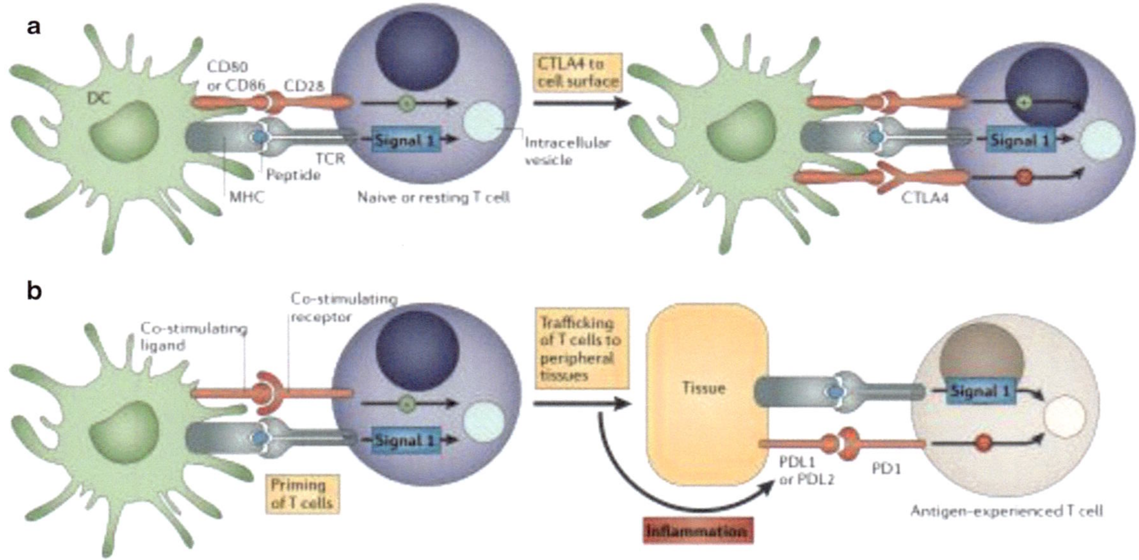

Fig. 2.4 (**a**) Cytotoxic T-lymphocyte-associated antigen-4 (CTLA-4)-mediated immune checkpoint is induced in T cells at the time of their initial response to antigen. The level of CTLA-4 induction depends on the amplitude of the initial T-cell receptor (TCR)-mediated signaling. High-affinity ligands induce higher levels of CTLA-4, which dampens the amplitude of the initial response. The key to the regulation of T-cell activation levels by the CD28–CTLA-4 system is the timing of surface expression. Naive and memory T cells express high levels of cell surface CD28 but do not express CTLA-4 on their surface. Instead, CTLA-4 is sequestered in intracellular vesicles. After the TCR is triggered by antigen encounter, CTLA-4 is transported to the cell surface. The stronger the stimulation through the TCR (and CD28), the greater the amount of CTLA-4 that is deposited on the T-cell surface. Therefore, CTLA-4 functions as a signal dampener to maintain a consistent level of T-cell activation in the face of widely varying concentrations and affinities of ligand for the TCR. (**b**) By contrast, the major role of the programmed cell death protein 1 (PD-1) pathway is not at the initial T-cell activation stage but rather to regulate inflammatory responses in tissues by effector T cells recognizing antigen in peripheral tissues. Activated T cells upregulate PD-1 and continue to express it in tissues. Inflammatory signals in the tissues induce the expression of PD-1 ligands, which downregulate the activity of T cells and thus limit collateral tissue damage in response to a microorganism infection in that tissue. The best characterized signal for PD-1 ligand 1 (PDL-1; also known as B7-H1) induction is interferon-γ (IFNγ), which is predominantly induced by T helper 1 (T1) cells, although many of the signals have not yet been defined completely. Excessive induction of PD-1 on T cells in the setting of chronic antigen exposure can induce an exhausted or anergic state in T cells. (Reprinted by permission from Springer Nature: Hwang et al. [88])

temporal and spatial levels and through different mechanisms (Fig. 2.4) [80–82]. CTLA-4 is expressed on T cells upon initial activation and competes with the CD28 for co-stimulatory ligands [83]. Consequently, CTLA-4 signaling undermines the early activation of T cells [82]. In addition, data suggests that CTLA-4 blockade decreases infiltration of regulatory T cells in tumor microenvironment; this, in turn, can further enhance cytotoxic T cell activity [84]. Contrastingly, PD-1 is expressed on activated T lymphocytes and contributes lymphocyte exhaustion [81]. Upon binding to its ligands, PD-1 lowers the threshold for apoptosis, promotes anergy, and leads to T cell depletion. Therefore, PD-1 decreases the cytotoxic activity of T cells engaged in an ongoing immune response in peripheral tissues [80].

Antibodies targeting the CTLA-4 and PD-1 axis are currently licensed as monotherapies or in combinations for various types of cancer [72, 74, 76–78, 80]. However, 50–80% of patients with tumors for which immune checkpoint inhibitors are indicated do not benefit from these drugs, suggesting that alternative or combined immunotherapeutic strategies should be considered. Rational combinations could also play an important role in improving clinical efficacy and outcomes in tumors such as triple-negative breast cancer, microsatellite-stable colon cancer, and prostate cancer, in which current immunotherapeutic approaches have demonstrated limited benefit to date. For example, the combination of radiation therapy and immunotherapy is an area of active investigation, in efforts to enhance the abscopal effect of radiation [85]. The term abscopal, coined in 1953, describes a radiation-triggered immune-mediated response to the cancer cells distant from the irradiated tumor [86]. In fact, radiotherapy has been shown to trigger the immune response by induction of immunogenic cell death – therefore broadening up the immune repertoire of T cells – recruitment of T cells toward the irradiated tumor, and increasing vulnerability toward T cell-mediated cell killing. Figure 2.5 highlights the mechanisms underlying the potential synergistic effects of radiation therapy and immune checkpoint inhibition, and there are numerous ongoing clinical trials investigating the optimal strategies for these combinations.

An additional area with promising results in contemporary cancer immunotherapy is that of adoptive cell-transfer-based therapies. Genetically engineered T cells constitute a powerful new class of therapeutic agents that offer hope for curative responses in patients with cancer [87]. CART cells were recently approved by the Food and Drug Administration (FDA) and are poised to enter the practice of medicine for the treatment of leukemia and lymphoma. Synthetic biology approaches for cellular engineering provide a broadly expanded set of tools to program immune cells for enhanced function. Advances in T cell engineering, genetic editing, the selection of the most functional lymphocytes, and cell manufacturing have the potential to broaden T-cell-based therapies and foster new applications beyond oncology in infectious diseases, organ transplantation, and autoimmunity [87].

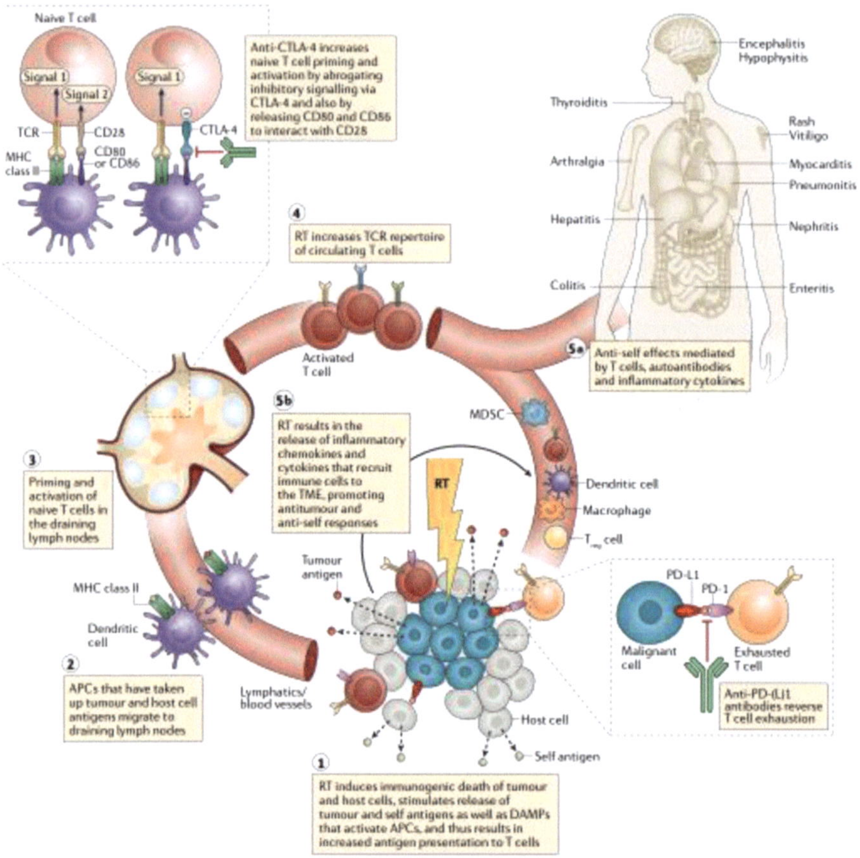

Fig. 2.5 This figure provides a stepwise overview of potential mechanisms of antitumor and anti-self responses to combination therapy, which occur owing to exposure of both malignant and nonmalignant tissues. In addition to the proposed role of T cells illustrated here, the mechanisms underlying the interplay between radiotherapy (RT) and immune checkpoint inhibition are likely far more complex than those depicted; humoral factors, cytokines, complement signaling pathways, and patient-specific factors are all likely to have important roles. (Reprinted by permission from Springer Nature: Pardoll [73])

Conclusion

In contemporary management of cancer, most patients will benefit from multidisciplinary expertise of physicians in medical oncology, surgical oncology, radiation oncology, and interventional radiology, among other specialties. Harmonious communication between members of multidisciplinary teams is essential for the optimization of local and systemic therapies and for the development of novel treatment strategies leading to improved patient outcomes. All these collaborative efforts may harness the basic and translational research efforts that may lead to more targeted treatment approaches toward the eradication of cancer. The ultimate focus should emphasize prevention strategies.

References

1. Tree AC, Harding V, Bhangu A, Krishnasamy V, Morton D, Stebbing J, et al. The need for multidisciplinarity in specialist training to optimize future patient care. Nat Rev Clin Oncol. 2016;14:508.
2. Rummans TA, Clark MM, Sloan JA, Frost MH, Bostwick JM, Atherton PJ, et al. Impacting quality of life for patients with advanced cancer with a structured multidisciplinary intervention: a randomized controlled trial. J Clin Oncol. 2006;24(4):635–42.
3. Fleissig A, Jenkins V, Catt S, Fallowfield L. Multidisciplinary teams in cancer care: are they effective in the UK? Lancet Oncol. 2006;7(11):935–43.
4. Saini KS, Taylor C, Ramirez AJ, Palmieri C, Gunnarsson U, Schmoll HJ, et al. Role of the multidisciplinary team in breast cancer management: results from a large international survey involving 39 countries. Ann Oncol. 2012;23(4):853–9.
5. Kesson EM, Allardice GM, George WD, Burns HJG, Morrison DS. Effects of multidisciplinary team working on breast cancer survival: retrospective, comparative, interventional cohort study of 13722 women. BMJ. 2012;344
6. Ely TP, Katrina S, Cameron P. Analysis of mortality in colorectal surgery in the Bi-National Colorectal Cancer Audit. ANZ J Surg. 2016;86(6):454–8.
7. Fisher B. Biological research in the evolution of cancer surgery: a personal perspective. Cancer Res. 2008;68(24):10007–20.
8. Wyld L, Audisio RA, Poston GJ. The evolution of cancer surgery and future perspectives. Nat Rev Clin Oncol. 2014;12:115.
9. Halsted WS. I. The results of operations for the cure of cancer of the breast performed at the Johns Hopkins Hospital from June, 1889, to January, 1894. Ann Surg. 1894;20(5):497–555.
10. Osborne MP. William Stewart Halsted: his life and contributions to surgery. Lancet Oncol. 2007;8(3):256–65.
11. Fisher B, Fisher ER. The organ distribution of disseminated ^{51}Cr-labeled tumor cells. Cancer Res. 1967;27(2 Part 1):412–20.
12. Fisher B. The revolution in breast cancer surgery: science or anecdotalism? World J Surg. 1985;9(5):655–66.
13. Fisher B, Jeong J-H, Anderson S, Bryant J, Fisher ER, Wolmark N. Twenty-five-year follow-up of a randomized trial comparing radical mastectomy, total mastectomy, and total mastectomy followed by irradiation. N Engl J Med. 2002;347(8):567–75.
14. Killelea BK, Yang VQ, Mougalian S, Horowitz NR, Pusztai L, Chagpar AB, et al. Neoadjuvant chemotherapy for breast cancer increases the rate of breast conservation: results from the National Cancer Database. J Am Coll Surg. 2015;220(6):1063–9.
15. Wong SL, Faries MB, Kennedy EB, Agarwala SS, Akhurst TJ, Ariyan C, et al. Sentinel lymph node biopsy and management of regional lymph nodes in melanoma: American Society of Clinical Oncology and Society of Surgical Oncology Clinical Practice Guideline Update. J Clin Oncol. 2017;36(4):399–413.
16. Krag DN, Weaver DL, Alex JC, Fairbank JT. Surgical resection and radiolocalization of the sentinel lymph node in breast cancer using a gamma probe. Surg Oncol. 1993;2(6):335–40.
17. Aklilu M, Eng C. The current landscape of locally advanced rectal cancer. Nat Rev Clin Oncol. 2011;8:649.
18. van der Valk MJM, Hilling DE, Bastiaannet E, Meershoek-Klein Kranenbarg E, Beets GL, Figueiredo NL, et al. Long-term outcomes of clinical complete responders after neoadjuvant

treatment for rectal cancer in the International Watch & Wait Database (IWWD): an international multicentre registry study. Lancet. 2018;391(10139):2537–45.
19. Dossa F, Chesney TR, Acuna SA, Baxter NN. A watch-and-wait approach for locally advanced rectal cancer after a clinical complete response following neoadjuvant chemoradiation: a systematic review and meta-analysis. Lancet Gastroenterol Hepatol. 2017;2(7):501–13.
20. Kuerer HM, Rauch GM, Krishnamurthy S, Adrada BE, Caudle AS, DeSnyder SM, et al. A clinical feasibility trial for identification of exceptional responders in whom breast cancer surgery can be eliminated following neoadjuvant systemic therapy. Ann Surg. 2018;267(5):946–51.
21. van der Noordaa M, van Duijnhoven FH, Loo CE, van Werkhoven E, van de Vijver KK, Wiersma T, et al. Identifying pathologic complete response of the breast after neoadjuvant systemic therapy with ultrasound guided biopsy to eventually omit surgery: Study design and feasibility of the MICRA trial (*M*inimally *I*nvasive *C*omplete *R*esponse *A*ssessment). The Breast. 2018;40:76–81.
22. Kuerer HM, Vrancken Peeters M-JTFD, Rea DW, Basik M, De Los SJ, Heil J. Nonoperative management for invasive breast cancer after neoadjuvant systemic therapy: conceptual basis and fundamental international feasibility clinical trials. Ann Surg Oncol. 2017;24(10): 2855–62.
23. Parsons R, Li GM, Longley M, Modrich P, Liu B, Berk T, et al. Mismatch repair deficiency in phenotypically normal human cells. Science. 1995;268(5211):738.
24. Kulik L. Criteria for liver transplantation in hepatocellular carcinoma. Clin Liver Dis. 2015;6(4):100–2.
25. Raymond TM, Dastur JK, Khot UP, Parker MC. Hospital stay and return to full activity following laparoscopic colorectal surgery. JSLS. 2008;12(2):143–9.
26. Fujii S, Tsukamoto M, Fukushima Y, Shimada R, Okamoto K, Tsuchiya T, et al. Systematic review of laparoscopic vs open surgery for colorectal cancer in elderly patients. World J Gastrointest Oncol. 2016;8(7):573–82.
27. Yun JE, Lee NR, Kwak C, Rha KH, Seo SI, Hong S-H, et al. Clinical outcomes and costs of robotic surgery in prostate cancer: a multiinstitutional study in Korea. Prostate Int. 2018;
28. Kim CW, Baik SH, Roh YH, Kang J, Hur H, Min BS, et al. Cost-effectiveness of robotic surgery for rectal cancer focusing on short-term outcomes: a propensity score-matching analysis. Medicine. 2015;94(22):e823e.
29. Karakitsos D, El Barbary M, Gillman LM, Papalois A, Shiloh A. Critical care and perioperative monitoring. Sci World J. 2014;2014:737628.
30. Rodgers A, Walker N, Schug S, McKee A, Kehlet H, van Zundert A, et al. Reduction of postoperative mortality and morbidity with epidural or spinal anaesthesia: results from overview of randomised trials. BMJ. 2000;321(7275):1493.
31. Atun R, Jaffray DA, Barton MB, Bray F, Baumann M, Vikram B, et al. Expanding global access to radiotherapy. Lancet Oncol. 2015;16(10):1153–86.
32. Thompson MK, Poortmans P, Chalmers AJ, Faivre-Finn C, Hall E, Huddart RA, et al. Practice-changing radiation therapy trials for the treatment of cancer: where are we 150 years after the birth of Marie Curie? Br J Cancer. 2018;119(4):389–407.
33. Radvanyi P, Villain J. The discovery of radioactivity. C R Phys. 2017;18(9):544–50.
34. Rontgen WC. On a new kind of rays. Science. 1896;3(59):227–31.
35. Nutting C, Dearnaley DP, Webb S. Intensity modulated radiation therapy: a clinical review. Br J Radiol. 2000;73(869):459–69.
36. Brown JM, Carlson DJ, Brenner DJ. The tumor radiobiology of SRS and SBRT: are more than the 5 R's involved? Int J Radiat Oncol Biol Phys. 2014;88(2):254–62.
37. Goodman CR, Seagle BL, Friedl TP, et al. Association of circulating tumor cell status with benefit of radiotherapy and survival in early-stage breast cancer. JAMA Oncol. 2018;4(8):e180163.
38. Payne MM. Charles Theodore dotter: the father of intervention. Tex Heart Inst J. 2001;28(1):28–38.
39. Gupta S, Wallace MJ, Cardella JF, Kundu S, Miller DL, Rose SC. Quality improvement guidelines for percutaneous needle biopsy. J Vasc Interv Radiol. 2010;21(7):969–75.

40. Barile A, Arrigoni F, Bruno F, Palumbo P, Floridi C, Cazzato RL, et al. Present role and future perspectives of interventional radiology in the treatment of painful bone lesions. Future Oncol. 2018;4(28):2945–55.
41. Krokidis M, Spiliopoulos S, Jarzabek M, Fotiadis N, Sabharwal T, O'Brien T, et al. Percutaneous radiofrequency ablation of small renal tumours in patients with a single functioning kidney: long-term results. Eur Radiol. 2013;23(7):1933–9.
42. Zhang W, Luo E, Gan J, Song X, Bao Z, Zhang H, et al. Long-term survival of hepatocellular carcinoma after percutaneous radiofrequency ablation guided by ultrasound. World J Surg Oncol. 2017;15(1):122.
43. Raval M, Bande D, Pillai AK, Blaszkowsky LS, Ganguli S, Beg MS, et al. Yttrium-90 radioembolization of hepatic metastases from colorectal cancer. Front Oncol. 2014;4:120.
44. Yamada R, Sato M, Kawabata M, Nakatsuka H, Nakamura K, Takashima S. Hepatic artery embolization in 120 patients with unresectable hepatoma. Radiology. 1983;148(2):397–401.
45. Bettmann MA, Perlmutt L, Finkelstein J, Meyerovitz MF, Richie JP. Percutaneous placement of soft, indwelling ureteral stent. Radiology. 1985;157(3):817–8.
46. Ferrucci JT, Mueller PR, Harbin WP. Percutaneous transhepatic biliary drainage: technique, results, and applications. Radiology. 1980;135(1):1–13.
47. Gupta S, Ahmed Para S, Pal D. Complications of ultrasound guided percutaneous nephrostomy- A hospital based study; 2017. 2383–7 p.
48. Rousseau H, Dahan M, Lauque D, Carré P, Didier A, Bilbao I, et al. Self-expandable prostheses in the tracheobronchial tree. Radiology. 1993;188(1):199–203.
49. Goodman LS, Wintrobe MM, Dameshek W, Goodman MJ, Gilman A, Mc LM. Nitrogen mustard therapy: use of methyl-bis(beta-chloroethyl)amine hydrochloride and tris(beta-chloroethyl) amine hydrochloride for hodgkin's disease, lymphosarcoma, leukemia and certain allied and miscellaneous disorders. J Am Med Assoc. 1946;132(3):126–32.
50. Farber S. Some observations on the effect of folic acid antagonists on acute leukemia and other forms of incurable cancer. Blood. 1949;4(2):160.
51. Cremolini C, Loupakis F, Antoniotti C, Lupi C, Sensi E, Lonardi S, et al. FOLFOXIRI plus bevacizumab versus FOLFIRI plus bevacizumab as first-line treatment of patients with metastatic colorectal cancer: updated overall survival and molecular subgroup analyses of the open-label, phase 3 TRIBE study. Lancet Oncol. 2015;16(13):1306–15.
52. Clarke DN, Jones PF, Needham CD. Outcome in colorectal carcinoma: seven-year study of a population. Br Med J. 1980;280(6212):431–5.
53. Bonadonna G, Brusamolino E, Valagussa P, Rossi A, Brugnatelli L, Brambilla C, et al. Combination chemotherapy as an adjuvant treatment in operable breast cancer. N Engl J Med. 1976;294(8):405–10.
54. Jácome AA, Sankarankutty AK, dos Santos JS. Adjuvant therapy for gastric cancer: what have we learned since INT0116? World J Gastroenterol. 2015;21(13):3850–9.
55. André T, Boni C, Mounedji-Boudiaf L, Navarro M, Tabernero J, Hickish T, et al. Oxaliplatin, fluorouracil, and leucovorin as adjuvant treatment for Colon cancer. N Engl J Med. 2004;350(23):2343–51.
56. Tolaney SM, Barry WT, Dang CT, Yardley DA, Moy B, Marcom PK, et al. Adjuvant paclitaxel and trastuzumab for node-negative, HER2-positive breast cancer. N Engl J Med. 2015;372(2):134–41.
57. Sagaster P, Flamm J, Flamm M, Mayer A, Donner G, Oberleitner S, et al. Neoadjuvant chemotherapy (MVAC) in locally invasive bladder cancer. Eur J Cancer. 1996;32(8):1320–4.
58. Dugger SA, Platt A, Goldstein DB. Drug development in the era of precision medicine. Nat Rev Drug Discov. 2017;17:183.
59. O'Brien SG, Guilhot F, Larson RA, Gathmann I, Baccarani M, Cervantes F, et al. Imatinib compared with interferon and low-dose cytarabine for newly diagnosed chronic-phase chronic myeloid Leukemia. N Engl J Med. 2003;348(11):994–1004.
60. Hochhaus A, Larson RA, Guilhot F, Radich JP, Branford S, Hughes TP, et al. Long-term outcomes of imatinib treatment for chronic myeloid leukemia. N Engl J Med. 2017;376(10):917–27.

61. Marquart J, Chen EY, Prasad V. Estimation of the percentage of us patients with cancer who benefit from genome-driven oncology. JAMA Oncol. 2018;4(8):1093–8.
62. Chapman PB, Hauschild A, Robert C, Haanen JB, Ascierto P, Larkin J, et al. Improved survival with vemurafenib in melanoma with BRAF V600E mutation. N Engl J Med. 2011;364(26):2507–16.
63. Casali PG, Zalcberg J, Le Cesne A, Reichardt P, Blay J-Y, Lindner LH, et al. Ten-year progression-free and overall survival in patients with unresectable or metastatic GI stromal tumors: long-term analysis of the European Organisation for Research and Treatment of Cancer, Italian Sarcoma Group, and Australasian Gastrointestinal Trials Group Intergroup Phase III Randomized Trial on Imatinib at Two Dose Levels. J Clin Oncol. 2017;35(15):1713–20.
64. Slamon D, Eiermann W, Robert N, Pienkowski T, Martin M, Press M, et al. Adjuvant trastuzumab in HER2-positive breast cancer. N Engl J Med. 2011;365(14):1273–83.
65. Mok TS, Wu Y-L, Thongprasert S, Yang C-H, Chu D-T, Saijo N, et al. Gefitinib or carboplatin–paclitaxel in pulmonary adenocarcinoma. N Engl J Med. 2009;361(10):947–57.
66. Zhou C, Wu Y-L, Chen G, Feng J, Liu X-Q, Wang C, et al. Erlotinib versus chemotherapy as first-line treatment for patients with advanced *EGFR* mutation-positive non-small-cell lung cancer (OPTIMAL, CTONG-0802): a multicentre, open-label, randomised, phase 3 study. Lancet Oncol. 2011;12(8):735–42.
67. Kosaka T, Yatabe Y, Endoh H, Yoshida K, Hida T, Tsuboi M, et al. Analysis of *epidermal growth factor receptor* gene mutation in patients with non–small cell lung cancer and acquired resistance to gefitinib. Clin Cancer Res. 2006;12(19):5764–9.
68. Soria J-C, Ohe Y, Vansteenkiste J, Reungwetwattana T, Chewaskulyong B, Lee KH, et al. Osimertinib in untreated EGFR-mutated advanced non–small-cell lung cancer. N Engl J Med. 2017;378(2):113–25.
69. Beck A, Goetsch L, Dumontet C, Corvaïa N. Strategies and challenges for the next generation of antibody–drug conjugates. Nat Rev Drug Discov. 2017;16:315.
70. Krop IE, Kim S-B, Martin AG, LoRusso PM, Ferrero J-M, Badovinac-Crnjevic T, et al. Trastuzumab emtansine versus treatment of physician's choice in patients with previously treated HER2-positive metastatic breast cancer (TH3RESA): final overall survival results from a randomised open-label phase 3 trial. Lancet Oncol. 2017;18(6):743–54.
71. Coley WB II. Contribution to the knowledge of sarcoma. Ann Surg. 1891;14(3):199–220.
72. Allard CB, Gelpi-Hammerschmidt F, Harshman LC, Choueiri TK, Faiena I, Modi P, et al. Contemporary trends in high-dose interleukin-2 use for metastatic renal cell carcinoma in the United States. Urol Oncol. 2015;33(11):496.e11–6.
73. Pardoll DM. The blockade of immune checkpoints in cancer immunotherapy. Nat Rev Cancer. 2012;12(4):252–64.
74. Mellman I, Coukos G, Dranoff G. Cancer immunotherapy comes of age. Nature. 2011;480:480.
75. Reck M, Rodríguez-Abreu D, Robinson AG, Hui R, Csőszi T, Fülöp A, et al. Pembrolizumab versus chemotherapy for PD-L1–positive non–small-cell lung cancer. N Engl J Med. 2016;375(19):1823–33.
76. Wolchok JD, Kluger H, Callahan MK, Postow MA, Rizvi NA, Lesokhin AM, et al. Nivolumab plus ipilimumab in advanced melanoma. N Engl J Med. 2013;369(2):122–33.
77. Motzer RJ, Tannir NM, McDermott DF, Arén Frontera O, Melichar B, Choueiri TK, et al. Nivolumab plus ipilimumab versus sunitinib in advanced renal-cell carcinoma. N Engl J Med. 2018;378(14):1277–90.
78. El-Khoueiry AB, Sangro B, Yau T, Crocenzi TS, Kudo M, Hsu C, et al. Nivolumab in patients with advanced hepatocellular carcinoma (CheckMate 040): an open-label, non-comparative, phase 1/2 dose escalation and expansion trial. Lancet. 2017;389(10088):2492–502.
79. Moskowitz CH, Zinzani PL, Fanale MA, Armand P, Johnson NA, Radford JA, et al. Pembrolizumab in relapsed/refractory classical Hodgkin lymphoma: primary end point analysis of the phase 2 keynote-087 study. Blood. 2016;128(22):1107.
80. Khalil DN, Smith EL, Brentjens RJ, Wolchok JD. The future of cancer treatment: immunomodulation, CARs and combination immunotherapy. Nat Rev Clin Oncol. 2016;13(5):273–90.

81. Boussiotis VA. Molecular and biochemical aspects of the PD-1 checkpoint pathway. N Engl J Med. 2016;375(18):1767–78.
82. Son C-H, Bae J, Shin D-Y, Lee H-R, Choi Y-J, Jo W-S, et al. CTLA-4 blockade enhances anti-tumor immunity of intratumoral injection of immature dendritic cells into irradiated tumor in a mouse colon cancer model; 2014. 1–7 p.
83. Roh W, Chen P-L, Reuben A, Spencer CN, Prieto PA, Miller JP, et al. Integrated molecular analysis of tumor biopsies on sequential CTLA-4 and PD-1 blockade reveals markers of response and resistance. Sci Transl Med. 2017;9(379):eaah3560.
84. Simpson TR, Li F, Montalvo-Ortiz W, Sepulveda MA, Bergerhoff K, Arce F, et al. Fc-dependent depletion of tumor-infiltrating regulatory T cells co-defines the efficacy of anti–CTLA-4 therapy against melanoma. J Exp Med. 2013;210(9):1695–710.
85. Ngwa W, Irabor OC, Schoenfeld JD, Hesser J, Demaria S, Formenti SC. Using immunotherapy to boost the abscopal effect. Nat Rev Cancer. 2018;18(5):313–22.
86. Mole RH. Whole body irradiation—radiobiology or medicine? Br J Radiol. 1953;26(305):234–41.
87. June CH, Sadelain M. Chimeric antigen receptor therapy. N Engl J Med. 2018;379(1):64–73.
88. Hwang WL, Pike LRG, Royce TJ, Mahal BA, Loeffler JS. The blockade of immune checkpoints in cancer immunotherapy. Nat Rev Cancer. 2012;12(4):252–64. https://doi.org/10.1038/nrc3239.

Chapter 3
Cancer Radiotherapy: General Considerations and Human Radiobiology

Alison K. Yoder, Matthew S. Ning, Melissa M. Joyner, and Lilie L. Lin

Radiobiology

Radiobiology is the field of medical science concerned with the study of ionizing radiation and its effect on living tissues. Radiation induces damage to cells by hindering their ability to reproduce. While other causes are still under investigation, the primary theory of cell damage is that radiation causes double-strand DNA breaks in the cells causing them to lose their reproductive capabilities [1]. This eventually leads to death of the cell during mitosis. Contributing to such DNA damage is ionizing radiation, which causes free-radical intermediates to form in the cells (such as H2O+ or OH●), which in turn cause further damage to cellular structures.

Survival Curves

Cell survival after radiation exposure is a logarithmic function dependent on radiation dose (see Fig. 3.1) [2]. There are two components: linear (α) and quadratic (β). The linear component (α) is caused by initial, irreparable damage to the cell

A. K. Yoder · M. S. Ning · L. L. Lin (✉)
Department of Radiation Oncology, The University of Texas MD Anderson Cancer Center, Houston, TX, USA
e-mail: ayoder@mdanderson.org; msning@mdanderson.org; lllin@mdanderson.org

M. M. Joyner
Department of Radiation Oncology, The University of Texas MD Anderson Cancer Center, Houston, TX, USA

Department of Radiation Oncology, The University of Texas Medical Branch, Galveston, TX, USA
e-mail: mmjoyner@mdanderson.org

F. C. L. Wong (ed.), *Locoregional Radionuclide Cancer Therapy*,
https://doi.org/10.1007/978-3-030-56267-0_3

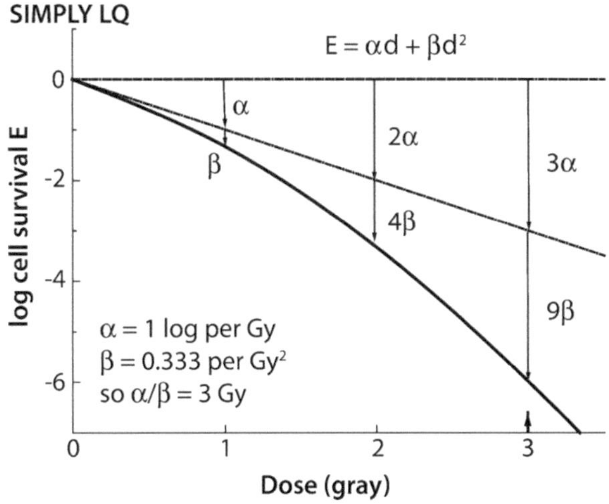

Fig. 3.1 The simple cell survival curve for linear quadratic cell kill versus radiation dose, for a single dose of radiation delivered within a few minutes. The alpha component increases as shown linearly with dose. The beta component is added to this in a curving pattern, increasing with the square of the dose. This example is numerically correct for the *α*/*β* ratio of 3 Gy

and forms the initial shoulder on the logarithmic survival curve, which is proportional to the dose of radiation. The quadratic component is proportional to the dose squared and represents damage caused by radiation that was not initially sufficient to result in cell kill. In equation form, the survival (S) is represented as follows:

$$S = e^{-\alpha D + \beta D^2}$$

where D is the dose of radiation in Gray (Gy), α is the cell kill per dose (Gy) of the initial linear component, and β is the cell kill per dose squared (Gy^2). A larger α indicates a steeper slope for the initial curve, and a larger β indicates a more curvature in the quadratic portion of the survival curve.

The individual linear and quadratic components intersect at the dose where $\alpha D = \beta D^2$ or when $D = \alpha/\beta$. Since the units for α are 1/Gy, and for β are 1/Gy^2, α/β is expressed in units of Gy. A small α/β will result in a curve with a large shoulder and a large curve, while a large α/β will have a steep, short shoulder with minimal curvature.

The slope of the shoulder is indicative of the repair capacity of a specific tissue. A tissue with a small α/β will have a greater repair capacity than a tissue with large α/β. In general, tissues that are highly mitotically active, such as malignant tumors, the GI tract, etc., have large α/β, while tissues that are less mitotically active such as the brain and nerves have a smaller α/β and are sometimes deemed late responding tissues.

Fractionation

We have taken advantage of this difference in α/β between the mitotically active neoplastic cells and late responding tissues by separating radiation treatments into fractions, or multiple small doses (see Fig. 3.2). Fractionating radiation can help to selectively spare the late effects on the surrounding tissues by allowing them to repair between radiation doses while continuing to kill neoplastic cells. The rationale for fractionation is based on the "four Rs" of radiobiology: *repair* of sublethal injury, *reoxygenation* of the tumor, *redistribution* of the cell cycle, and *regeneration* of surviving cells between dose fractions (see Fig. 3.3). These were originally defined by HR Withers in 1975 [3] and continue to define our understanding of radiobiology today [4].

Repair After a dose of radiation, cells have the ability to repair sublethal damage. This is dependent on the shoulder in the low-dose region of the survival curve. Elkind et al. [5] showed that a single dose of radiation kills more cells than the same dose split over two fractions. This is due to the ability of cells to repair in the time between the two fractions of radiation, which is dependent on the properties of the tissue itself, and the associated α/β ratio.

Reoxygenation A cell's responsiveness to radiation is dependent on oxygen supply [6]. As tumors increase in size, their centers can outgrow their blood supply and thus become hypoxic which can result in radiation resistance. Fractionation can help to overcome chronic hypoxia centrally within tumors. Cells with their oxygen supply at the peripheral edge of the tumor die first; thus debulking the tumor and thereby allowing the blood supply to return to the cells closer to the center can increase their susceptibility to radiation.

Redistribution of the cell cycle A cell's sensitivity to radiation is also dependent on where it is in the cell cycle. There are four phases of the cell cycle: mitosis (M), DNA synthesis (S), and two phases of cell growth (G1 and G2). Radiation is most

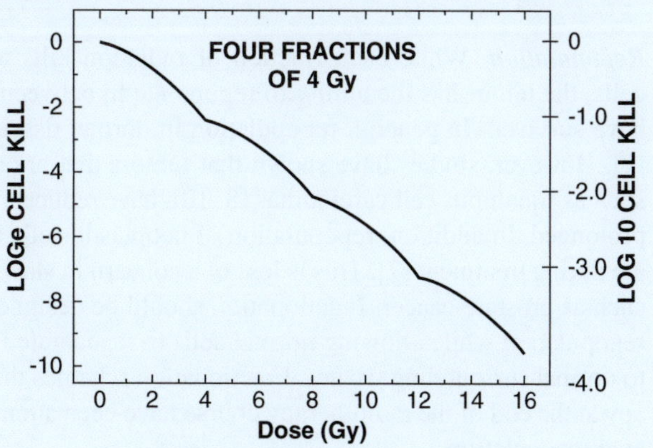

Fig. 3.2 The survival curve for four equal radiation doses given sequentially, with sufficient time – at least 6 h – between them to allow complete repair of the beta component of radiation damage. Since the shape of each is then a repetition of the previous dose, the track of the result after each dose fraction is a straight line when plotted as log cell kill against dose as shown

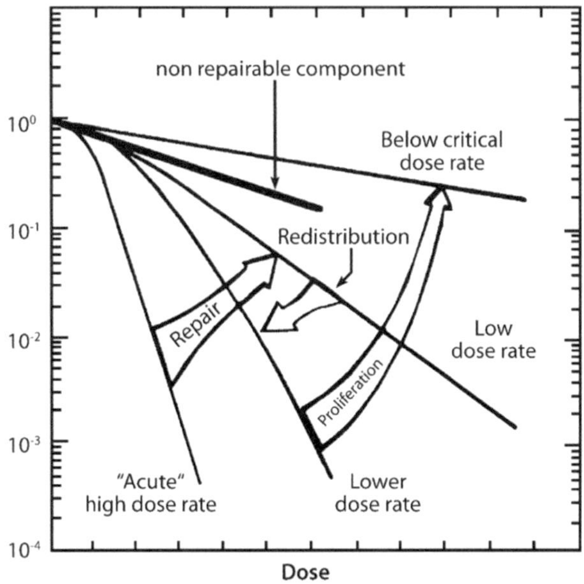

Fig. 3.3 The dose-rate effect due to repair of sublethal damage, redistribution in the cycle, and cell proliferation. The dose-response curve for acute exposures is characterized by a broad initial shoulder. As the dose rate is reduced, the survival curve becomes progressively shallower as more and more sublethal damage is repaired but cells are "frozen" in their positions in the cycle and do not progress. As the dose rate is lowered further and for a limited range of dose rates, the survival curve steepens again because cells can progress through the cycle to pile up at a block in G_2, a radiosensitive phase but still cannot divide. A further lowering of dose rate allows cells to escape the G_2 block and divide; cell proliferation may then occur during the protracted exposure, and survival curves become shallower as cell birth from mitosis offsets cell killing from the irradiation. (Based on the ideas of Dr. Joel Bedford)

effective on cells in the M and G2 phases. Fractionation increases the effectiveness of radiation as the chance that radiation is delivered to a cell while it is in a radiosensitive phase is increased.

Repopulation While each fraction of radiation kills a portion of the neoplastic cells, the tumor has the ability to repopulate in between fractions via the cells that have survived. In general, repopulation in normal tissue occurs faster than tumors [7]. However, studies have shown that tumors that are able to quickly repopulate, such as squamous cell carcinomas [8–10], have reduced local control if treatment is prolonged. In addition, repopulation of neoplastic cells has been shown to accelerate during treatment [7]. This is less of a concern in slowly repopulating neoplasms, such as prostate cancer. Fractionation should be designed so as to minimize tumor repopulation while allowing normal cells to regenerate in order to reduce toxicities to normal surrounding tissues. Fractionation schemes that include twice-daily therapy at the end of the radiotherapy course have been attempted to counteract accelerated repopulation.

Radiation Techniques

External Beam Radiation

As its name suggests, external beam radiation therapy (EBRT) is radiation delivered from a source outside of the body. Photons are the most commonly used modality, though electrons and protons are also frequently used. As imaging technologies have advanced, the ability to deliver conformal radiation has also progressed. Originally, orthogonal megavoltage imaging was used to align the patient daily for radiotherapy in addition to skin markings. However, this only allowed for alignment to bony anatomy. With the advent of CT imaging, we are now able to align and make shifts based on soft tissue anatomy. In addition, improvements in radiation treatment planning systems and linear accelerators themselves have increased our ability to deliver tailored radiotherapy with reduced margins to account for setup uncertainties and organ motion.

Electron Therapy

Electrons as particles are largely used to treat superficial lesions. This is due to their dose distribution, as electrons deposit the majority of their dose within 1–3 cm of the skin [11] (see Fig. 3.4). They also have a steep dose falloff, which means that they spare internal organs better than photons (see Fig. 3.5) [12], particularly at low energies. Common applications of electron therapy include skin ailments such as mycosis fungoides or cutaneous T-cell lymphoma [13], breast cancer to boost the

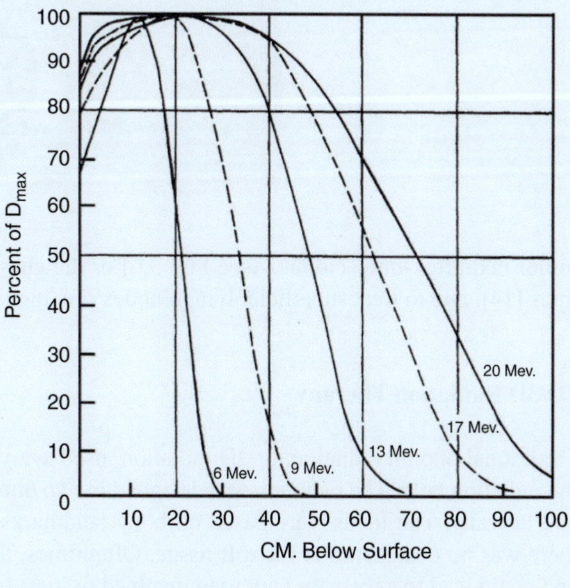

Fig. 3.4 Central axis percentage depth dose as a function of beam energy from 4 MeV to 20 MeV

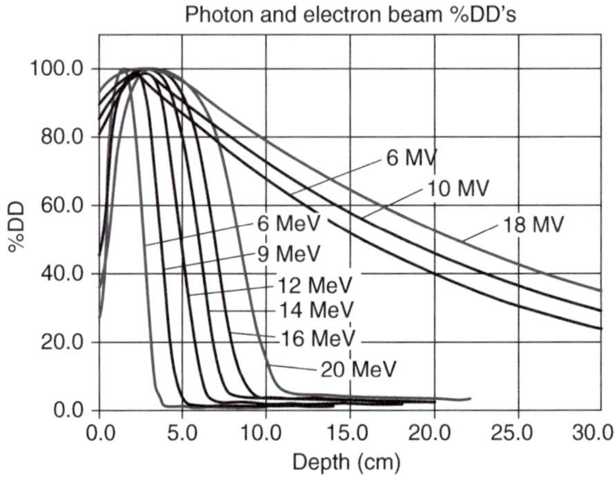

Fig. 3.5 Examples of typical photon beam and electron beam central axis percent depth dose curves for a 10 × 10-cm field for selected energies

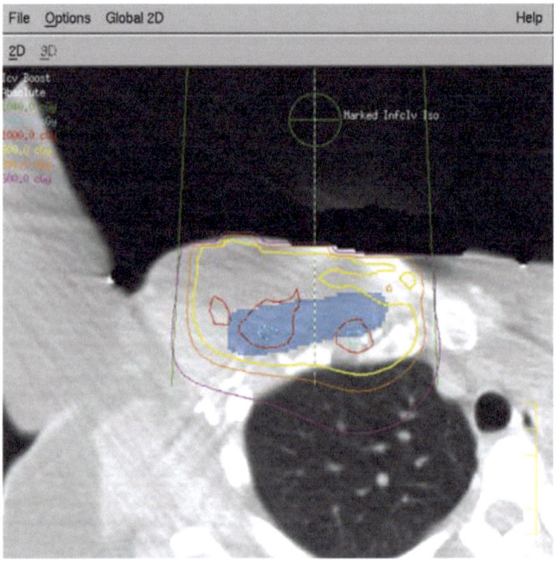

Fig. 3.6 Electron planning of an infraclavicular boost. The target is encompassed within the distal 90% isodose line. Electrons are typically prescribed at the 100% isodose line

tumor bed after lumpectomies (see Fig. 3.6) or the chest wall scar after mastectomies [14], and to treat superficial lymph nodes (i.e. inguinal region).

2D/3D Radiation Therapy

Traditional photon radiation, or 2D radiation, used x-ray films (plain films) to plan the radiation field. The radiation was designed in two dimensions, anterior-posterior and laterally. The fields were based on bony landmarks determined by x-ray, and there was no consideration for soft tissue. Oftentimes, this resulted in a large field and could lead to excess toxicity to uninvolved tissues. In addition, there have been studies showing that this type of treatment planning could result in missing the target tumor itself due to anatomical heterogeneity [15].

3D conformal radiation quickly became the standard of treatment for most disease sites when CT imaging became commonplace. For 3D radiation, the patient is placed in treatment position and immobilized. A CT scan is then performed with the patient in the treatment position (see Fig. 3.7). This is commonly referred to as a "CT simulation scan" because it "simulates" the treatment position. With this simulation scan, the treating physician can visualize both the tumor or regions at risk and the organs at risk (OAR). The scan is transferred into radiation planning software, and from there the physician can begin the planning process (see Fig. 3.8).

First, the gross tumor volume (GTV) is identified and delineated in the planning system. The clinical target volume (CTV), which takes into account microscopic extension of the neoplasm or areas at risk (i.e., draining lymph nodes that may be uninvolved), is then demarcated based on the disease location and histology. For sites with concern for significant internal target motion (e.g., breathing motion in thoracic, bladder or rectal filling variations for pelvic, etc.) an internal target volume (ITV) is sometimes warranted (see Fig. 3.9). This ITV typically expands upon the CTV to ensure that major location shifts (anterior-posterior, superior-inferior, lateral) due to internal target motion are accounted for (see Fig. 3.10). To aid this process, sometimes additional CT simulation scans are warranted. For example, a 4D-CT capturing an entire breathing cycle is often obtained for peripheral lung cancers (see Fig. 3.11), and the target volumes encompass tumor motion on each phase of the breathing cycle (see Fig. 3.12). For pelvic malignancies, multiple scans with variations of bladder and/or rectal fullness (emptiness) can help assist in accounting for this internal target motion. Finally, a planning target volume (PTV) adds further margin onto the CTV (or ITV) to account for daily variations in treatment setup and other expected variabilities in target motion. The organs at risk (OAR) are also outlined (see Fig. 3.13).

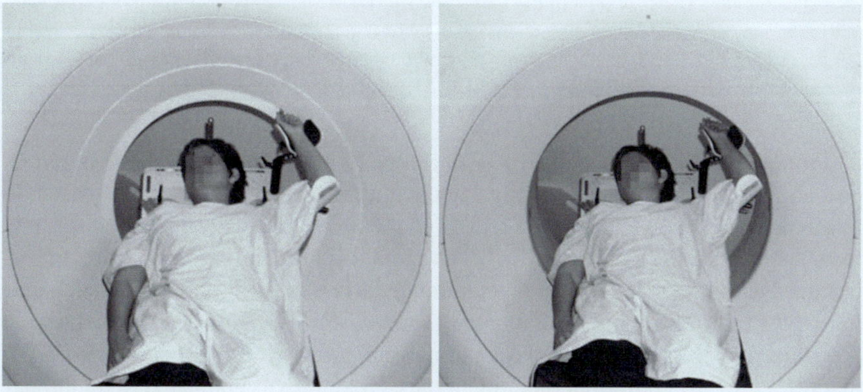

Fig. 3.7 Complex treatment techniques, such as tangential breast irradiation, can be problematic to set up on diagnostic CT scanners or older CT simulators (70-cm bore) because of bore size limitations. The modern large-bore (85-cm) CT scanner developed by Marconi (now part of Philips) designed specifically for radiation oncology applications has solved this problem

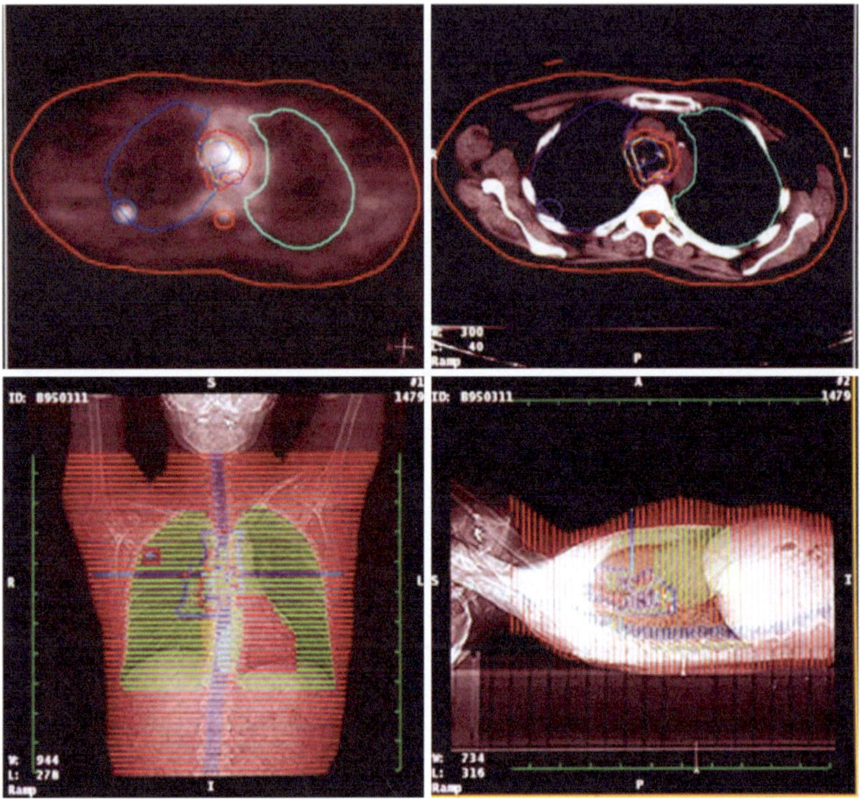

Fig. 3.8 Three-dimensional treatment planning system (TPS) image segmentation software provides effective tools for radiation oncologists and treatment planners to delineate critical structures, tumor, and target volumes for 3D planning. The CT data are displayed, and contours are drawn by the treatment planner/radiation oncologist around the tumor, target, and normal tissues on a slice-by-slice basis, as seen in the *upper right panel.* At the same time, planar images from both anteroposterior and lateral projections are displayed in the *bottom right and left panels. Upper left* panel shows PET scan data with overlying contours after image registration with the CT data

From these outlines, a treatment plan can be designed by the dosimetrist, physicist, and treating physician to ensure that the tumor is receiving adequate dose while minimizing radiation to the OARs and staying within defined dosimetric constraints to protect the OARs (see Fig. 3.14). The radiation plan for 2D or 3D radiation is designed using static fields positioned around the patient in a configuration depending on the tumor location, patient habitus, and OARs. Beam dose and weighting is determined by the planning team to optimize radiation delivery. Studies have shown that the use of 3D conformal radiation reduces toxicities as compared to traditional 2D radiation which does not typically take into account the placement of organs [16, 17]. In addition, because of the ability to avoid OARs and their ensuing radiation toxicities, physicians may be able to escalate the dose to the tumor itself.

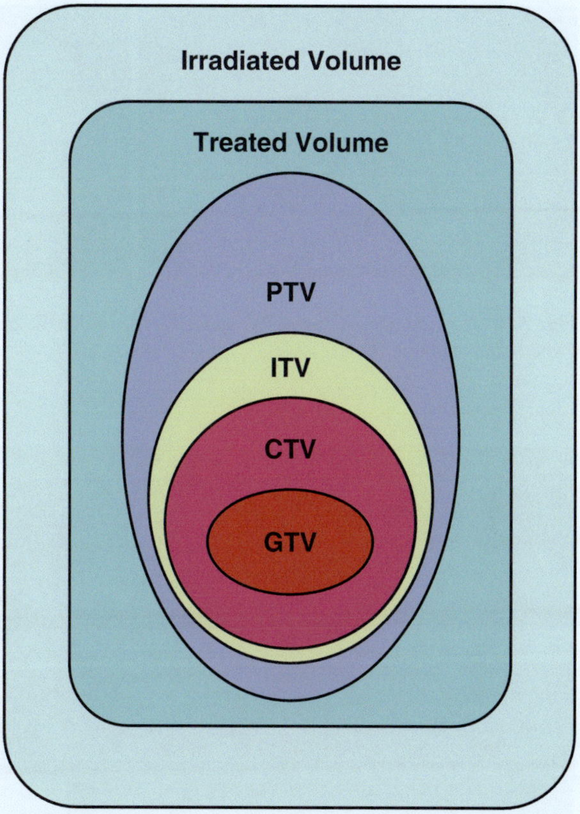

Fig. 3.9 International Commission on Radiation Units and Measurements (ICRU) reports 50 and 62 volumes used in 3D treatment planning. Gross tumor volume (GTV) is the volume(s) of known tumor. Clinical target volume (CTV) is the volume(s) of suspected microscopic tumor infiltration. Planning target volume (PTV) is the volume containing the CTV/GTV with enough margin necessary to account for setup variations and organ and patient motion. Internal target volume (ITV) represents the movements of the CTV referenced to the patient coordinate system by internal and external reference points

Intensity-Modulated Radiation Therapy

Intensity-modulated radiation therapy, or IMRT, provides an even more conformal delivery method compared to standard 3D radiation (see Fig. 3.15). The main difference between IMRT and 3D radiation is that the beams in IMRT have varying intensity, while those used in 3D radiation have uniform intensities [18]. This is made possible with increased computing capabilities as well as advancements in the linear accelerators themselves. The radiation beam is modulated, or varied in intensity, by separating each beam into smaller "beamlets." Multileaf collimators (MLC) are used to create these smaller beamlets. The MLCs can be moved in and out of the radiation field during treatment in order to shape and modulate the radiation beam [19].

IMRT uses the same CT simulation scan as 3D conformal radiation, but instead of placing beams manually, the computer planning system is tasked with inverse planning, or back-calculating the optimal beam locations, intensity, and MLC placement. The inverse planning is done with both target and OAR minimum and/or maximum dose and coverage as determined by the treatment team. With the use of MLCs and inverse planning, the radiation dose is able to be sculpted around normal

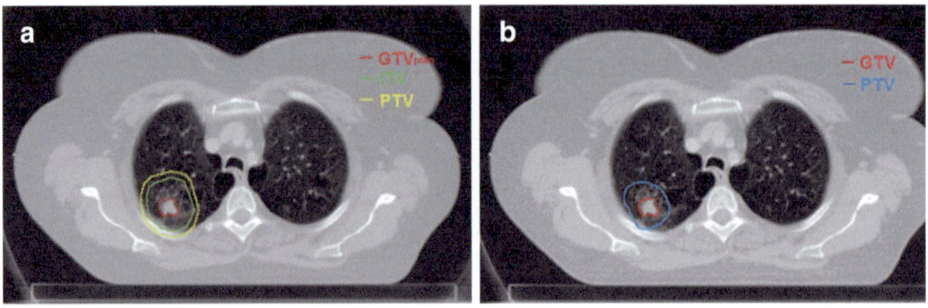

Fig. 3.10 An example of the GTV and PTV definition in one patient for 3D-CRT (**a**) and CyberKnife planning (**b**)

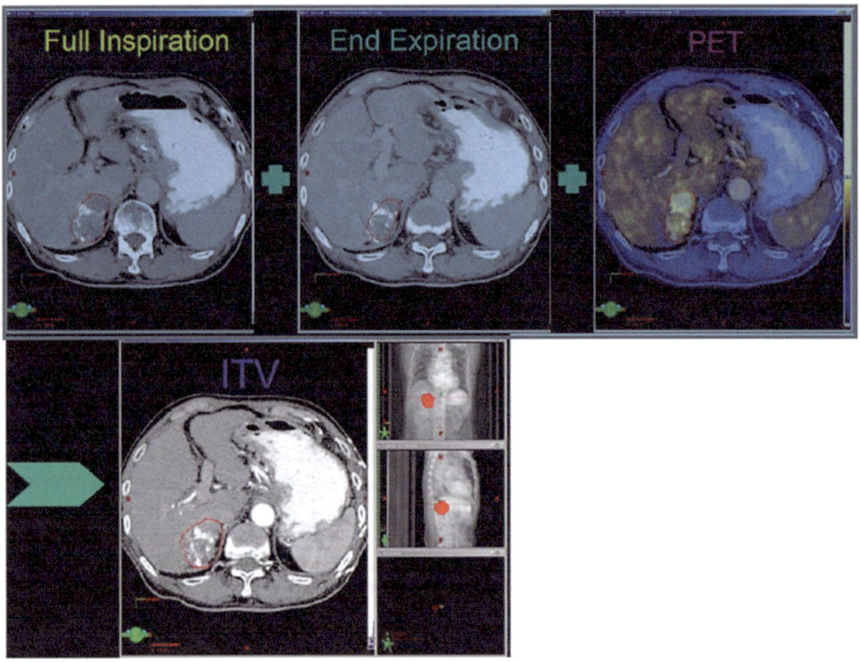

Fig. 3.11 Internal target volume (ITV) definition based on 4D-CT using the full inspiratory phase CT, full expiratory phase CT, and PET information. The final ITV combines the GTV's contoured on inspiration and expiration, taking into consideration the PET information

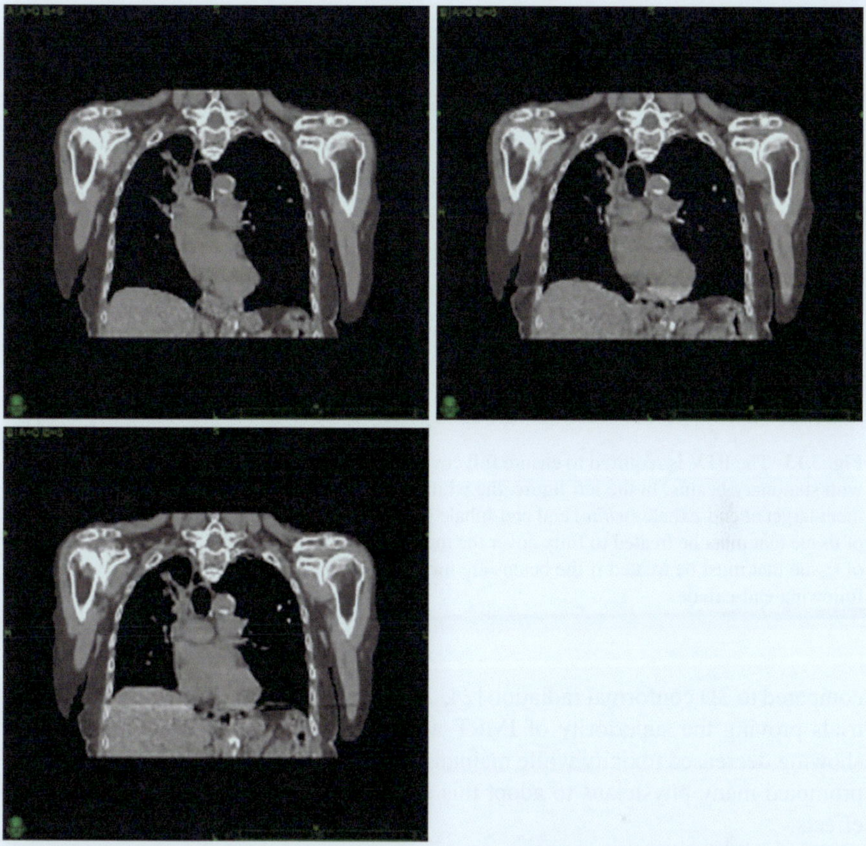

Fig. 3.12 Coronal slices through three individual 3D-CT images in a 4D-CT image study. Each individual 3D-CT image represents a different phase of the patient's breathing cycle. The movement of the diaphragm during the breathing cycle is substantial

organs in a way not previously attainable with the use of standard 3D radiation alone (see Fig. 3.16).

Much like with the increased conformality when transitioning from 2D to 3D treatment, IMRT gives physicians the ability to further escalate the dose to the target tissue while minimizing dose to OARs [20]. In general, radiation dose is limited by maximum dose to OARs in order to minimize toxicities. With the increased conformality achieved using IMRT, the dose to nearby structures is decreased, thereby allowing physicians to increase the overall total dose to the patient and the tumor. Dosimetric comparisons have shown improved conformality to the target and decreased radiation dose to OARs using IMRT in multiple studies [21–23]. Importantly, randomized studies have shown decreased toxicities with IMRT as

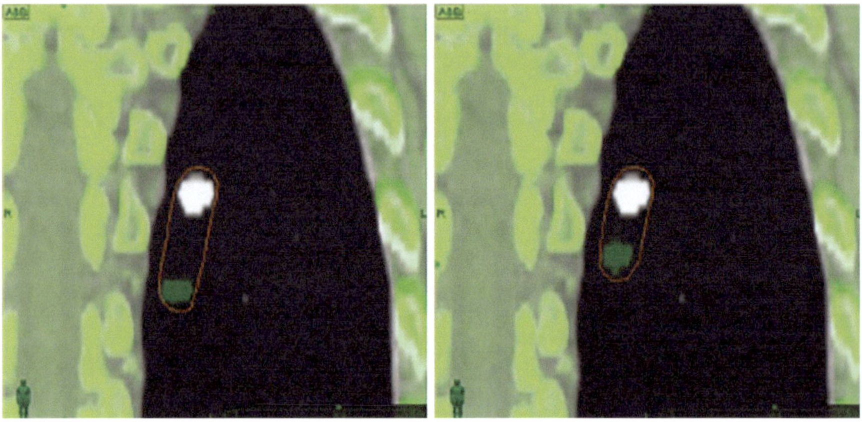

Fig. 3.13 The PTV is required to ensure full coverage of the CTV for a radiation delivery system with stationary beams. In the left figure, the white and green blobs show the position of the treatment target at end-exhale (*white*) and end-inhale (*green*), and the orange contour shows the region of tissue that must be treated to fully cover the moving target. In the right figure, we show the area of tissue that must be treated if the beams are turned on only for the 20% of the respiratory cycle following end-exhale

compared to 3D conformal radiation [24, 25]. While there have been no randomized trials proving the superiority of IMRT with respect to disease outcomes, studies showing decreased toxicity while maintaining adequate coverage of the target have prompted many physicians to adopt this technology because of less resultant side effects.

There are disadvantages with IMRT as compared to traditional 3D radiation. Of note, there is an increased risk of secondary malignancies due to longer "beam-on" times with IMRT than 3D [26]. In addition, because the treatment is so tightly conformal around the target, there is a higher chance for setup error when treating with IMRT [27]. This error can result in a tumor "miss" if adequate margins are not included in the plan. This is especially important to consider when treating a mobile target, such as tumors in the abdomen/pelvis [28, 29].

In order to ensure that the target is receiving the intended dose, image-guided IMRT (IG-IMRT) has been widely adopted for mobile tumors. Image guidance can be performed using cone-beam CT, where the CT scan is taken using the linear accelerator with the patient on the treatment table, or with a CT-on-rails, where the patient is on the treatment table and a diagnostic CT scan is performed in the treatment room. In both cases, daily CTs are done in order to ensure that the tumor is being correctly targeted and alignment is confirmed. As imaging and technology continues to advance, we have been able to further improve target localization with techniques such as correcting for respiratory motion [30].

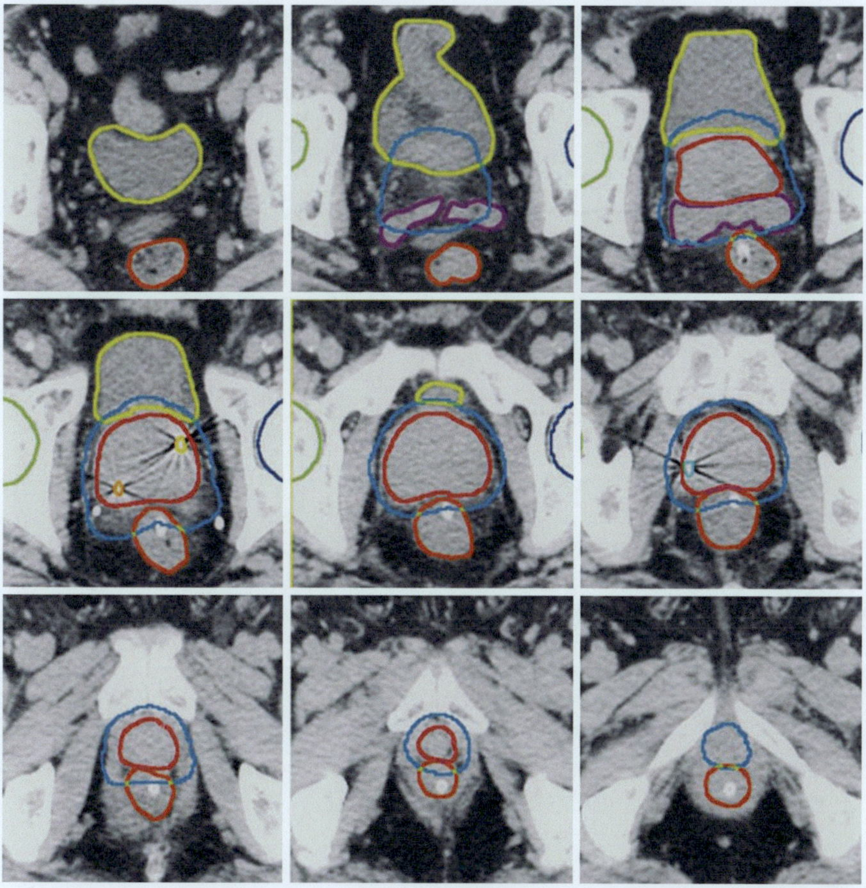

Fig. 3.14 Target volumes and organs at risk are defined on serial images of a treatment planning CT scan. For illustration purposes, only every fourth CT image is displayed. The bladder (*yellow*) and rectum (*orange*) are contoured as solid organs; prostate (*red*) is contoured from its base superiorly to the apex at the genitourinary diaphragm. In this patient, the first 1 cm of seminal vesicle tissue (*violet*) is included with the CTV and no attempt is mad e to treat them above this level. The PTV (*cyan*) margin is 7 mm from the prostate border. In this example, the fiducial markers are seen inside the prostate gland

Stereotactic Radiation Therapy

Another radiation technique that was made possible with the improvement of linear-accelerator technology, treatment planning, treatment delivery, and imaging quality is stereotactic body radiation therapy (SBRT). Originally, stereotactic radiosurgery was developed for intracranial lesions and utilized very focused,

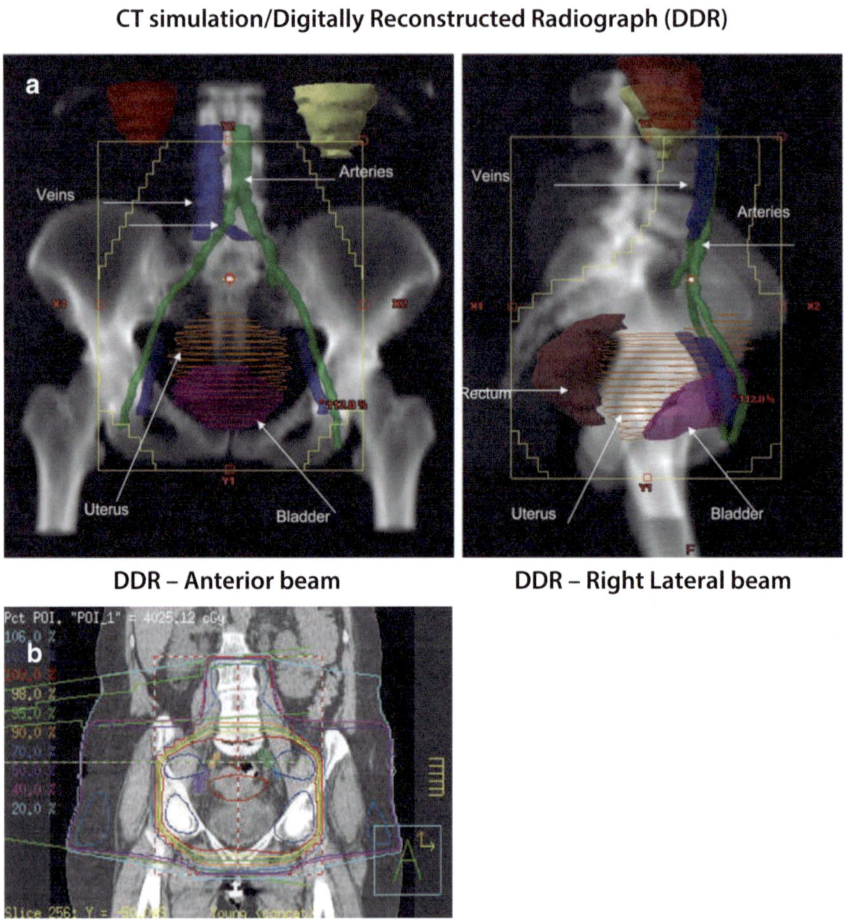

Fig. 3.15 Digitally reconstructed radiograph computed tomography (CT) scan with contours of external and internal iliac vessels outlined as well as the small bowel, bladder, and rectum. In general, a 2-cm margin on the vessels will encompass the associated lymph nodes and can be considered the clinical target volume (CTV). A margin placed around this volume for day-to-day setup variation can be considered the planning target volume (PTV)

high-dose per fraction radiation to treat brain lesions [31]. This treatment modality evolved to include lesions outside of the brain including tumors in the lung and liver [32].

Today, SBRT is widely utilized for sites throughout the entire body. When it was originally being transitioned from intracranial to extracranial sites, frames like those used for brain lesions were employed to immobilize patients [33]. For extracranial sites, these earlier immobilization devices have been largely replaced with image-guided treatment that verifies the location of the tumor before the patient is treated.

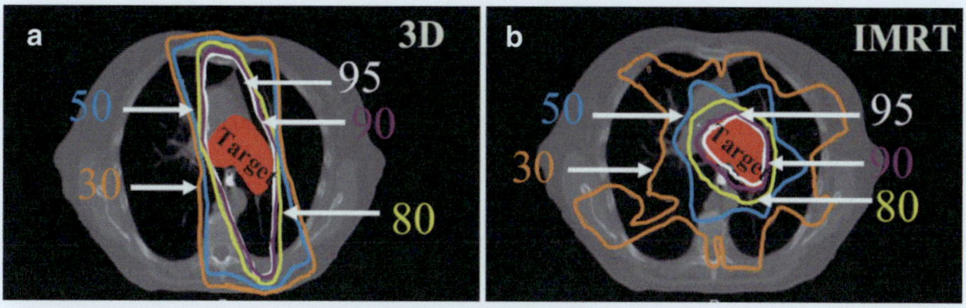

Fig. 3.16 Percent relative isodose distributions for the 3DCRT plan (**a**) and IMRT-2 plan (**b**). The dose distributions show that the IMRT-2 plan is more conformal than the 3DCRT plan at the cost of slightly losing target coverage. Unlike the UTCP plan values, the $UTCP_{QALY}$ values, which incorporate clinically realistic quality of life data, suggest that the $UTCP_{QALY}$ formalism provides better differentiation between plans

One complicating aspect of stereotactic treatment to the body as opposed to intracranial sites is internal organ motion induced by respiration. Due to the high dose per fraction and minimal margins around the tumor, there is even less margin for error when using SBRT than with other radiation treatment modalities [34]. As such, accounting for respiratory motion is critical. There are multiple ways to execute this including abdominal binders, deep inspiration breath hold, and respiratory gating. Utilization of each technique is institution- and physician-dependent. In addition, internal and/or external fiducials can be used to track the target during treatment which allows for potentially smaller margins around the tumor. While still a relatively new technology, the use of SBRT continues to expand in both its utility and frequency throughout the radiation community.

Proton Therapy

The use of protons to irradiate tissues was first discussed in a laboratory setting in 1946 [35] and was first used clinically to irradiate pituitary tumors in 1958 [36]. Proton therapy utilization has since increased with a wide array of tumor treatments/applications, and the number of patients treated with protons continues to increase [37, 38].

The advantage of proton therapy as compared to traditional photons is in its dose distribution, which is a function of the physical properties of protons themselves. Protons deposit their maximum dose over the last few millimeters of the proton's range, which is known as the Bragg peak [39]. As such, protons do not penetrate completely through a tissue. This is in comparison to photons, which deposit their maximum dose at a few centimeters of depth into tissue (this depth depends on the starting energy of the photons) and then continue to deposit energy as they penetrate through the tissue. Therefore, the use of protons can lead to minimal exit dose and increased precision when compared to photons.

This increased dose conformality therefore generates plans with decreased dose to nearby healthy tissue [40], which in turn means potentially fewer side effects and subsequent unwanted toxicities [41]. While there is an obvious theoretic advantage to protons, and studies thus far have been promising in terms of survival and reduced toxicities [42, 43], there have been no randomized clinical trials comparing proton and photon therapy. Continued research is needed to explore the feasibility and cost-effectiveness of protons.

Brachytherapy

Brachytherapy is a radiation treatment that places radioactive sources in direct contact with or adjacent to a tumor (see Fig. 3.17). The main advantage of brachytherapy is that it can deliver much higher doses of radiation to the tumor with very minimal doses to nearby tissues due to rapid dose falloff (see Fig. 3.18). It has multiple uses including for the treatment of gynecologic malignancies, prostate cancer, ocular cancers, and some head and neck tumors. The placement of sources can be temporary or permanent, depending on location and physician preference.

Dose distribution is largely described by the inverse square law, which is expressed as:

$$\text{dose} = 1/\text{distance}^2$$

Practically, this results in the dose decreasing by a factor of four when the distance from the source doubles.

Radium-226 was discovered by the Curies in 1898 and was the first brachytherapy source used by physicians. The use of radium was eventually replaced by Cesium-137 due to the fact that Ra-226 leaks radon gas which has detrimental effects. Today, Iridium-192, Iodine-125, and Palladium-103 are all common sources for brachytherapy treatment. These sources have differing energies and half-lives, and their use is dictated by physician preference.

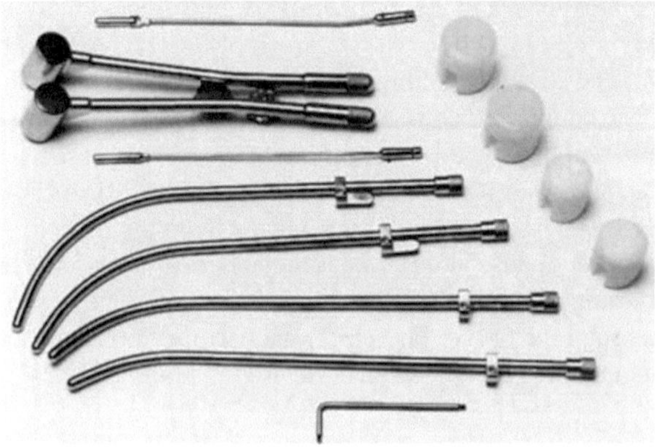

Fig. 3.17 Fletcher-Suit low-dose-rate cervix applicator set. (Best Medical, Springfield, Virginia)

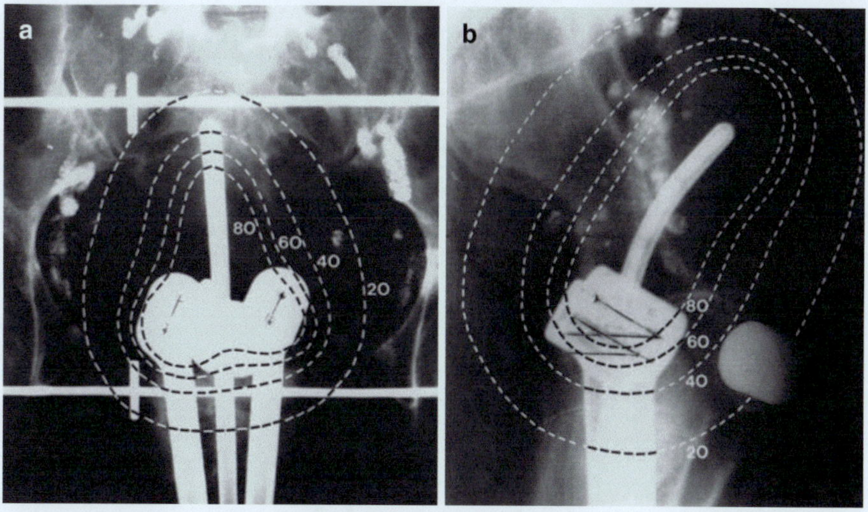

Fig. 3.18 (**a**) Anteroposterior view of intracavitary insertion for carcinoma of the uterine cervix. (**b**) Lateral view of same implant. Isodose curves (cGy/h) are superimposed

Brachytherapy is described based on the time required to complete the treatment. Low-dose radiation, or LDR brachytherapy, takes an average of 2–3 days to deliver treatment such as with temporary sources in gynecologic brachytherapy, while high-dose radiation, or HDR brachytherapy, generally lasts only a few minutes based on the dose prescribed (see Fig. 3.19).

LDR is used for both gynecologic and prostate cancer treatment. In gynecologic cancers, there are multiple modalities including tandem and ovoid, tandem and cylinder, vaginal cuff, and interstitial needles. Radioactive sources can be manually loaded into these devices to treat gynecological cancers including vulvar, vaginal, cervical, or uterine depending on the device and physician preference.

In general, LDR brachytherapy uses sources that decay at a rate of 0.4–2 Gy/hr. As such, these devices are generally left inside the patient for 2–3 days if temporary. Patients are kept in the hospital and immobilized during treatment. After the appropriate dose has been delivered, the devices are removed from the patient.

Another form of LDR brachytherapy is used to treat early-stage prostate cancer using radioactive Iodine-125 or Palladium-103 permanent seeds. For this modality, radioactive seeds are inserted into the prostate while the patient is under anesthesia which is typically an outpatient procedure. The seeds release radiation over a few weeks to months dependent on the source used, at a very low energy, thus reducing the risk of exposure to others.

For tumors involving the orbit, ocular plaques can be utilized to treat the tumor. In these cases, sources are manually loaded into the plaque. The plaque is then left on the eye for a set duration to deliver the desired dose.

HDR can also be used for gynecologic and prostate cancers. When utilizing HDR, the same treatment modalities for gynecologic cancers can be used. For gynecologic malignancies, the main difference is that the procedure is done as an

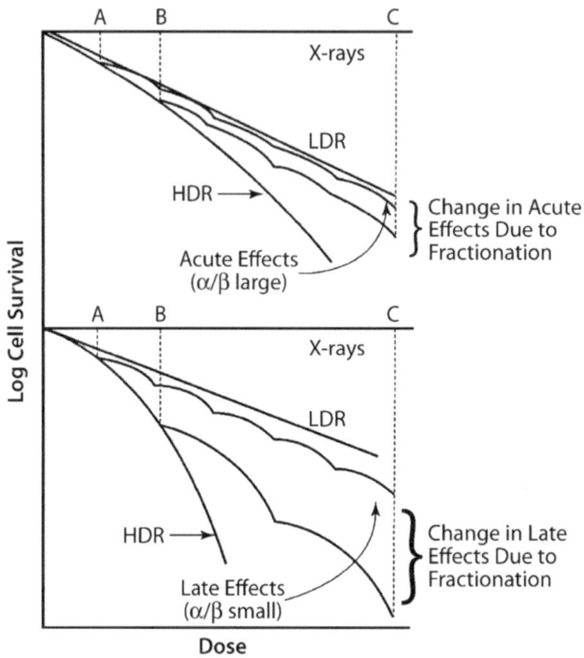

Fig. 3.19 For X-rays, late-responding tissues have a much more curved dose-response relationship and consequently show a much greater sparing in a multifraction regimen than early-responding tissues. Low dose rate (*LDR*) is, effectively, an infinite number of infinitely small doses. LDR therefore gives the maximum differential in sparing late-responding normal tissues compared with early-responding tissues, which includes tumors

outpatient and the device is typically in place for only 2–4 hours, while the treatment is planned and then delivery of dose takes a few minutes versus multiple days in the case of LDR brachytherapy. With HDR, the device is removed, and the patient goes home the same day.

When HDR is utilized for prostate cancers, interstitial needles are placed transperineally into the prostate. The devices are then connected to a mobile radiation source, known as an afterloader that will allow radiation to move through the device at a calculated rate in order to deposit the prescribed dose. Radiation is deposited at a rate of over 12 Gy/hr., and so the sources are only in the device for minutes at a time. The device can then be removed from the patient.

Investigational/Research Applications

As technology continues to advance, the uses for radiation also continue to evolve. An exciting new frontier is the use of radiation for consolidative treatment of oligometastatic disease. Emerging literature over the past decade has supported the existence of a distinct "oligometastatic" biologic state for malignancies [44–50]. First mentioned in a review by Weichselbaum et al. [44], the term "oligometastatic" disease has been broadly defined over time as a disease involving a limited number of distant regions [45].

Within this subset of metastatic patients, there may still be potential for disease control and prolonged survival with definitive local treatment (radiation or surgery) to disease sites [45]. Indeed, SBRT can be effective in the setting of oligometastatic melanoma [46], and definitive RT for patients with oligometastatic breast cancer may also yield better survival outcomes [47]. In the setting of oligometastatic cervical cancer, definitive RT can result in excellent local control of treated sites and contribute to long-term survival for carefully selected patients [48].

However, the most convincing literature for consolidation in the setting of oligometastatic disease can be attributed to non-small-cell lung cancer (NSCLC). Indeed, following several retrospective reports of consolidation in metastatic NSCLC [45], Gomez et al. published the first multi-institutional randomized phase II study comparing the role of aggressive local therapy in patients with NSCLC and ≤3 metastases who did not progress on standard frontline chemotherapy [49]. This study demonstrated that local consolidative therapy significantly improved progression-free survival for these patients when compared to maintenance therapy alone. Since then, these results have been further supported by other phase II randomized studies examining the role of consolidative RT in oligometastatic disease [50].

Taken together, these emerging data indicate that for patients with Stage IV cancer and limited numbers of metastatic sites, there may still be a role for local consolidative therapy (including RT) in improving disease outcomes through ablation or cytoreduction of active sites of disease [45]. Given these exciting implications, the benefit of consolidative RT in the oligometastatic setting merits further investigation extended to other sites in the setting of randomized controlled trials, particularly to elucidate which subgroups of patients are most likely to benefit from this aggressive approach.

References

1. Nunez MI, et al. Relationship between DNA damage, rejoining and cell killing by radiation in mammalian cells. Radiother Oncol. 1996;39(2):155–65.
2. Hall EJ, Giaccia AJ. Radiobiology for the radiologist. 6th ed. Philadelphia: Lippincott Williams & Wilkins; 2006. ix, 546 p.
3. Withers HR. The four R's of radiotherapy. Adv Radiat Biol. 1975;5:241–71.
4. Marcu LG. The first Rs of radiotherapy: or standing on the shoulders of giants. Australas Phys Eng Sci Med. 2015;38(4):531–41.
5. Elkind MM et al.; Radiation Response of Mammalian Cells Grown in Culture. V. Temperature dependence of the repair of x-ray damage in surviving cells (aerobic and hypoxic). Radiat Res. 1965:25;359–76.
6. Gray LH, et al. The concentration of oxygen dissolved in tissues at the time of irradiation as a factor in radiotherapy. Br J Radiol. 1953;26(312):638–48.
7. Withers HR, Taylor JM, Maciejewski B. The hazard of accelerated tumor clonogen repopulation during radiotherapy. Acta Oncol. 1988;27(2):131–46.

8. Bentzen SM, et al. Clinical radiobiology of squamous cell carcinoma of the oropharynx. Int J Radiat Oncol Biol Phys. 1991;20(6):1197–206.
9. Barton MB, et al. The effect of treatment time and treatment interruption on tumour control following radical radiotherapy of laryngeal cancer. Radiother Oncol. 1992;23(3):137–43.
10. Fyles A, et al. The effect of treatment duration in the local control of cervix cancer. Radiother Oncol. 1992;25(4):273–9.
11. Brengues M, et al. Method for validating radiobiological samples using a linear accelerator. EPJ Tech Instrum. 2014;1(1)
12. Funk RK, Stockham AL, Laack NNI. Chapter 3 – Basics of radiation therapy. In: Herrmann J, editor. Clinical cardio-oncology: Elsevier; 2016. p. 39–60.
13. Mazzeo E, et al. The current management of mycosis fungoides and Sézary syndrome and the role of radiotherapy: principles and indications. Rep Pract Oncol Radiotherap. 2013;19(2):77–91.
14. Haviland JS, et al. The UK Standardisation of Breast Radiotherapy (START) trials of radiotherapy hypofractionation for treatment of early breast cancer: 10-year follow-up results of two randomised controlled trials. Lancet Oncol. 2013;14(11):1086–94.
15. Kantzou I, et al. Conventional versus virtual simulation for radiation treatment planning of prostate cancer: final results. J BUON. 2011;16(2):309–15.
16. Soffen EM, et al. Conformal static field radiation therapy treatment of early prostate cancer versus non-conformal techniques: a reduction in acute morbidity. Int J Radiat Oncol Biol Phys. 1992;24(3):485–8.
17. Koper PC, et al. Acute morbidity reduction using 3DCRT for prostate carcinoma: a randomized study. Int J Radiat Oncol Biol Phys. 1999;43(4):727–34.
18. Bortfeld T. IMRT: a review and preview. Phys Med Biol. 2006;51(13):R363–79.
19. Young MR, Yu JB. Intensity modulated radiotherapy and image guidance. In: Mydlo JH, Godec CJ, editors. Prostate cancer: Academic Press; 2016. p. 413–26.
20. D'Souza WD, et al. Feasibility of dose escalation using intensity-modulated radiotherapy in posthysterectomy cervical carcinoma. Int J Radiat Oncol Biol Phys. 2005;61(4):1062–70.
21. Roeske JC, et al. Intensity-modulated whole pelvic radiation therapy in patients with gynecologic malignancies. Int J Radiat Oncol Biol Phys. 2000;48(5):1613–21.
22. Beriwal S, et al. Intensity-modulated radiotherapy for the treatment of vulvar carcinoma: a comparative dosimetric study with early clinical outcome. Int J Radiat Oncol Biol Phys. 2006;64(5):1395–400.
23. Wu VW, Kwong DL, Sham JS. Target dose conformity in 3-dimensional conformal radiotherapy and intensity modulated radiotherapy. Radiother Oncol. 2004;71(2):201–6.
24. Salama JK, et al. Preliminary outcome and toxicity report of extended-field, intensity-modulated radiation therapy for gynecologic malignancies. Int J Radiat Oncol Biol Phys. 2006;65(4):1170–6.
25. Michalski JM, et al. Preliminary toxicity analysis of 3-dimensional conformal radiation therapy versus intensity modulated radiation therapy on the high-dose arm of the Radiation Therapy Oncology Group 0126 prostate cancer trial. Int J Radiat Oncol Biol Phys. 2013;87(5):932–8.
26. Kry SF, et al. The calculated risk of fatal secondary malignancies from intensity-modulated radiation therapy. Int J Radiat Oncol Biol Phys. 2005;62(4):1195–203.
27. Haslam JJ, et al. Setup errors in patients treated with intensity-modulated whole pelvic radiation therapy for gynecological malignancies. Med Dosim. 2005;30(1):36–42.
28. Yoder AK, et al. Hitting a moving target: successful management of diffuse large B-cell lymphoma involving the mesentery with volumetric image-guided intensity modulated radiation therapy. Clin Lymphoma Myeloma Leuk. 2019;19(1):e51–61.
29. Dabaja B, et al. Successful treatment of a free-moving abdominal mass with radiation therapy guided by cone-beam computed tomography: a case report. J Med Case Rep. 2010;4:329.
30. Dzyubak O, et al. Evaluation of tumor localization in respiration motion-corrected cone-beam CT: prospective study in lung. Med Phys. 2014;41(10):101918.

31. Kavanagh BD, Timmerman RD. Chapter 24 – Stereotactic body irradiation: extracranial tumors. In: Gunderson LL, Tepper JE, editors. Clinical radiation oncology. 4th ed. Philadelphia: Elsevier; 2016. p. 427–431.e1.
32. Blomgren H, et al. Stereotactic high dose fraction radiation therapy of extracranial tumors using an accelerator. Clinical experience of the first thirty-one patients. Acta Oncol. 1995;34(6):861–70.
33. Lee SW, et al. Stereotactic body frame based fractionated radiosurgery on consecutive days for primary or metastatic tumors in the lung. Lung Cancer. 2003;40(3):309–15.
34. Solberg TD, et al. Quality and safety considerations in stereotactic radiosurgery and stereotactic body radiation therapy: executive summary. Pract Radiat Oncol. 2012;2(1):2–9.
35. Wilson RR. Radiological use of fast protons. Radiology. 1946;47(5):487–91.
36. Lawrence JH, et al. Pituitary irradiation with high-energy proton beams: a preliminary report. Cancer Res. 1958;18(2):121–34.
37. Hartsell WF, et al. Proton therapy in the USA from 2012 to 2014; increasing treatment of pediatric, lung, head and neck, gastrointestinal, and breast cancers, but no increase in prostate cancer treatments: a Study From the National Association for Proton Therapy. Int J Radiat Oncol Biol Phys. 2016;96(2):S136–7.
38. Tian X, et al. The evolution of proton beam therapy: current and future status. Mol Clin Oncol. 2018;8(1):15–21.
39. Delaney T, Kooy H. Proton and charged particle radiotherapy. Philadelphia: Lippincott Williams & Wilkins; 2008.
40. Milby AB, et al. Dosimetric comparison of combined intensity-modulated radiotherapy (IMRT) and proton therapy versus IMRT alone for pelvic and para-aortic radiotherapy in gynecologic malignancies. Int J Radiat Oncol Biol Phys. 2012;82(3):e477–84.
41. St Clair WH, et al. Advantage of protons compared to conventional X-ray or IMRT in the treatment of a pediatric patient with medulloblastoma. Int J Radiat Oncol Biol Phys. 2004;58(3):727–34.
42. Grutters JPC, et al. Comparison of the effectiveness of radiotherapy with photons, protons and carbon-ions for non-small cell lung cancer: a meta-analysis. Radiother Oncol. 2010;95(1):32–40.
43. Kagei K, et al. Long-term results of proton beam therapy for carcinoma of the uterine cervix. Int J Radiat Oncol Biol Phys. 2003;55(5):1265–71.
44. Hellman S, Weichselbaum RR. Oligometastases. J Clin Oncol. 1995;13:8–10.
45. Ning MS, Gomez DR, Heymach JV, Swisher SG. Stereotactic ablative body radiation for oligometastatic and oligoprogressive disease. Transl Lung Cancer Res. 2018;8:97.
46. Sarnaik AA, et al. Multidisciplinary management of special melanoma situations: oligometastatic disease and bulky nodal sites. Curr Oncol Rep. 2007;9:417–27.
47. Wong AC, et al. Clinical and molecular markers of long-term survival after oligometastasis-directed stereotactic body radiotherapy (SBRT). Cancer. 2016;122:2242–50.
48. Ning MS, et al. Outcomes and patterns of relapse after definitive radiation therapy for oligometastatic cervical cancer. Gynecol Oncol. 2018;148(1):132–8.
49. Gomez DR, et al. Local consolidative therapy versus maintenance therapy or observation for patients with oligometastatic non-small-cell lung cancer without progression after first-line systemic therapy: a multicentre, randomised, controlled, phase 2 study. Lancet Oncol. 2016;17(12):1672–82.
50. Iyengar P, Wardak Z, Gerber DE, et al. Consolidative radiotherapy for limited metastatic non-small-cell lung cancer: a phase 2 randomized clinical trial. JAMA Oncol. 2018;4:e173501.

Chapter 4
Radionuclide Cancer Therapy: Unsealed Alpha- and Beta-Emitters

A. Cahid Civelek and Franklin C. L. Wong

Introduction: Theranostics

The continuing advents in science, resulting in medical and technical advances, are allowing more and more treatment options to become available to patients with cancer. Such treatment selections include surgery, chemotherapy, radiation therapy, or their various types of combination. More recently, the use of targeted therapies in nuclear medicine has gained quite a recognition in cancer treatment as a viable option using radiopharmaceuticals with α-, β-, and γ-emitting unsealed radionuclides.

Radiation therapy or external radiotherapy utilizing ionizing radiations (such as high-energy X-rays) is the most frequently used type of radiation treatment. However, along with the targeted primary tumor, a limited amount of surrounding tissue around the tumor is also irradiated with high-energy X-rays, causing varying degrees of morbidities.

The use of targeted radionuclide therapy on the other hand involves the administration of radionuclide substances to patients, aiming for an organ-based tumor or the whole body of the patient. They reach targeted cells via the blood supply, as it happens in chemotherapy. Conversely, though, since these radioactive substances are explicitly aiming for specified malignant cells, the potential risk of systemic side effects is significantly reduced [1].

A. C. Civelek (✉)
Department of Radiology, Division of Nuclear Medicine and Molecular Imaging, Johns Hopkins Medicine, Baltimore, MD, USA
e-mail: acivele1@jhmi.edu

F. C. L. Wong
Department of Nuclear Medicine, University of Texas, M. D. Anderson Cancer Center, Houston, TX, USA
e-mail: fwong@mdanderson.org

F. C. L. Wong (ed.), *Locoregional Radionuclide Cancer Therapy*,
https://doi.org/10.1007/978-3-030-56267-0_4

One of the conditions for radiopharmaceuticals to be suited for therapeutic purposes is its ability to strongly bind with the tumor, that is, the high tumor affinity. Those radiopharmaceuticals with high affinity or high binding power to the specific tumor can transport intended doses of radiation directly to the tumors and its metastases, sparing the surrounding healthy tissue from radiation toxicity. One may direct such radiopharmaceuticals to a tumor's specific molecular moiety, such as antigens, receptors, or peptides. The various types of ionizing radiation emitted by radionuclides connected to the carrier can destroy or impair cancer cells by inflicting damage to their DNA resulting in targeted tumor suppression.

In addition to a very high affinity to malignant tumor cells, desired properties of an ideal radiopharmaceutical include the ability to distribute throughout the cells of the cancerous tumors and, while carrying the maximum doses of radiation to targeted tumor cells to destroy, spare the healthy cells.

The form of ionizing radiation emitted by the radionuclide determines the destructive biological effect of a radiopharmaceutical. In nuclear medicine, imaging procedures require radionuclides that emit gamma (γ) radiation, which can penetrate the body, and to reach the detector of the imaging device. For radionuclide therapy, however, radionuclides having optimal relative biological effectiveness are needed. Examples are those radionuclides emitting ionizing radiation with short tissue penetration, such as alpha (α)- or beta (β)-emitting radionuclides (Table 4.1).

In nuclear medicine, the term "theranostics" refers to the use of specific targeting molecules labeled with diagnostic radionuclides with gamma or positron emitters or labeled with therapeutic radionuclides such as beta, alpha, or internal conversion electrons, X-ray emitters, so that the diagnosis and treatment of a particular malignancy is accomplished (Fig. 4.1). It means that in molecular imaging, following the successful diagnosis of the disease can result in an effective treatment utilizing the same targeting molecule.

"Theranostics" is the combination of the words *thera*peutics and diag*nostics* which intends to link a diagnostic to therapeutic [2]. Since its beginning in 1940, theranostics has been fostering personalized medicine and targeted therapy and may well provide a cost-effective and specific successful treatment protocols. John Funkhouser, the President and CEO of PharmaNetics, was credited as the pioneer of the term theranostics [3].

Table 4.1 Types of therapeutic radionuclides

Types of therapeutic radionuclides	The range of emitted particle radiation into the tissue	Therapy effect inflicted if
β^--Emitter	From 1.0 mm	Therapy effect – if reaching the cell environment
Alpha-emitter	0.1 mm (100 μm)	Therapy effect – if reaching cell membrane
Auger electron emitter	0.01 mm (10 μm)	Therapy effect – if reaching cell nucleus
Internal conversion electron emission	0.2–0.55 mm (200–550 μm)	Therapy effect – if reaching cell nucleus

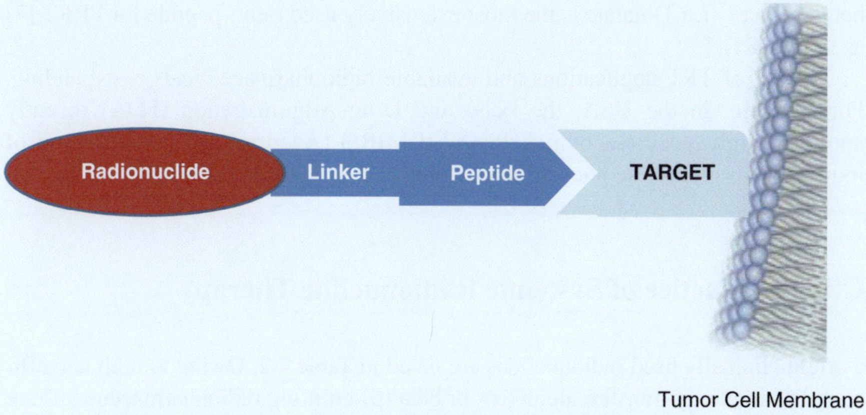

Radionuclide	Linker	Peptide	Target
^{111}In	DTPA	Octreotide	SSTR3 & 5
^{90}Y	DOTA	TOC	SSTR2
^{177}Lu	DOTA	TATE	SSTR2
^{68}Ga	DOTA	TATE	SSTR2
^{68}Ga	DOTA	NOC	SSTR3 & 5
^{68}Ga	DOTA	TOC	SSTR5

Fig. 4.1 Theranostics – definition: *thera*peutics + diag*nostics*. Schematic representation of how a radionuclide is linked to a peptide by means of a linker (chelator) for imaging or therapy of specific agents

It is complimentary to personalized medicine which is achieved by correctly identifying and appropriately selecting patients with a specific molecular phenotype indicative of positive response to treatment [4]. Thus, theranostic approach is predictive, preventive, personalized, and participatory. It identifies the right drug for the right patient at the right time and increases the quality of clinical care and treatments and will ultimately save costs [5].

Theranostic approaches in oncology have opened a new era in nuclear medicine [6]. Recent successful examples of theranostics are peptide receptor scintigraphy (PRS) and "peptide receptor radionuclide therapy" (PRRT), also called "radioligand therapy" (RLT) of neuroendocrine tumors. From its start since the early 1990s, these modalities with radiolabeling of somatostatin analogs by various radionuclides have led to significant advances in patient management resulting in a growth of the theranostic principle into other oncology indications.

Targeted radionuclide therapies (TRTs) utilize unsealed radionuclide sources, for example, a beta (β)-emitting radiopharmaceutical to target peptide receptors to deliver localized or targeted treatment, thus sparing as much the healthy cells as possible. Currently, PRRT is used for treating neuroendocrine tumors. A beta-emitter ^{177}Lu-Dotatate is the most extensively used radio-peptide for PRRT [7] as in Fig. 4.1.

The list of TRT applications and available radiopharmaceuticals is expanding. For example, in the USA, the Food and Drug Administration (FDA) recently approved high-specific-activity (HSA) ^{131}I-MIBG (Azedra®) for the treatment of inoperable or metastatic pheochromocytoma and/or paraganglioma (PPGL) [8].

Clinical Practice of Systemic Radionuclide Therapy

Current clinically used radionuclides are listed in Table 4.2. Owing to high and efficient linear energy transfer, alpha (α)- or beta (β)-emitting radiopharmaceuticals are more efficacious in therapy, while gamma-emitters would allow localization and quantification of the molecule. Radionuclides such as ^{131}I which emit beta as well as gamma radiations have the advantages of being able to ablate abnormal tissues and be imaged for localization and quantification. Since ^{131}I has been used to treat thyroid cancer since 1947, much clinical experience has been culminated. Following clinical cancer therapy sections on α-emitting (a) and β-emitting (b) radiopharmaceuticals, an additional section (c) is dedicated to thyroid cancer radioiodine therapy with requisite considerations to illustrate complexities of radionuclide cancer therapy.

Alpha-Emitters for Clinical Cancer Therapy (Table 4.2)

α-Particles are helium nuclei with the ability of deposition of considerable energy, approximately 100 keV/μm, along their straight, short path (5–10 cell diameters). Because of their high linear energy transfer (LET), they are very efficient at killing viable cells. Relatively few alpha particles 'travels across' that is needed to kill the cell, and this killing effect is minimally dependent on oxygen [9, 10]. An α-particle deposits >1500 times more energy per unit path length than a β-particle. The goal in cancer therapy is to target malignant cells while sparing normal cells. The use of appropriate radionuclide carrier may confine alpha radiation to the targeted cells with minimal "healthy tissue" damage. However, the lack of such targeting capability may result in excessively high doses to normal tissues that may provoke mutations and secondary cancers.

Targeted alpha-therapy (TAT) In May 2013, a pharmaceutical-grade radium-223 chloride solution was the first α-emitting radiopharmaceutical approved in the USA for clinical use in the treatment of metastatic bone disease. Radium-223 is a unique α-emitting radiopharmaceutical and may be used in ionic form as "simple" chloride salt. Since its approval, it is being marketed by a major pharmaceutical company as "Xofigo" (radium-223 chloride) and successfully demonstrated the clinical feasibility of TAT. Xofigo shows a favorable efficacy profile and good tolerance to treat

Table 4.2 Commonly used α- and β^--emitting therapeutic radionuclides – physical characteristics

	β^--Emitter						Alpha-emitter			
	^{32}P Phosphorus-32	^{89}Sr Strontium-89 (Metastron)	^{90}Y Yttrium-90	^{153}Sm Samarium-153	^{131}I Iodine-131	^{177}Lu Lutetium-177	^{223}Ra Radium-223 (Xofigo)	^{211}At Astatine-211	^{225}Ac Actinium-225	^{213}Bi Bismuth-213
Emission type (β^-, α, γ, EC)	β^-	β^-	β^-	β^- and γ	β^- and γ, e–	β^- and γ	α (95.3%) β^- (3.6%) 0.4 MeV γ (1.1% 0.01–1.27MeV	α, γ	α	α, β^-
Physical T1/2 (Hr/ Day)	14.3 days	50.5 days	2.67 days	1.9 days	8.1 days	6.71 days	11.43 days	7.2 h	10 days	46.5 min
Average energy (meV)	0.70 MeV	0.58 MeV	0.934 MeV	810 MeV (γ emission −103 kev 28%)	0.182 MeV	353 MeV	5.65 MeV (5–7.5 MeV)		28 MeV-cumulative α Two beta disinte-grations of 1.6 and 0.6 MeV γ 218 and 440 keV	
Maximum energy (meV)	1.71 MeV	1.49 MeV	2.28 MeV	0.23 MeV	0.606 MeV (γ emission: 364 keV 81%)	498 MeV (γ emission: 208 keV 11% 113 keV 6%)	7.5 MeV	5.87 (42%) (γ emission: 670 keV 0.03%)	28 MeV cummulative	8.4 and 5.8 MeV
Average range in tissue (mm)	3 mm	2.4 mm	2.5 mm	0.6 mm	0.4 mm	0.28 mm	<0.1 mm (<100 μm)	0.06 mm	Successive α-emission, thus, no clear range	α: 0.076 mm β^-: 2.1 mm

(continued)

Table 4.2 (continued)

	β^--Emitter						Alpha-emitter			
	^{32}P Phosphorus-32	^{89}Sr Strontium-89 (Metastron)	^{90}Y Yttrium-90	^{153}Sm Samarium-153	^{131}I Iodine-131	^{177}Lu Lutetium-177	^{223}Ra Radium-223 (Xofigo)	^{211}At Astatine-211	^{225}Ac Actinium-225	^{213}Bi Bismuth-213
Maximum range in tissue (mm)	8 mm	6.7 mm	11.0 mm		2.9 mm	2.0 mm			Successive α-emission, thus, no clear range	
R_{95} (mm)			5.94 mm							
In therapeutic use; X% of the radiation is delivered in X days			94% of the radiation delivered in 11 days						Its relatively long half-life of 10 days and the multiple alpha particles generated in the rapid decay chain render 225Ac a particularly cytotoxic radionuclide	
Utilized for	Bone mets PV Leukemia Intracavitary	Bone mets	Targeted therapy SIRT NH lymphoma NSCLC Intracavitary Rx for glioblastoma Radionuclide synovectomy for RA		Hyperthyroid and thyroid cancer treatment. Intracavitary Rx	Treatment of NETs, multiple other tumors	Metastatic bone disease	Hyperthyroid treatment mAbs in cancer Rx	Therapy of metastatic castration-resistant prostate cancer AML	RIT myelogenous leukemia Lymphoma Glioma Breast cancer Metastases NET Melanoma

Typical dose	12.0 mCi – -fractionated	4.0 mCi i.v., over 1–2 min	27 mCi of 90Y delivers a total absorbed radiation dose of 50 Gy/kg	0.5–1.0 mCi/kg	Variable	Variable	1.49 microcurie per kg body weight, given at 4-week intervals for six injections		0.023–0.39 mCi (0.004 mCi/kg) The current worldwide production is approximately 1.7 Ci/year	27.0–202.7 mCi injected in fractions of 13.5–40.5 arterial catheter in the tumor feeding vessel
Site of deposit	Skeleton: 85% Muscle, L/S:15%	Sites of new bone formation	Delivered organ	Skeletal mets	Thyroid and metastasis	SSReceptor guided	Bone	Delivered organ	Delivered organ	Delivered organ
Excretion route	Urine and feces: 5–10%/24 h 20%/1 week	Urine > fecal	–	Blood stream, urinary excretion	Promptly excreted by the kidneys: 35–75% in 24 h	Blood stream, urinary 44% in 5 h 58% in 24 h 65% in 48 h >99% in 14 days	Intestine 15 min–20% in blood 4 h–4% 24 h <1%			

e− internal conversion – electrons, X-rays, *SIRT* selective internal radiotherapy, *R95* the distance β-particle transfers 95% of its energy to the target tissue male patients with symptoms of advanced prostate cancer that has only bone metastases. Xofigo therapy assumes that α-emitting radionuclides can destroy cancer cells while sparing nearby healthy cells, thus reducing toxicity.

^{223}Ra has a half-life of 11.4 days and emits alpha, beta, and gamma radiation. The standard Nuclear Pharmacy and Nuclear Medicine instrumentation may detect its gamma and beta radiation. Xofigo®, as calcium does, forms complexes with the bone mineral hydroxyapatite at areas of increased bone turnover, such as bone metastases. The high linear energy transfer of its alpha rays leads to a high frequency of double-stranded DNA breaks in adjacent cells, resulting in its antitumor effect. The α-particle range from radium-223 is less than 100 micrometers that are less than ten cell diameters, which limits damage to the surrounding tissue. Xofigo (radium Ra 223 dichloride) injection, for intravenous use [prescribing information] [11].

Although no dedicated pharmacokinetic study in patients with renal impairment conducted because the excretion in urine is minimal and the primary route of elimination is via the feces, renal impairment is not expected to affect the pharmacokinetics of radium-223 dichloride. Treatment dose range is 50 kBq (1.35 microcurie) per kg body weight, given at 4-week intervals for six injections [12, 13].

The primary evidence of treatment efficacy of 223Ra (Xofigo®) in patients who had metastatic castration-resistant prostate cancer (mCRPC) and only bone metastases is based on a randomized, double-blind, placebo-controlled phase III study with a cohort of 921 patients [14].

This study showed not only improvement of overall survival in treated patients but also a 30% reduction in mortality, compared with placebo, with median overall survival of 14 months in the treated group versus 11.2 months in the placebo group.

Beta-Emitters for Clinical Cancer Therapy (Table 4.2)

^{131}I–NaI for Thyroid Cancer and ^{131} I-MIBG for Pheochromocytoma

^{131}I emits radiations of β^- & γ, e^- (internal conversion electrons) with half-life of 8.1 days. Its principal particulate emission is β^- with average energy of 0.182 MeV and maximum range of 2.9 mm that is suitable for ablation, while the principal γ emission of 364 keV (81%) is suitable for imaging. ^{131}I sodium iodide (NaI) has been used to treat thyroid cancer with typical oral doses between 30 and 250 mCi. ^{131}I MIBG is for the treatment of refractory pheochromocytoma and neuroblastoma with typical dose of 500 mCi. High-specific-activity 131 I MIBG was recently approved by the FDA for the treatment of inoperable metastatic pheochromocytoma [8].

^{89}Sr-Metastron and ^{153}Sm-Quadramet for Painful Osseous Metastasis

Strontium-89 (^{89}Sr) has a half-life of 50.5 days and emits $\beta^-$with average energy of 0.58 MeV and maximum range of 6.7 mm. ^{89}Sr chloride (Metastron) has been approved for palliation of pain from osseous metastasis. ^{89}Sr is a calcium analog that binds to hydroxyapatite in newly formed bones (osteoblastic activity on bone scan). A fixed intravenous dose of 4 mCi is typically administered. The general requirements are adequate hematologic function and the confirmation of no impending spinal cord compression by osseous metastasis in the vertebra to avoid direct irradiation of the spinal cord.

Samarium-153 ^{153}Sm has half-life of 1.9 days and emits β^- with average energy of 710 Mev and maximum range of 3 mm and γ emission at 103 kev (28%) that is also amenable for scintigraphy. ^{153}Sm-lexidronam (EDTMP or Quadramet) also binds to newly formed bones, in similar locations when metastasis is revealed on bone scans. The FDA-approved dosage is 1 mCi/kg. Dosages as high as 4–6 mCi/kg have been used in clinical trials without report of acute toxicity. The general requirements for ^{153}Sm-lexidronam are similar to those of ^{89}Sr chloride. Because of the shorter half-life of 1.9 days, half of the radiation-absorbed dose from ^{153}Sm is expected to deposit in the metastasis in 2 days (compared to 50 days for ^{89}Sr) to provide faster relief of pain. Unlike ^{223}Ra, neither ^{89}Sr chloride (Metastron) nor ^{153}Sm-lexidronam (Quadramet) has been demonstrated to confer survival benefits in phase III trials. Therefore, these two radiopharmaceuticals targeting osteoblastic activities have remained second choices in treating prostate osseous metastasis. Multiple trials have been performed in treating other cancer types using ^{89}Sr chloride (Metastron) or ^{153}Sm-lexidronam (Quadramet) or in combination with other cancer treatment modalities to enlarge therapeutic windows. Often, these endeavors are limited by additive hematotoxicity [15, 16].

^{90}Y-Zevalin and ^{131} I-Bexxar for CD20+ Lymphoma

Yttrium-90 ^{90}Y emits β^- with half-life of 2.67 days and average energy of 0.934 MeV and maximum range of 11.0 mm. 90Y-labeled anti-CD20 monoclonal murine antibody, Zevalin (ibritumomab tiuxetan) has been approved by the FDA for treating refractory lymphomas. Upon histologic confirmation of CD20 positivity, the patient undergoes an optional ^{111}In-labeled anti-CD20 monoclonal antibody for whole-body imaging (bioscan) to confirm proper biodistribution before treatment. On the treatment day, the patient initially receives infusion of non-labeled Zevalin to mask the low-affinity binding sites in the body. Patients will then receive infusion of ^{90}Y-Zevalin at doses of 0.4 mCi/kg up to 32 mCi. The limiting factor would be hematologic toxicity and allergic reactions. Its application has been tested in trials to different types of hematologic malignancies including chronic lymphocytic leukemia [17, 18].

Similar strategy is applied to the FDA-approved ^{131}I-Bexxar (tositumomab) with an initial low dosage to conduct the bioscan to confirm biodistribution and to derive the whole-body radiation-absorbed dose in order to optimize the injected treatment dosage which is typically between 50 and 120 mCi [19, 20]. The anti-CD20 monoclonal antibody therapy using ^{90}Y-Zevalin or ^{131}I-Bexxar is restricted to refractory lymphoma. With more nonradioactive competing therapeutic modalities against lymphomas, such as targeted therapies, immunotherapies, stem cell transplants, and cellular, the use of ^{90}Y-Zevalin has been decreasing over the last decade in spite of initial good results. ^{131}I-Bexxar is no longer commercially available in the USA.

^{32}P-Phosphate for Chronic Leukemia and Polycythemia Vera

Phosphorus-32 (^{32}P) has a physical half-life of 14.3 days and emits a β^- particle with average energy of 0.70 MeV. The maximum particle range in soft tissue is 8.0 mm. With the development of nuclear reactors, radiophosphorus is produced from bombarding $^{16}S_{32}$ with fast neutrons, which results in a carrier-free product. ^{32}P was the first radionuclide introduced many decades ago for the palliation of bone pain from bone metastases and used until the 1980s. Phosphorus-32 sodium phosphate has also been approved by FDA in 4 ml intravenous injection for the treatment of chronic leukemia (at dosage of 6–15 mCi) and polycythemia vera (at dosage of 1–8 mCi) [21, 22].

^{111}In-Octreotide as a Potential Theranostic Radiopharmaceutical

Indium-111 (^{111}In) is produced by cyclotron. The radioactive ^{111}In decays to ^{112}Cd with a physical half-life of 2.83 days. Its gamma photon energies of 150.8 keV, 171.3 keV, and 245.4 keV allow imaging using multiple photopeaks to assure good image quality. The multitude of Auger electrons delivers large radiation payload to surrounding tissues within short ranges.

Neuroendocrine tumors (NETs) are characterized by a high expression of somatostatin receptors (SSTR) [23]. Based on the published European study results of about 350 patients with gastroenteropancreatic neuroendocrine tumors (GEP-NETs), the Food and Drug Administration of the USA approved ^{111}In-Octreotide (pentetreotide) as an imaging radiopharmaceutical in 1994. In that study, the sensitivity and specificity of the ^{111}In-pentetreotide in patients with GEP-NETs were higher than those obtained using computed tomography or magnetic resonance imaging, making the ^{111}In-pentetreotide the first approved receptor-targeted, peptide-based imaging radiopharmaceutical [24].

There is an overexpression of the somatostatin receptors (types 2 and 5) at the surface of the NET cancer cells. ^{111}In-octreotide is bounded to the somatostatin inhibitors and transferred into the cancer cell. Auger electrons emitted from ^{111}In can damage the DNA of the cancer cell [25]. Either with planar or SPECT scintigraphic images, one may calculate the dosimetry of ^{111}In-octreotide therapy.

Inspired by the use of radioactive iodine in thyroid cancer diagnosis and treatment, investigators used high doses of ^{111}In-pentetreotide to treat GEP-NET trial patients in the US and European clinical trials which was limited by nephrotoxicity which necessitated the use of nonradioactive kidney protection tracer blocking agent. Subsequently, radionuclides with better physical characteristics and a more extended range of tissue penetration, such as yttrium-90 (^{90}Y-) and lutetium-177 (^{177}Lu-), were used as a therapeutic agent [26].

^{68}Ga-DOTA(0)-Tyr(3)-octreotate (^{68}Ga-Dotatate) positron emission tomography (PET)/CT is found to be superior to most imaging modalities, including ^{111}In SSTR scintigraphy, in the detection of NETs [27]. ^{68}Ga-Dotatate or ^{111}In-SSTR scintigraphy has the added advantage of allowing the assessment of somatostatin receptor status of the tumors, which becomes essential for the selection of these patients for treatment with cold SSAs or "peptide receptor radionuclide therapy," especially in metastatic patients.

^{177}Lu-Lutathera for the Treatment of Neuroendocrine Tumors

Lutetium-177 (^{177}Lu-) has a half-life of 6.7 days emitting $\beta^{-}$with average energy of 0.353 Mev and maximum range of 2 mm along with γ emissions at 208 keV (11%) and 113 keV (6%) [28].

The therapy agent ^{177}Lu-DOTATATE (Lutathera) [L-Lysine Hydrochloride, L-Arginine Hydrochloride] has a diagnostic imaging pair; ^{68}Ga-DOTATATE. Manufacturer of these agents is Advanced Accelerator Applications (AAA).

The ^{177}Lu-labeled Dotatate was first used in clinical studies in 2000, forming the basis of the NETTER-1 multinational phase III trial [7]. Later in 2003, Strosberg et al. published the results of their study in 35 patients treated with ^{177}Lu-Dotatate for GEP-NETs that demonstrated complete remission in 1 patient (3%), partial remission in 12 patients (35%), stable disease in 14 patients (41%), and progressive disease in 7 patients (21%); three patients died of disease-related reasons during their treatments [29].

In 2012, a critical multinational phase III (NETTER-1) study was initiated at 41 sites worldwide. By 2015, this study reached its primary endpoint of assessing progression-free survival and demonstrated that ^{177}Lu-Dotatate significantly improved progression-free survival compared with high-dose octreotide acetate injection in patients with advanced midgut NETs, and the results were published [7]. Additionally NETTER-1 data demonstrated that in patients with progressive midgut neuroendocrine tumors, clinically relevant improvement of ^{177}Lu-Dotatate treatment and significantly longer time to deterioration quality of life measures achieved compared to octreotide LAR alone [7].

The efficient and patient-centric theranostic approach helps physicians to identify those patients who are better responders to a specific therapy, ensuing effective disease management. Theranostics not only enhances our ability to diagnose, stage, and select best-fit therapies; it also enables physicians to better monitor treatment response or disease progression, hence providing better health outcomes to their patients.

^{131}I Ablation of Thyroid Cancer: Complexities of Radionuclide Cancer Therapy

Over the last 70 years, the worldwide use of ^{131}I sodium iodide in treating thyroid cancer has uncovered critical issues important to clinical care of oncologic patients. These issues involve the cancer cell type vulnerabilities, detection of tumor response by biomarkers and by imaging, patient comforts, radiation exposure and safety concerns, stimulation and return of iodide uptakes by tumor, and radiation dosimetry in estimation of efficacy and toxicity. Each of these typical oncologic patient care issues would deserve separate detailed coverage. Nevertheless, they are briefly discussed below to draw due attention that would be needed when dealing with other radionuclide theranostic therapies.

Therapeutic use of radioiodine Robley Evans, while at the physics faculty at the Massachusetts Institute of Technology in Boston, Massachusetts, together with Dr. Saul Hertz and Dr. Arthur Roberts, helped to build the field of nuclear medicine: Using ^{128}I, they demonstrated that the thyroid of a rabbit would accumulate radioactive iodine in a reproducible and quantitative way. Later, they showed that the uptake of a hyperactive thyroid was several times that of a healthy thyroid [30]. Subsequently, they proceeded to diagnostic thyroid uptake studies in humans and, beginning in early1941, the application of ^{130}I to the treatment of thyroid disorders. Later, ^{131}I would replace ^{130}I. Later, in the late 1980s with more suitable physical characteristics, ^{123}I became accessible as the diagnostic radionuclide. Thus, the use of ^{123}I-^{131}I pair has become the first "theranostic" agents in nuclear medicine.

The types of thyroid cancers The papillary- and follicular-type differentiated thyroid cancers (DTC) have a more favorable prognosis than other types of thyroid malignancies, with an overall risk of relapse $\leq$20% [31]. Distant metastases develop in 10–15% of patients. Although DTC cells concentrate ^{131}I, along the course, two-thirds of the patients become refractory to radioactive iodine, and these patients have a poor prognosis, with 10-year survival rates of 29–38% [32]. The incidence of DTC in the USA is possibly increasing. Tumors presenting with locoregional extension, distant metastases, or more aggressive variant of tumors, such as the tall cell, columnar, and solid/trabecular (insular) variant and the hobnail variant of papillary thyroid carcinomas, are considered at higher risk for recurrence and death. The initial optimal management of patients with high-risk DTC which have clinically involved central or lateral neck lymph nodes consists of total thyroidectomy with therapeutic neck dissection. Similarly, prophylactic central compartment neck dissection is considered in patients with advanced papillary thyroid cancer tumors.

As DTC cells dedifferentiate, they lose their iodine-concentrating ability, and their cellular glucose metabolism become activated, which facilitates ^{18}F-FDG uptake. ^{18}F-FDG PET/CT is used to localize recurrent cancer foci in patients with elevated serum thyroglobulin (Tg) and negative whole-body ^{131}I scans. The meta-analysis-based pooled sensitivity of ^{18}F-FDG PET/CT to detect recurrence in patients with negative ^{131}I scans and elevated serum thyroglobulin (Tg) is 79% [33]. The "flip-Flop phenomenon" describes this pattern of differential radiotracer uptake, although both radioiodine-avid and ^{18}F-FDG-avid cells can coexist in the same patient [34, 35].

Thyroid cancers with ^{18}F-FDG uptake usually do not concentrate ^{131}I. Tumor hypoxia is associated with relative radio- and chemoresistance in several types of cancers, including DTC. Evidence for hypoxia in DTC is documented by immunohistochemistry for the hypoxia-inducible factor (HIF); increased expression of HIF 1 α may be associated with lymph node and distant metastases [36]. Metastatic thyroid cancers with high ^{18}F-FDG uptake usually behave aggressively. In metastatic thyroid cancer patients, ^{18}F-FDG PET/CT after ^{131}I therapy may be useful in predicting short-term progression. ^{18}F-FDG-SUVmax is an independent factor for short-term progression. For example, in one study, although 77% of patients with a negative ^{18}F-FDG PET/CT scan had an elevated level of normalized Tg, 81% of the patients with positive ^{18}F-FDG PET/CT scan still displayed elevated Tg levels at short-term follow-up after ^{131}I therapy.

Detecting recurrence following thyroidectomy or lobectomy: Tg and TgAb In patients with DTC who underwent total thyroidectomy and radioiodine ablation of the remnant thyroid tissue, the use of serum thyroglobulin (Tg) and thyroglobulin antibody (TgAb) measurements for detecting disease recurrence is well-validated, and later, a subsequent rise in serum Tg indicates the disease recurrence. The assessment of the Tg and TgAb is the main reasoning for the use of radioiodine ablation of the remnant thyroid tissue after total thyroidectomy. However, limited data is available on the efficacy of the application of such measurement in patients treated with thyroid lobectomy, rather than thyroidectomy. One recent study with a cohort of 167 patients evaluated the role of Tg and TgAb to detect recurrence of the papillary thyroid cancer following lobectomy. Patients were followed for more than 1 year, with sufficient data on Tg and TgAb, including subgroup analysis for Hashimoto's thyroiditis and contralateral nodules. The authors concluded, "Serum thyroglobulin" used independently is of limited value for predicting or detecting disease recurrence following thyroid lobectomy. Further study should be needed to evaluate the other potential roles of Tg, such as detecting distant metastases following lobectomy [37].

Safety Practice in I-131 Therapy Dose Administration All women of childbearing age must have a pregnancy test before undergoing imaging with ^{123}I or treatment with radioactive iodine (^{131}I). This policy will ensure the prevention of potential fetal exposure. Exceptions include any patient who has had a hysterectomy or is at least 1 year postmenopausal or 1 year post-tubal ligation and sexually active.

To ensure that the patient is not pregnant, usually, the patient's serum quantitative HCG is drawn at the time of the clinic visit before the scheduled imaging procedure or treatment. In cases where the clinic visit is longer than 1 week from the planned imaging procedure or treatment or where "procedures" are arranged over the telephone, the patient will be required to have the test performed at a local laboratory the week of the procedure (Fig. 4.2).

Before all therapy procedures, double-checking the name and history number of the patient, the dose, and the type of radiopharmaceutical agents might prevent misadministration. All incidents of misadministration and radioactive contamination must be reported immediately to the chief technologist and the attending physician for proper management and official reporting.

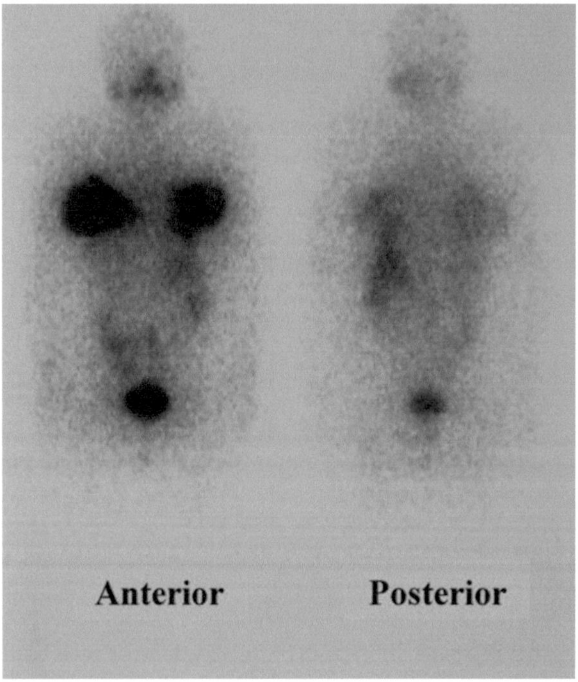

Fig. 4.2 Anterior and posterior 48 h. Whole-body planar ^{131}I images of a thyroid cancer metastatic survey study. A significant degree of ^{131}I activity is present throughout both breasts of this 28-year-old patient who is 4 month postpartum. Based on personal reasons, she chose to postpone the treatment of her thyroid cancer until after her child's birth. The radiation burden both from ^{123}I and especially ^{131}I to the breasts, which are radiosensitive, is quite high and easily be avoidable by proper timing of the imaging with patients' menses and pregnancy status. To minimize or avoid the patient's radiation burden to the breasts, lactating females should not receive ^{131}I imaging procedures or therapies, unless medically crucial. Usually, during the ovulatory and secretory phases of menstruation, the breast tracer uptake is higher and much lower during the late follicular and luteal phases of the menstrual cycle

Patient Stimulation Before the Administration of ^{131}I- Patient stimulation before the administration of ^{123}I for imaging or ^{131}I for treatment is necessary and can be achieved either by hormone withdrawal (deprivation) or by rhTSH stimulation. rhTSH stimulation is the method of choice because of better patient tolerance and comfort, alleviating potentially severe hypothyroid symptoms of the patients. The efficacy of ^{131}I administrated either after thyroid hormone withdrawal or after rhTSH is similar.

Schematic diagrams of patient preparations for ^{123}I imaging and ^{131}I therapy depicted in Fig. 4.3a–c.

A standard dose activity of 3.7 GBq or 100 mCi ^{131}I can be considered efficient and certainly safe in treating thyroid cancer patients with distant metastases.

However, in patients with renal failure and diffuse miliary lung metastases, using an empiric ^{131}I dose may result in an increased risk of toxicity, which might be alleviated by calculating individual maximal tolerable therapy ^{131}I dose.

Future studies employing accurate measurements of lesional dosimetry by the use of whole-body and blood dosimetry studies are likely to define a subset of patients in whom the necessary administered effective therapeutic dose does not exceed safety limits.

Reprogramming the biology of metastatic thyroid cancer cells by restoring the expression of genes required for iodide uptake and accumulation might improve the efficacy of definitive RAI therapy [38].

Finally, when reprogramming of the biology of metastatic thyroid cancer cells coupled with the whole body-blood clearance dosimetry-based approach as well as lesional dosimetry approaches, both the RAI treatment efficacy and the safety are better optimized.

Association of Radioactive Iodine Treatment with Cancer Mortality in Patients with Hyperthyroidism Using data from 18,805 patients with hyperthyroidism who were treated with radioactive iodine, Kitahara et al. investigated the association of organ- or tissue absorbed dose- and site-specific cancer death. At the time, their study was the world's largest cohort and the first study to characterize the dose-response relationship between RAI treatment and site-specific cancer mortality in patients with hyperthyroidism using reliable estimates of absorbed dose to exposed organs or tissues [39].

The authors reported a statistically significant positive dose-response relationship for risk of death for all solid cancers (6% increase in risk per 100 mGy dose to the stomach), breast cancer (12% increase in risk per 100 mGy dose to the breast), and all solid cancers excluding breast (5% increase in risk per 100 mGy dose to the stomach).

Their reported findings suggest a modest positive association between higher organ absorbed doses of radioactive iodine and risk of solid cancer death. The authors concluded that hyperthyroid treatment decisions should take into consideration the balance of risks with the benefits of each available treatment option as well as patient preference, health status, and access to these options. The risk of death

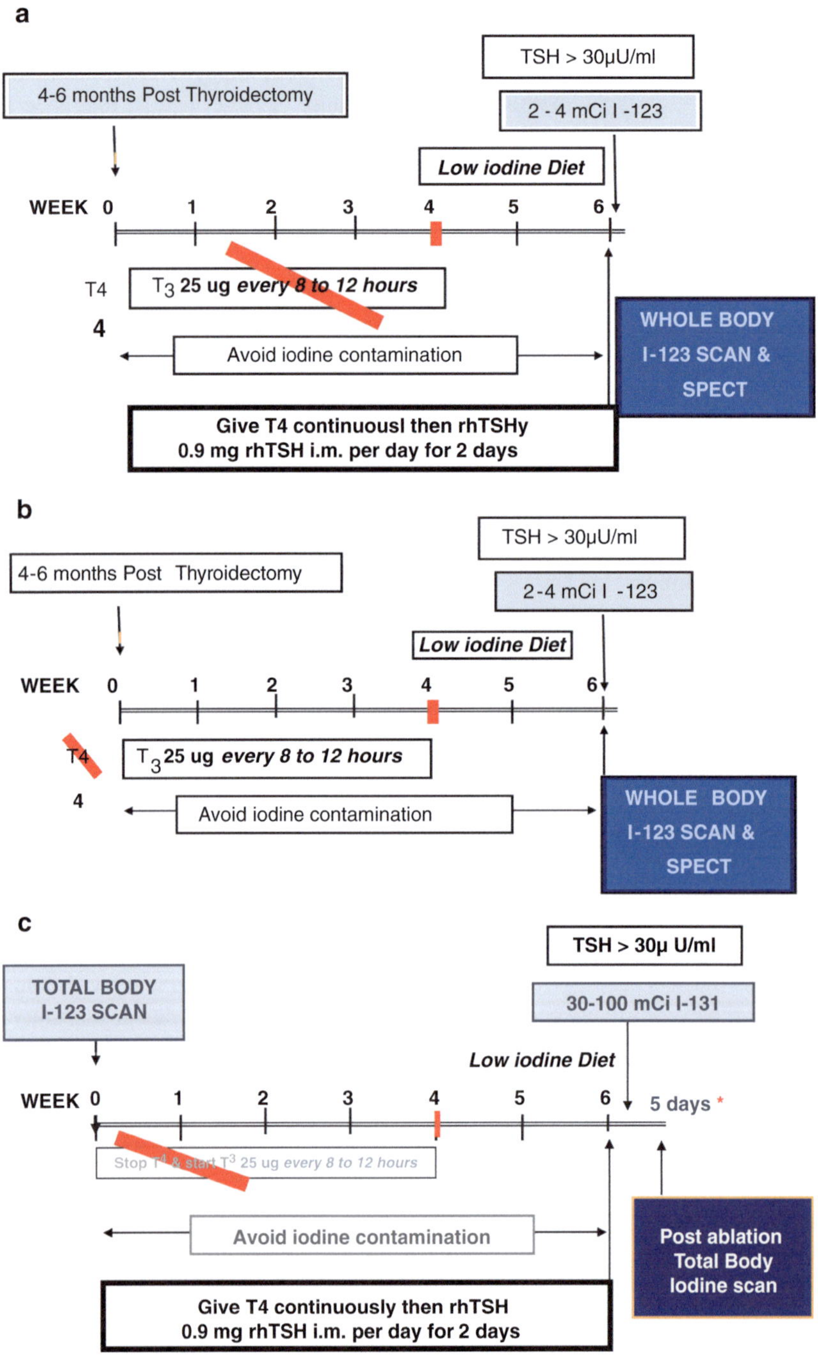

Fig. 4.3 (**a**) Patient preparation for a diagnostic whole-body iodine scan with rhTSH stimulation. (**b**) Patient preparation for a diagnostic whole-body iodine scan with hormonal withdrawal. (**c**) Patient preparation for radioiodine ablation of thyroid remnant

from solid cancer (including breast cancer) increases with the higher absorbed dose to exposed organs and tissues. How to minimize or avoid breast radiation burden is summarized in Fig. 4.2 legend.

Nevertheless, additional studies might be needed to adequately estimate the risks and advantages of radioactive iodine and other treatment options available for patients with hyperthyroidism. The readers are encouraged to read the "Strengths and Limitations" section of the manuscript by Kitahara [39].

Are the incidence and associated mortality of thyroid cancer in the USA rising? Yan KL et al., in his June 2020 publication utilizing a retrospective analysis of all thyroid cancers in the California Cancer Registry (2000–2017), reported a rising incidence and incidence-based mortality of thyroid cancer in California. In the registry, the authors identified 69,684 patients with thyroid cancer with a median age of 50 years. Over the study period, the incidence of thyroid cancer increased from 6.43 to 11.13 per 100,000 person-years, accounting for an average increase of 4% per year. The rise in the prevalence of thyroid cancer is observed in all sizes and not limited to small papillary thyroid cancers. The study also demonstrated increased incidence-based mortality more so in men and patients with larger tumors, suggesting a real increase in clinically significant disease [40].

There are, however, contenders of such opinions. The invited commentary, appearing on the same journal, for example, stated that "The steady, worldwide increase in the incidence of differentiated thyroid cancers are largely the result of the increasing diagnosis of less than 1 cm in diameter—the so-called microcarcinomas, small 'papillary' malignancies" [41].

The question on necessity of screening for thyroid cancer The existence of small, clinically silent thyroid cancers is already known from autopsy studies [42]. Most endocrinologists accept that the vast majority of thyroid microcarcinomas are indolent intrathyroidal tumors. They rarely metastasize, and when it happens, they tend to be locoregional in the neck. Furthermore, although rare, the occurrence of locoregional lymph node metastasis has virtually no impact on patient survival. Moreover, such locoregional disease, as residual foci of cancer left behind or metastatic lymph nodes, can safely be managed without difficulty, such as surgically or with nonsurgical ways, such as laser, radiofrequency, or microwave ablation or with observation alone [41].

The authors of the above referenced commentary suggested halting the practice of thyroid cancer screening for individuals with no symptoms or signs of the disease and no known risk factors such as exposure to neck radiation or a family history of thyroid cancer in the general population. They advocated that those small, subclinical cancers incidentally detected by diagnostic imaging studies during the workup of non-thyroid reasons could be stratified by a careful ultrasound assessment of the nodule, rather than an FNA cytology, and then with simple surveillance [43]. Likewise, when thyroid microadenomas incidentally detected on postoperative thyroid tissue are removed for benign disease, instead of using aggressive diagnostic or therapeutic procedures, one may consider utilizing clinical and pathological criteria to identify those tumors with "a very low risk" of recurrence [44]. Such an algorithm may enable alleviating postoperative radioactive iodine administration and thyroid hormone suppression therapies and allowing patients followed with more relaxed protocols involving a simple physical examination and assays of serum thyroglobulin and thyroglobulin antibody levels at least every 2 years [45].

In patients with differentiated thyroid cancer who underwent total thyroidectomy and radioiodine ablation of the remnant thyroid tissue, the use of serum thyroglobulin (Tg) and thyroglobulin antibody (TgAb) measurements for detecting disease recurrence is well-validated, but not in patients with partial thyroidectomy. Please refer to the section "Detecting recurrence following thyroidectomy or lobectomy: Tg and TgAb" on page 11. Other potential roles of Tg, such as detecting distant metastases following lobectomy, should be further studied [37, 43].

Dosimetry-Based Versus Empiric Prescribed Activity of ^{131}I for Therapy of Differentiated Thyroid Cancer (DTC) [46] Usually, ^{131}I ablation therapy follows surgical treatment. Depending on the individual patient, the primary goal of the first dose of the postsurgical radioactive iodine (RAI) ablation therapy may be for ablation of the remnant thyroid tissue or to decrease the risk of recurrence and disease-specific mortality by destroying the suspected, but the unproven, metastatic disease (as adjuvant therapy) or to treat the known persistent disease (as RAI therapy). The administered RAI dose is determined either by use of the arbitrary, empirically prescribed activity of ^{131}I as is employed at most treatment centers or by use of whole body-blood clearance dosimetry-based approach, with the patient-specific prescribed activity of ^{131}I [47].

Klubo-Gwiezdzinska et al. demonstrated the clinical benefit of dosimetry-based treatment in the subgroup of patients with locally advanced differentiated thyroid cancer. The complete response (CR) rate in patients after dosimetry-based treatment was significantly higher than the patients who received standard empiric fixed prescribed activity of ^{131}I. On the other hand, the advantage of dosimetry-based treatment was not apparent for patients with distant metastasis [46].

More recently, Deandreis et al., in a large cohort of iodine-avid distant metastatic thyroid cancer patients, compared the empiric dose radioactive iodine (^{131}I) treatment approach to the whole body-blood clearance dosimetry-based approach (without measuring lesional dosimetry) and found similar overall survival (OS) of the groups. The safety profile on the dosimetric method compared with the empiric approach was identical to the study of Klubo-Gwiezdzinska et al. [48].

The whole body-blood clearance dosimetry-based approach calculates the maximum tolerated activity of ^{131}I using blood as a surrogate for the bone marrow and aims to deliver a radiation dose of 200 rad (2 Gy) or less, thus diminishing the likelihood of an adverse bone marrow effect while providing the highest radiation dose to the tumor. However, this approach does not consider the magnitude of ^{131}I activity uptake by the individual metastatic lesions.

Several studies with small patient cohorts demonstrated that identification and quantification of the ^{131}I-derived radiation-absorbed dose to the metastatic lesion, e.g., lymph nodes, is feasible and the likelihood of cure be increased from 20% to approximately 90% by increasing the prescribed activity delivered to a lesion from 40 to 80 rad (cGy) [49].

The "hybrid dosimetric approach" combines whole body-blood clearance dosimetry-based approach with targeted lesional quantification dosimetry. Using this approach, Dorn et al. achieved CR with tumor doses ranging from 10,000 to 15,000 rad (100–150 Gy) [50].

Some studies reported that the addition of PET technology and using ^{124}I PET-guided lesional dosimetry could provide more improved absorbed lesion doses and help to calculate the safest and the most effective ^{131}I activity to be administered [51]. Similarly, recent SPECT/CT camera quantification algorithms also make the calculation of absorbed dose in normal organs and tumoral lesions possible [52].

Sestamibi uptake of the thyroid gland The evidence suggests that thyroid sestamibi uptake is likely due to nonspecific binding of sestamibi and is not primarily due to free Tc-99m pertechnetate or a metabolic by-product of the Tc-99m sestamibi. However, strong evidence suggests that the mechanism of Tc-99m sestamibi uptake by normal and malignant thyroid tissue is not purely blood flow-dependent and may reflect its substitution for potassium by the ATPase-dependent sodium-potassium pump. Although the actual mechanism remains unclear, there is evidence that Tc-99m sestamibi tissue uptake is related to its sequestration within the cytoplasm and mitochondria of cells in response to the electrical potentials generated across the membrane bilayers [53]. Low-level thyroidal sestamibi uptake is not suppressible with potassium perchlorate ($KCLO_4$) and not mediated by the gland's iodine trapping mechanism [54]. This observation inspired the reasoning for "delayed only ^{99m}Tc sestamibi SPECT scintigraphy technique" for preoperative localization of primary hyperparathyroidism [55].

Practical challenging circumstances in ^{131}I therapy Most thyroid cancer patients with or without metastases may receive ^{131}I therapy on an outpatient basis. However, ^{131}I therapy for ablation of postoperative thyroid remnants or treatment of residual differentiated thyroid cancer and its metastasis may become a challenging task in patients with special needs. Example cases representing such challenging patients include a quadriplegic patient with draining, wet decubitus ulcers; a renal failure patient dependent on three dialyses a week; and a gastric feeding tube-dependent, chronically bedridden patient who cannot swallow. Possible treatment complications and side effects, therapeutic alternatives, expected patient outcome, proper handling of the liquid ^{131}I use for the patient who cannot swallow, ways of obtaining a legally valid written informed consent from a quadriplegic patient, calculating the optimum ^{131}I therapy dose in renal failure patients, logistics of delivering radiation safety, minimizing procedure-related radiation dose burden to the caregivers, and administrative and legal aspects of such therapies are essential discussion topics among the team members of the multi-modality care team [56]. An acceptable approach to such a situation is to form a team to include the referring physician, the nuclear medicine physician, the radiation safety officer, the nuclear medicine technologist, and nursing managers. Such a team may come up with a treatment plan with division of assignments and responsibilities for the involved caregivers.

To obtain an accurate total body count of a bedridden patient, one might need to modify the "total body counting" technique. The additional training with all shifts of the nursing staff on the patient's floor provided by the radiation safety officer and nuclear medicine manager would significantly decrease the apprehension of the team regarding their perceived radiation burden. The emphasis of this training would be radiation safety for both the nurse and patient during the administration of nursing care. Second, the referring physician and the nursing staff may develop a modified patient care plan that would minimize bedside nursing as much as possible. Third, the radiation safety officer provides additional radiation waste containers that could be removed from the patient room daily to help minimize nursing exposure to stored ^{131}I-contaminated dressings. The upfront involvement of the physician, management, nursing, and technical staff may help nuclear medicine to prepare for and successfully conduct these therapies and keep everyone safe and everyone's radiation burden within ALARA concepts [57].

Clinical Practice Using Locoregional Radionuclide Therapy

^{32}P-Chromic Phosphate for Intracavitary Therapy of Tumors

Treatment of intracerebral cystic neoplasms using ^{32}P has been proposed and utilized. Direct instillation of colloidal phosphorus-32 into intracranial cystic tumors can be an effective means of controlling cyst growth and fluid production. Several techniques of administering the radioisotope are available, with rigorous pre- and post-instillation assessments applied [58].

The imaging of ^{32}P, a pure beta-emitter, although challenging, is achievable by imaging bremsstrahlung rays. One could improve the delivery and verify the post-instillation location of ^{32}P utilizing both pre- and posttreatment imaging assessments. A pretreatment computed tomography produces a more accurate volume estimation of the cystic lesion by injecting an iodine contrast agent into the cyst via an Ommaya system, which also helps to assess the patency of the Ommaya, leakage of the cyst, and cyst loculation if present, thus determining the appropriateness of ^{32}P treatment.

^{32}P administered with a small amount of iodine contrast is injected into the cyst. ACT scan done after instillation can locate the iodine contrast by inference, the ^{32}P. Scintigraphic imaging can provide further confirmation of the presence of the ^{32}P within the cyst. Iodine intensifies the ^{32}P bremsstrahlung, thereby enhancing scintigraphic imaging for verification of isotope location. The posttreatment evaluations through CT and scintigraphy determine the effective instillation of ^{32}P.

Other applications of Phosphorus-32 therapy: Intrapleural administration of ^{32}P-chromic phosphate colloids could treat the suspected residual local chest, chest wall disease in patients with Ewing sarcoma, Askin tumor (tumor of the chest wall) [59].

^{90}Y-Microspheres (Theraspheres and SIRSpheres) for Liver Cancers

Yttrium-90 (^{90}Y) emits β^- with half-life of 2.67 days and average energy of 0.934 MeV and maximum range of 11.0 mm. Under neutron activation schemes using glass or polymer microspheres, ^{90}Y-Theraspheres and ^{90}Y-SIRSpheres are manufactured, respectively [60, 61]. They have gained approval by the FDA as devices under the IDE pathway to treat hepatocellular and metastatic liver cancers, respectively. They are typically injected intra-arterially via the common hepatic artery, or it branches under interventional radiology guidance to result in embolization of arterioles in the tumor territory to deliver locoregional irradiation of the liver cancer. The dosage ranges between 50 and 150 mCi. The explicit intent is to deliver 80–150 Gy to the whole liver. With better interventional technology to reliably deliver the microspheres in the more distal territory for specific irradiation of the tumors, the dosage could be fractionated according to the vascular territories. One of the prerequisites for the therapy is a low pulmonary shunting fraction (<20%) that can be detected by a perfusion scan of the lungs. Recent advances in imaging have allowed detection of ^{90}Y from its Bremsstrahlung radiations using SPECT-CT or imaging of pair production from ^{90}Y using PET-CT [62, 63]. Image-based dosimetric analyses may enable robust correlation between outcomes and radiation-absorbed doses of hepatic lobes to allow prediction of outcome and decision to modify therapy [64].

With the use of sealed radiolabeled microspheres in an unsealed manner, the distinction between sealed and unsealed radiopharmaceuticals has been blurred. However, with locoregional applications, the unsealed microspheres are literally confined to the targeted region.

Clinical Trials of Radionuclide Therapy

The approval of gallium ^{68}Ga-Dotatate and edotreotide for the localization of NETs by PET/CT and the use of lutetium ^{177}Lu-Dotatate and oxodotreotide as treatment agents by the US and European regulatory bodies have significantly changed the management of the NETs in oncology (Fig. 4.1).

Currently, using novel targets and targeting molecules, multiple research projects are exploring the use of theranostics in the management of many other cancers. For example, the investigation of radiolabeled compounds targeting prostate-specific membrane antigen (PSMA) for both diagnostic and therapeutic applications in the management of patients with castration-resistant prostate cancer, and investigations of PSMA Radioligand Therapy (RLT) with use of several PSMA compounds. The use of radiolabeled gastrin-releasing peptide receptor (GRPR) antagonist in prostate cancer treatment is another recent application of theranostics in oncology [65]. Peptide receptor radionuclide therapy of treatment-refractory metastatic thyroid cancer using ^{90}Yttrium- and ^{177}Lutetium-labeled somatostatin analogs has also gained attention but needs to consider toxicity, response, and survival analysis [66].

The treatment options of metastatic castration-resistant prostate cancer are also expanding. For instance, the use of ^{177}Lu as a radiopharmaceutical in ^{177}Lu-PSMA-617 to treat metastatic castration-resistant prostate cancer is another example of a new application in PRRT. ^{177}Lu-PSMA-617 has high affinity for prostate-specific membrane antigen (PSMA), enabling targeted β-irradiation of prostate cancer [67]. A recent prospective phase II study demonstrated high therapeutic efficacy and low toxicity for 177Lu-PSMA in men with metastatic castration-resistant prostate cancer who have progressed after standard therapies. The study further provided evidence of improvement in the quality of life. However, despite the high response rates in patients rechallenged with 177Lu-PSMA on progression, their "therapy responses" were less durable [68].

The utility of 223Ra therapy in non-prostate cancers, either alone or in combination with other therapies, needs to be further investigated, and such studies are underway (ClinicalTrials.gov identifier NCT02283749). Other α-emitting radionuclides that are medically relevant and currently available for potential therapeutic application include astatine-211 (^{211}At), bismuth-212 (^{212}Bi), bismuth-213 (^{213}Bi), actinium-225 (^{225}Ac), radium-223 (^{223}Ra), lead-212 (^{212}Pb), thorium-227 (^{227}Th), and terbium-149 (^{149}Tb). Production technologies for these radionuclides range from nuclear reactors to cyclotrons and generator systems. Of those radionuclides, bismuth-213, actinium-225, thorium-227, and astatine-211 are likely more suitable for such therapies, since they cover most or all applications from small-molecular-weight carriers to antibodies for systemic and local injections [Technical Meeting on "Alpha emitting radionuclides and radiopharmaceuticals for therapy" June 24–28, 2013 IAEA Headquarters, Vienna, Austria].

Currently, targeted alpha-therapy is an emerging option for cancer treatment. After many years of research, several other products are in the development lines for a variety of indications. Recent clinical trials are encouraging, and preclinical studies will provide even more candidates for TAT. Several newer α-emitting drugs are in human clinical development for different solid cancer types and groups of leukemia [69, 70].

The alpha-emitters ^{225}Ac and ^{213}Bi can be reliably produced from established radionuclide generator systems with high specific activity and high radionuclide purity. Their availability in clinical settings independent from local reactor or cyclotron facilities and their favorable chemical properties allow the synthesis of stable radio-conjugates using established chelate molecules. Consequently, a large number of preclinical studies and several pioneering clinical trials have been conducted, showing that targeted alpha-therapy with ^{225}Ac and ^{213}Bi is feasible and safe and may provide new therapeutic options to patients who are refractory to standard therapies. In particular, peptide receptor alpha-therapy with ^{225}Ac and ^{213}Bi using fast-diffusible, low-molecular-weight peptides such as DOTATOC, Dotatate, and substance P as carrier molecules is promising and can be expected to play an increasing role in future clinical application.

More schemes of theranostics have been explored for cancer therapy. The ability to use the same or analog targeting molecule for diagnostic and therapeutic purposes is the basis of theranostics. Attaching β^+-emitter radionuclides like fluorine-18 (F-18), gallium-68 (^{68}Ga), or copper-64 (^{64}Cu-) to the targeting molecule allows imaging of ^{177}Lu-, Y-90, or alpha-emitters to guide therapy. Another novel approach is illustrated in Chap. 8 by animal tumor models. Tumor suppression is noted by injection of positrons (β^+) [71] which dissipate potent energies in mm ranges inside the tumor before their annihilation with an electron (β^-) to produce pairs of 0.511 Mev photons (γ) that are detectable by PET scans. These β^+-emitting radionuclides by themselves may be used to design radiopharmaceuticals for theranostic purpose.

Discussion

The solo radionuclide therapy or in their combination has been gaining popularity as an alternative means to conventional treatment options in oncology, namely, chemotherapy and external beam radiation therapy.

The ability to diagnose and subsequently treat a disease, cancer, by utilizing proper isotopes of a radiotracer is quite desirable and commonly practiced in nuclear medicine for many decades, which started with the efforts of Robley Evans, at the Massachusetts Institute of Technology in Boston, together with Dr. Saul Hertz and Dr. Arthur Roberts, when they began diagnostic and subsequently therapeutic applications in thyroid disease and cancer. The start of their practice precedes several decades the adaptation of the term theranostics.

Today, some of the previously used therapeutic radiotracers and their applications have been replaced by the newer, more sophisticated radionuclides targeting specific molecules, receptors, or organ-specific tumors with increased specificity and accuracy. Peptide receptor radionuclide therapy (PRRT) is an example. The list of available therapeutic agents is growing, and there are many new agents present in the pipeline getting closer for their approval by the FDA in the USA.

At the times of "precision medicine," theranostics became an essential component of the patient care, by helping to select patients for targeted therapy utilizing the advanced imaging diagnostics. Theranostics continue to make a significant impact on patient outcomes. The complexity of the process created awareness for the need for multimodality, multidisciplinary approach, in which nuclear medicine is one of the most crucial components. Today, theranostics in nuclear medicine has progressed far beyond its initial endocrine radiotherapy application to become an integral part of the oncologic radiotherapy. With that, nuclear medicine training programs are welcoming such needs and adjusting their training curriculum to provide the necessary knowledge and skills for their learners so that they could successfully maintain their important role in multimodality, multidisciplinary boards in their practice.

References

1. Bagheri MH, Ahlman MA, Lindenberg L, et al. Advances in medical imaging for the diagnosis and management of common genitourinary cancers. Urol Oncol. 2017;35(7):473–91.
2. Pene F, Courtine E, Cariou A, Mira JP. Toward theranostics. Crit Care Med. 2009;37:S50–8.
3. Jeelani S, Reddy RC, Maheswaran T, Asokan GS, Dany A, Anand B. Theranostics: a treasured tailor for tomorrow. J Pharm Bioallied Sci. 2014;6(Suppl 1):S6–8. https://doi.org/10.4103/0975-7406.137249.
4. Chan IS, Ginsburg GS. Personalized medicine: progress and promise. Annu Rev Genomics Hum Genet. 2011;12:217–44. https://doi.org/10.1146/annurev-genom-082410-101446.
5. Sairamesh J, Michael R. An economic perspective on personalized medicine. HUGO J. 2013;7:1.
6. Levine R, Krenning EP. Clinical history of the theranostic radionuclide approach to neuroendocrine tumors and other types of cancer: historical review based on an interview of Eric P. Krenning by Rachel Levine. J Nucl Med. 2017;58:3S–9S.
7. Strosberg J, El-Haddad G, Wolin E, et al. Phase 3 trial of ^{177}Lu-dotatate for midgut neuroendocrine tumors. N Engl J Med. 2017;376:125–35.
8. Pryma DA, Chin BB, Noto RB, et al. Efficacy and safety of high-specific-activity I-131 MIBG therapy in patients with advanced pheochromocytoma or paraganglioma. J Nucl Med. 2019;60:623–30.
9. Kassis AI, Adelstein SJ. Therapeutic potential of internally administered radionuclides. In: Black PMcL, Schoene WC, Lampson LA, eds. Contemporary issues in neurological surgery. Astrocytomas: diagnosis, treatment, and biology. Special Supplement of Medical Physics on radiolabeled antibody tumor dosimetry. Med Phys. 1993;20:497.
10. Macklis RM, Kinsey BM, Kassis AI, Ferrara JLM, Atcher RW, Hines JJ, Coleman CN, Adelstein SJ, Burakoff SJ. Radio immunotherapy with alpha – particle-emitting immune conjugates. Science. 1988;240:1024–6.
11. Bayer NJ. Xofigo (radium Ra 223 dichloride) injection [prescribing information]. Bayer HealthCare Pharmaceuticals, Inc; May 2013.
12. Poeppel TD, Handkiewicz-Junak D, Andreeff M, et al. EANM guideline for radionuclide therapy with radium-223 of metastatic castration-resistant prostate cancer. Eur J Nucl Med Mol Imaging. 2018;45:824–45. https://doi.org/10.1007/s00259-017-3900-4.
13. Hoskin P, Sartor O, O'Sullivan JM, Johannessen DC, Helle SI, Logue J, Bottomley D, Nilsson S, Vogelzang NJ, Fang MW, Aksnes A-K, Parker C. Efficacy and safety of radium-223 dichloride in patients with castration-resistant prostate cancer and symptomatic bone metastases with or without previous docetaxel use: a pre-specified subgroup analysis from the randomized, double-blind, phase 3 ALSYMPCA trial. Lancet Oncol. 2014;15(12):1397–406, ISSN 1470-2045.
14. Parker C, Nilsson S, Heinrich D, et al. Alpha emitter radium-223 and survival in metastatic prostate cancer. N Engl J Med. 2013;369:213–23.
15. Tu SM, Kim J, Pagliaro LC, Vakar-Lopez F, Wong FC, Wen S, General R, Podoloff DA, Lin SH, Logothetis CJ. Therapy tolerance in selected patients with androgen-independent prostate cancer following strontium-89 combined with chemotherapy. J Clin Oncol. 2005;23(31):7904–10.
16. Tu SM, Mathew P, Wong FC, Jones D, Johnson MM, Logothetis CJ. Phase I study of concurrent weekly docetaxel and repeated samarium-153 lexidronam in patients with castration-resistant metastatic prostate cancer. J Clin Oncol. 2009;27(20):3319–24.
17. Jain N, Wierda W, Ferrajoli A, Wong F, Lerner S, Keating MK, O'Brien S. A phase 2 study of yttrium-90 ibritumomab tiuxetan (Zevalin) in patients with chronic lymphocytic leukemia. Cancer. 2009;115(19):4533–9.
18. Witzig TE, Gordon LI, Cabanillas F, et al. Randomized controlled trial of yttrium-90-labeled ibritumomab tiuxetan radioimmunotherapy versus rituximab immunotherapy for patients with relapsed or refractory low-grade, follicular, or transformed B-cell non-Hodgkin's lymphoma. J Clin Oncol. 2002;20:2453–63.

19. Kaminski MS, Estes J, Zasadny KR, et al. Radioimmunotherapy with iodine (131)I tositumomab for relapsed or refractory B-cell non-Hodgkin lymphoma: updated results and long-term follow-up of the University of Michigan experience. Blood. 2000;96:1259–66.
20. Wahl RL. The clinical importance of dosimetry in radioimmunotherapy with tositumomab and iodine I 131 tositumomab. Semin Oncol. 2003;30(Suppl 4):31–8.
21. Abbatt JD. Experiences of management and treatment of polycythemia using P32 as a therapeutic weapon. J Fac Radiol. 1953;5(2):141–7.
22. Tennvall J, Brans B. EANM procedure guideline for ^{32}P phosphate treatment of myeloproliferative diseases. Eur J Nucl Med Mol Immaging. 2007;34(8):1324–7.
23. Papotti M, Bongiovanni M, Volante M, et al. Expression of somatostatin receptor types 1-5 in 81 cases of gastrointestinal and pancreatic endocrine tumors. A correlative immunohistochemical and reverse-transcriptase polymerase chain reaction analysis. Virchows Arch. 2002;440:461–75.
24. Krenning EP, Kwekkeboom DJ, Bakker WH, et al. Somatostatin receptor scintigraphy with [^{111}In-DTPA-D-Phe1]- and [123ITyr3]-octreotide: the Rotterdam experience with more than 1000 patients. Eur J Nucl Med. 1993;20:716–31.
25. Limouris GS, Dimitropoulos N, Kontogeorgakos D, et al. Evaluation of the therapeutic response to ^{111}In-DTPA-octreotide based targeted therapy in liver metastatic neuroendocrine tumors according to CT/MRI/US findings. Can Bio Rad. 2005;20(2):215–7.
26. Waldherr C, Pless M, Maecke HR, Haldemann A, Mueller-Brand J. The clinical value of [90Y-DOTA]-D-Phe1-Tyr3-octreotide (^{90}Y-DOTATOC) in the treatment of neuroendocrine tumours: a clinical phase II study. Ann Oncol. 2001;12:941–5.
27. Dromain C, Déandréis D, Scoazec JY, et al. Imaging of neuroendocrine tumors of the pancreas. Diagn Interv Imaging. 2016;97:1241–57.
28. Lyra ME, Andreou M, Georgantzoglou A, Kordolaimi S, Lagopati N, Ploussi A, Salvara A-L, Vamvakas I. Radionuclides used in nuclear medicine therapy – from production to dosimetry. Curr Med Imaging Rev. 2013;9(1):51–75.
29. Strosberg J, Wolin E, Chasen B, et al. Health related quality of life in patients with progressive midgut neuroendocrine tumors treated with 177Lu-Dotatate in the phase III NETTER-1 trial. J Clin Oncol. 2018;36(25):2578–84.
30. Evans RD. Early history (1936–1946) of nuclear medicine in thyroid studies at Massachusetts General Hospital. Med Phys. 1975;2(3):105–9.
31. Tuttle RM, Tala H, Shah J, Leboeuf R, Ghossein R, Gonen M, Brokhin M, Omry G, Fagin JA, Shaha A. Estimating risk of recurrence in differentiated thyroid cancer after total thyroidectomy and radioactive iodine remnant ablation: using response to therapy variables to modify the initial risk estimates predicted by the new American Thyroid Association staging system. Thyroid. 2010;20(12):1341–9.
32. Durante C, Haddy N, Baudin E, Leboulleux S, Hartl D, Travagli JP, Caillou B, Ricard M, Lumbroso JD, De Vathaire F, Schlumberger M. Long-term outcome of 444 patients with distant metastases from papillary and follicular thyroid carcinoma: benefits and limits of radioiodine therapy. J Clin Endocrinol Metab. 2006;91(8):2892–9.
33. Haslerud T, Brauckhoff K, Reisæter L, Küfner Lein R, Heinecke A, Varhaug JE, Biermann M. F18-FDG-PET for recurrent differentiated thyroid cancer: a systematic meta-analysis. Acta Radiol. 2016;57(10):1193–200.
34. Kim SJ, Lee TH, Kim IJ, Kim YK. Clinical implication of F-18 FDG PET/CT for differentiated thyroid cancer in patients with negative diagnostic iodine-123 scan and elevated thyroglobulin. Eur J Radiol. 2009;70(1):17–24.
35. Bertagna F, Bosio G, Biasiotto G, Rodella C, Puta E, Gabanelli S, Lucchini S, Merli G, Savelli G, Giubbini R, Rosenbaum J, Alavi A. F-18 FDG-PET/CT evaluation of patients with differentiated thyroid cancer with negative I-131 total body scan and high thyroglobulin level. Clin Nucl Med. 2009;34(11):756–61.
36. Klaus A, Fathi O, Tatjana TW, Bruno N, Oskar K. Expression of hypoxia-associated protein HIF-1α in follicular thyroid cancer is associated with distant metastasis. Pathol Oncol Res. 2018;24(2):289–96.

37. Ritter A, Mizrachi A, Bachar G, Vainer I, Shimon I, Hirsch D, Diker-Cohen T, Duskin-Bitan H, Robenshtok E. Detecting recurrence following lobectomy for thyroid cancer: role of thyroglobulin and thyroglobulin antibodies. J Clin Endocrinol Metab. 2020;105:1–7.
38. Ho AL, Grewal RK, Leboeuf R, et al. Selumetinib-enhanced radioiodine uptake in advanced thyroid cancer. N Engl J Med. 2013;368:623–32.
39. Kitahara CM, et al. Association of radioactive iodine treatment with cancer mortality in patients with hyperthyroidism. JAMA Intern Med. 2019;179(8):1034–42. https://doi.org/10.1001/jamainternmed.2019.0981.
40. Yan KL, Li S, Tseng C-H, Kim J, Nguyen DT, Dawood NB, Livhits MJ, Yeh MW, Leung AM. Rising incidence and incidence-based mortality of thyroid cancer in California, 2000–2017. J Clin Endocrinol Metab. 2020;105(6):1–8. https://doi.org/10.1210/clinem/dgaa121.
41. McLeod DSA, Zhang L, Durante C, Cooper DS. Contemporary debates in adult papillary thyroid cancer management. Endocr Rev. 2019;40(6):1481–99.
42. Harach HR, Franssila KO, Wasenius VM. Occult papillary carcinoma of the thyroid. A "normal" finding in Finland. A systematic autopsy study. Cancer. 1985;56(3):531–8.
43. Brito JP, Ito Y, Miyauchi A, Tuttle RM. A clinical framework to facilitate risk stratification when considering an active surveillance alternative to immediate biopsy and surgery in papillary microcarcinomas. Thyroid. 2016;26(1):144–9.
44. Durante C, Attard M, Torlontano M, Papillary Thyroid Cancer Study Group, et al. Identification and optimal postsurgical follow-up of patients with very low-risk papillary thyroid microcarcinomas. J Clin Endocrinol Metab. 2010;95(11):4882–8.
45. Grani G, Ramundo V, Falcone R, et al. Thyroid cancer patients with no evidence of disease: the need for repeat neck ultrasound. J Clin Endocrinol Metab. 2019;104(11):4981–9.
46. Klubo-Gwiezdzinska J, Van Nostrand D, Atkins F, et al. Efficacy of dosimetric versus empiric prescribed activity of ^{131}I for therapy of differentiated thyroid cancer. J Clin Endocrinol Metabol. 2011;96(10):3217–25. https://doi.org/10.1210/JC.2011-0494.
47. Deandreis D, Rubino C, Tala H, Leboulleux S, Terroir M, Baudin E, Larson S, Fagin JA, Schlumberger M, Tuttle RM. Comparison of empiric versus whole-body/-blood clearance dosimetry-based approach to radioactive iodine treatment in patients with metastases from differentiated thyroid cancer. J Nucl Med. 2017;58(5):717–22.
48. Deandreis D, Rubino C, Tala H, Leboulleux S, Terroir M, Baudin E, Larson S, Fagin JA, Schlumberger M, Tuttle RM. Comparison of empiric versus whole-body/-blood clearance dosimetry–based approach to radioactive iodine treatment in patients with metastases from differentiated thyroid cancer. J Nucl Med. 2017;58:717–22. https://doi.org/10.2967/jnumed.116.179606.
49. Thomas SR, Maxon HR, Kereiakes JG. In vivo quantitation of lesion radioactivity using external counting methods. Med Phys. 1976;3:253–5.
50. Dorn R, Kopp J, Vogt H, Heidenreich P, Carroll RG, Gulec SA. Dosimetry-guided radioactive iodine treatment in patients with metastatic differentiated thyroid cancer: largest safe dose using a risk adapted approach. J Nucl Med. 2003;44:451–6.
51. Sgouros G, Hobbs RF, Atkins FB, Van Nostrand D, Ladenson PW, Wahl RL. Three-dimensional radiobiological dosimetry (3D-RD) with 124I PET for ^{131}I therapy of thyroid cancer. Eur J Nucl Med Mol Imaging. 2011;38(suppl 1):S41–7.
52. Berker Y, Goedicke A, Kemerink GJ, Aach T, Schweizer B. Activity quantification combining conjugate-view planar scintigraphies and SPECT/CT data for patient-specific 3-D dosimetry in radionuclide therapy. Eur J Nucl Med Mol Imaging. 2011;38:2173–85.
53. Piwnica-Worms D, Holman LB. Noncardiac application of hexakis (alkylisonitrile) technetium-99m complexes. J Nucl Med. 1990;31:1166.
54. Civelek AC, Durski K, Shafique I, Matsumura K, Sostre S, Wagner HN Jr, Ladenson PW. Failure of perchlorate to inhibit Tc-99m isonitrile binding by the thyroid during myocardial perfusion studies. Clin Nucl Med. 1991;16(5):358–61.

55. Civelek AC, Ozalp E, Donovan P, Udelsman R. Prospective evaluation of delayed technetium-99m sestamibi SPECT scintigraphy for preoperative localization of primary hyperparathyroidism. Surgery. 2002;131(2):149–57.
56. Bhatt G, Li XF, Civelek AC. ^{131}I thyroid cancer therapy in chronically bedridden & dialysis patients with severe renal failure: challenges and solutions for determining the optimum therapy dose and how to minimize radiation dose to caregivers. J Nucl Med. 2014;55:1365–423.
57. Phegley D, Bjorklund A, Smith R, Petti M, Robichaux J, Civelek AC. Challenges and solutions for I-131 therapy in the complex inpatient with thyroid cancer: a technologist prospective. J Nucl Med. 2007;48(2):447.
58. Welsh JS, Yang NC, Civelek AC, Wharam MD, Williams JA. Treatment protocol for phosphorus-32 therapy for intracerebral cystic neoplasms: a preliminary report. J Brachyther Int. 1999;15(3–4):211–6.
59. Halperin E, Fallat M, Bond S, Crew J, Johnson R, Mills M, Bhatt G, Hughes SC, Civelek AC. Role of 32P-chromic phosphate colloids in the treatment of a skin tumors, Ewing's sarcoma. J Nucl Med. 2012;53:1079.
60. Carr BI, Kondragunta V, Buch SC, Branch RA. Therapeutic equivalence in survival for hepatic arterial chemoembolization and 90Yttrium microspheres (Y90) treatments in unresectable hepatocellular carcinoma: a 2 cohort study. Cancer. 2010;116(5):1305–14.
61. Wang EA, Broadwell SR, Bellavia RJ, Stein JP. Selective internal radiation therapy with SIR-Spheres in hepatocellular carcinoma and cholangiocarcinoma. J Gastrointest Oncol. 2017;8(2):266–78.
62. Tollefson C, Krause S, Nguyen B. Utility of SPECT/CT imaging in Y-90 microsphere therapy. J Nucl Med. 2015;56(suppl 3):2517.
63. Scott NP, McGowan DR. Optimising quantitative 90Y PET imaging: an investigation into the effects of scan length and Bayesian penalised likelihood reconstruction. EJNMMI Res. 2019;9:40.
64. Salem R, et al. Clinical and dosimetric considerations for Y90: recommendations from an international multidisciplinary working group. Eur J Nucl Med Mol Imaging. 2019;46:1695–704.
65. Nock BA, Kaloudi A, Lymperis E, et al. Theranostic perspectives in prostate cancer with the gastrin-releasing peptide receptor antagonist NeoBOMB1: preclinical and first clinical results. J Nucl Med. 2017;58(1):75–80.
66. Budiawan H, Salavati A, Kulkarni HR, Baum RP. Peptide receptor radionuclide therapy of treatment-refractory metastatic thyroid cancer using ^{90}Yttrium and ^{177}Lutetium labeled somatostatin analogs: toxicity, response and survival analysis. J Nucl Med Mol Imaging. 2014;4(1):39–52.
67. Violet J, Sandhu S, Iravani A, et al. Long-term follow-up and outcomes of retreatment in an expanded 50-patient single-center phase II prospective trial of 177Lu-PSMA-617 theranostics in metastatic castration-resistant prostate cancer. J Nucl Med. 2020;61:857–65.
68. Violet J, Sandhu S, Amir Iravani A, et al. Long-term follow-up and outcomes of retreatment in an expanded 50-patient single-center phase II prospective trial of 177Lu-PSMA-617 theranostics in metastatic castration-resistant prostate cancer. J Nucl Med. 2020;61:857–65.
69. Allen BJ. Future prospects for targeted alpha therapy. Curr Radiopharm. 2011;4:336–42.
70. Morgenstern A, Bruchertseifer F, Apostolidis C. Bismuth-213 and Actinium-225 – generator performance and evolving therapeutic applications of two generator-derived alpha-emitting radioisotopes. Curr Radiopharm. 2012;5(3):221–7.
71. Wong F, Naff K, Liu C, Ferguson A, Hwu P. Intratumoral positron emission cancer therapy (IPECT) using F-18 FDG, Cu-64 Cl and Ga-68 Cl. J Nucl Med. 2013;54(supplement 2):1400.

Chapter 5
Locoregional Therapy: Cancer Interventions with and Without Radionuclides

Steven Yevich and Armeen Mahvash

Abbreviations

^{90}Y	^{90}Yttrium
CT	Computed tomography
DEBIRI	Drug-eluting beads loaded with irinotecan
FDA	Food and Drug Administration
HCC	Hepatocellular carcinoma
MA	Microwave ablation
MAA	^{99m}Tc-macroaggregated albumin
MRI	Magnetic resonance imaging
RCC	Renal cell carcinoma
RFA	Radiofrequency ablation
TACE	Trans-arterial chemoembolization
TARE	Trans-arterial radioembolization

Introduction

Interventional oncology applies image guidance and low-profile devices to treat primary and metastatic cancer in a minimally invasive approach. The treatments encompass curative and palliative options and can be applied either alone or in concert with medical, surgical, and radiation oncology treatments. The rationale for targeted locoregional therapy is to maximize tumor damage and minimize systemic

S. Yevich (✉) · A. Mahvash
Department of Interventional Radiology, Division of Diagnostic Imaging, University of Texas MD Anderson Cancer Center, Houston, TX, USA
e-mail: syevich@mdanderson.org; armeen.mahvash@mdanderson.org

F. C. L. Wong (ed.), *Locoregional Radionuclide Cancer Therapy*,
https://doi.org/10.1007/978-3-030-56267-0_5

and same-organ toxicity. All treatments are performed through small incisions less than 0.5 cm in length, with needle or catheter advancement under direct image guidance. Treatment outcomes are followed by imaging and often can be repeated in the event of incomplete tumor response. In general, interventional oncology treatments can be categorized into endovascular catheter-delivered and percutaneous needle-guided approaches.

As pertaining to locoregional treatment, the most common endovascular treatments are hepatic arterial infusion of chemotherapy, transarterial chemoembolization, and radioembolization. These procedures begin with the advancement of a low-profile catheter through a peripheral artery into the hepatic artery under fluoroscopic guidance. For hepatic arterial infusion, the catheter is used to inject a high dose of chemotherapy directly to the liver tumor. Chemoembolization adds an additional step to embolize the tumor-feeding arteries after delivery of the chemotherapy. Radioembolization follows a similar principle to chemoembolization but instead achieves locoregional response through the delivery of radiation-loaded microembolic material.

In contrast, percutaneous thermal ablation is performed by the advancement of a small-caliber needle directly through the skin into the tumor. These needles, also known as electrodes or probes, are then activated to achieve a pronounced change in temperature at the needle tip. The thermal change is hyperthermic for radiofrequency ablation and microwave ablation and hypothermic for cryoablation. The thermal energy results in cellular death within a zone of ablation defined by the manufacturer.

High-quality, real-time imaging is a necessity for all of these interventional oncology techniques to achieve locoregional goals with minimal collateral damage to the surrounding structures. Real-time imaging is essential to ensure precise catheter or needle position, to prevent and monitor for immediate procedure-related complications, and to make immediate assessment for adequate ablation margins that completely encompass the tumor. Success relies upon operator experience, precise image guidance, understanding of the treatment technology, and the biology of the tumor in relation to the background tissue. In this chapter, we review the aforementioned locoregional cancer interventions for the treatment of primary and metastatic cancer in the liver, kidneys, lungs, and musculoskeletal system.

Intra-arterial Treatments for Hepatic Tumors

Common intra-arterial hepatic treatment options include infusion of high concentration chemotherapy alone or in combination with an embolic agent and injection of a radioembolic material. Regardless of the injected agent, the technique capitalizes on the difference in blood flow and oxygenation between normal hepatocytes and hepatic tumors. Normal hepatocytes obtain blood supply from both the hepatic artery and the portal vein, with the portal vein providing the majority of the blood flow and approximately half of the oxygen requirement. In contrast, the hepatic artery provides approximately 90% of the blood flow for both primary and metastatic hepatic tumors [1, 2]. Hence, selective injection into hepatic arteries will preferentially deliver the cytotoxic agent to the tumor compared to the surrounding normal liver.

Given the above principle, the techniques for locoregional hepatic intra-arterial treatments are similar. The hepatic tumor blood supply is identified through subselective angiography, followed by delivery of treatment directly into the tumor blood supply [3–5]. Selective catheterization of tumor blood supply requires advancement of a small caliber catheter into the arterial system, typically through the common femoral artery or the radial artery. New technologies that include hydrophilic catheter coatings and low-profile microcatheter systems have enabled subselection of small tumor-feeding arteries that measure less than 2 mm in diameter. Once the arterial anatomy has been delineated by selective angiograms, the catheter is advanced into the tumor-feeding arteries, and the treatment is delivered through the catheter.

Hepatic Intra-arterial Chemotherapy Infusion

Hepatic intra-arterial chemotherapy infusion is performed predominantly to treat colorectal liver metastases. The technique requires repetitive infusion of high concentration chemotherapy through the hepatic artery. This may be achieved by cannulation of the patient's liver artery at each infusion or by surgical placement of a hepatic arterial port catheter that can be accessed whenever infusions are indicated based on tumor progression and systemic toxicity assessment. Termed hepatic artery infusion chemotherapy (HAIC), this treatment has reported up to 60–90% objective response rate and 20–47% conversion rate for previously nonsurgical candidates with metastatic colorectal cancer to the liver [6–8].

While HAIC has demonstrated benefit for some patients with metastatic colorectal cancer to the liver, the practice is not ubiquitously performed as the procedure requires multiple treatments that expose the patient to arterial injury and chemotherapy toxicities. Due to the comorbidities from surgical placement of a hepatic artery port catheter, an interventional oncology deployed port has been developed. This port provides a less invasive means for permanent access to the hepatic artery with equivalent primary function to the surgically placed port; however, this infusion port device is not yet approved by the FDA for use in the USA [9–11].

Transarterial Chemoembolization

Transarterial chemoembolization (TACE) combines the direct intra-arterial injection of high concentration chemotherapy into the liver tumor with subsequent arterial embolization (Fig. 5.1). The combination of chemotherapy followed by embolization is thought to act synergistically through two primary mechanisms to

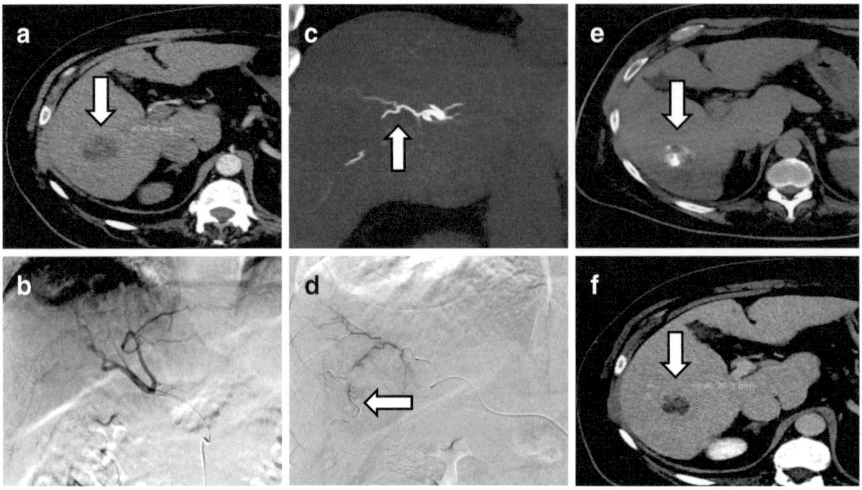

Fig. 5.1 A 52-year-old man with multifocal hepatocellular carcinoma deemed to not be a candidate for surgical resection due to four locations of disease in multiple liver segments. TACE treatments were performed, including right hepatic mass in segment 6 that measured approximately 3.5 cm on pre-procedure CT with contrast (**a**, arrow identifies mass). Initial procedural angiogram with injection through the common hepatic artery did not identify definitive tumor blush (**b**). A CT angiogram with injection of contrast through the common hepatic artery identified the tumor-feeding branch (**c**, arrow). A selective angiogram through the right hepatic artery demonstrated mild arterial architectural distortion with some tumor blush, and drug-eluting beads were injected through the catheter (**d**, arrow). A CT angiogram with injection of contrast through the right hepatic artery confirmed tumor blush in the region of treatment (**e**, arrow). A follow-up CT with contrast performed 2 months post-procedure demonstrates response to treatment with decreased diameter from approximately 3.5 cm to approximately 2.5 cm (**f**, arrow)

achieve a greater degree of tumor cellular death than HAIC. First, the exposure time of the chemotherapy to the tumor tissue is increased after embolization as a consequence of the reduced blood flow through the tumor [12–14]. Second, tumor absorption of chemotherapeutic agents is increased from the embolization-induced ischemic damage to tumoral transmembrane pumps [15, 16].

Various combinations of chemotherapeutic drugs and embolic materials have been advanced, without clear superiority of a particular combination [17]. Selection of chemotherapy is typically at the discretion of the operator, based upon experience, tumor type, and regional availabilities. For hepatocellular cancer, commonly used chemotherapeutic agents are doxorubicin, cisplatin, and mitomycin C. For colorectal liver metastases, the most common chemotherapeutic agents are irinotecan, cisplatin, mitomycin, and 5-fluorouracil. The chemotherapy may be loaded directly onto microspheres, termed drug-eluting beads (DEB-TACE), emulsified with iodized oil (lipiodol, Guerbet, France), termed conventional TACE. For DEB-TACE, the cytotoxic and ischemic effects are thought to occur at the location of bead lodgment. These drug-eluting beads are made from superabsorbent polymers that slowly release the chemotherapy over the course of hours to weeks. For conventional TACE, the emulsification provides a mechanism to concentrate the chemotherapy within tumor cells and also to prolong cytotoxic exposure [18–20]. Due to the absence of Kupffer cells in hepatic tumors, iodized oil accumulates and remains in tumor vasculature to a greater degree in comparison with the surrounding hepatocytes [21–24]. After injection of the emulsification, the cytotoxic effects are further potentiated by embolization using embolic material such as Gelfoam or particles. Gelatin sponge is a porous material made from purified pork skin that is cut to size and pressure injected through the catheter to provide temporary occlusion that typically reabsorbs after 2–6 weeks. The particles are supplied at multiple specified diameters and can be made from different material such as polyvinyl alcohol or trisacryl gelatin. Selection of embolic material is at the discretion of the operator, with no clear superiority in treatment outcome.

TACE may be performed for palliation of unresectable HCC as a treatment for intermediate-stage disease, as an adjunct to liver resection or thermal ablation, or as a bridge to liver transplantation [25, 26]. In patients with inoperable HCC, TACE has demonstrated efficacy to improve survival and offers the opportunity for conversion of some patients into operable candidates [27, 28]. For metastatic tumor, there is less data; however, some studies show promising response rates [29, 30]. TACE has also been applied for metastatic colorectal cancer to the liver, with recent use of drug-eluting beads loaded with irinotecan (DEBIRI). Preclinical trials showed some improved pharmacokinetic in comparison with irinotecan administered via a peripheral vein or even through slow hepatic intra-arterial infusion [31]. In clinical trials, patients had an improved median outcome survival (22 months vs. 15 months) and progression-free survival (7 months compared to 4 months) with DEBIRI treatment in comparison with systemic FOLFIRI, although early toxicity was significantly higher for DEBIRI treatments [32].

Regardless of the type of TACE performed, patients will often experience a temporary post-embolization syndrome that can include right upper abdominal pain, fever, nausea, fatigue, and elevated liver enzymes. Complications include liver abscess and sepsis, gallbladder infarction, and nontarget embolization that can lead to gallbladder, bowel, or diaphragmatic infarction [33, 34]. In patients with impaired liver function, the treatment can induce liver failure or hepatorenal syndrome. Contradictions to TACE include poor liver function, encephalopathy, low serum albumin level, impaired hepatopetal flow due to portal vein obstruction (particularly in the event of variceal bleeding), biliary obstruction, poor performance status, tumor burden involving more than 50% of the liver, extrahepatic metastases that cannot be controlled, thrombocytopenia, and tumor invasion into the portal vein or inferior vena cava. Pre-procedure antibiotics should be administered as prophylaxis for hepatic abscess in patient with compromise of the sphincter of Oddi from prior surgery, sphincterotomy, or internal biliary stents.

Transarterial Radioembolization

Hepatic transarterial radioembolization (TARE) may be performed for palliation of unresectable hepatic tumor, as an adjunct to liver resection or thermal ablation, or as a bridge to liver transplantation. The treatment is analogous to TACE, with radiation delivered internally to the tumor by injection through the appropriate hepatic artery branches. Glass microspheres and resin are loaded with a measured quantity of yttrium-90 (^{90}Y), a beta emitter. The two devices approved by the Food and Drug Administration are TheraSpere (glass microspheres) for the treatment of unresectable HCC and SIR-Spheres (resin) for the treatment of colorectal metastases to the liver.

Given the overall treatment similarities to TACE, there has been debate as to the superiority of one treatment to the other, with some recent prospective trials suggesting possible improved outcomes for HCC. For example, in one prospective cohort study of 1000 patients, the overall survival outcomes were noteworthy for patients stratified by baseline Child-Pugh class and Barcelona Clinic Liver Cancer (BCLC) staging [35]. For Child-Pugh A patients, overall survival was listed as 47.3 months in BCLC A patients, 25.0 months in BCLC B patients, and 15.0 months in BCLC C patients. For Child-Pugh B patients, overall survival was listed as 27 months for BCLC A patients, 15.0 months for BCLC B patients, and 8.0 months for BCLC C patients. Toxicity was low, with 5% of patients developing albumin toxicity and 11% of patients developing bilirubin toxicities. A randomized phase II study in the treatment of HCC found radioembolization to have a longer time to progression (>26 months) than TACE (6.8 months) [36].

Radioembolization is a two-part procedure, often performed in two separate days (Fig. 5.2). First, a diagnostic procedure is performed to identify tumor blood supply, occlude possible collateral flow to extrahepatic organs, and quantify any tumor shunting to the lungs. Due to the radioactive nature of the microspheres, administration to any hepatoenteric collaterals may result in inadvertent damage to extrahepatic organs including the stomach, duodenum, or pancreas. If appropriate, this collateral circulation is occluded. Next, appropriate catheter location for treatment injection is determined, and a measured dose of ^{99m}Tc-macroaggregated albumin (MAA) is administered through the catheter at this location. MAA is similar in size to the ^{90}Y microspheres, and hence the distribution of MAA can be used to approximate the distribution of ^{90}Y in the subsequent second procedure. The distribution of MAA is then assessed by either planar or single photon emission computed tomography (SPECT) gamma cameras. Several corrective measures can be pursued in the event of extrahepatic deposition to the bowel, gallbladder, or diaphragm. The catheter tip location can be modified to exclude an arterial branch responsible for extrahepatic administration. Alternatively, this arterial branch can be embolized if appropriate collateral circulation is present to prevent undesired end-organ damage. Finally, shunting of MAA to the lungs is measured as a fraction of the total MAA injected. Determination of lung shunting is important to minimize the risk of radiation pneumonitis during subsequent radioembolization treatment. At present

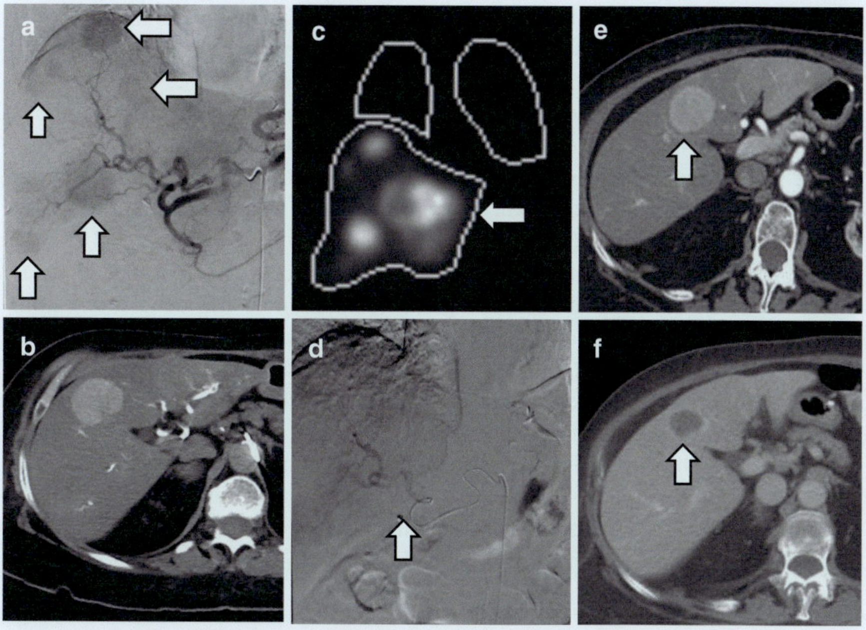

Fig. 5.2 A 72-year-old woman with multifocal metastatic neuroendocrine cancer to the liver. TARE treatment was performed to control enlarging metastases and palliate worsening diarrhea. Initial procedural angiogram with injection through the celiac artery demonstrates multiple metastases (**a**, arrows). A CT angiogram with injection of contrast through the common hepatic artery identified tumor-feeding branches and absence extrahepatic perfusion (**b**, arrow). Injection of MAA into the hepatic arteries demonstrated heterogeneous distribution of radiotracer consistent with sites of tumor (**c**, arrow) and minimal pulmonary shunt percentage (5.3%). A selective angiogram through the right hepatic artery was performed, and radioembolic material was injected (**d**, arrow). This same process was performed for the left hepatic artery. Comparison of pretreatment CT obtained 1 month prior to treatment and the posttreatment CT obtained 3 months postprocedure demonstrates decreased size of lesions, for example, a lesion in segment 4B decreased from approximately 3 cm to 2 cm (**e** and **f**, arrows)

for both devices, the maximum lung dose per treatment session is 30 Gy and the maximum cumulative lung dose is 50 Gy [37]. For the resin microsphere, treatment by TARE can typically be pursued if lung shunting is less than 20% as assessed by the MAA injection procedure. Specific shunt fraction limits for glass microspheres have not been established beyond the limits above. Once all shunting is accounted for, and the safety for radioembolization is determined, then the second procedure can be scheduled. The second procedure requires placement of the treatment microcatheter in the same way that the MAA was injected in the first procedure, followed by injection of the radioactive microspheres.

Similar to TACE, patients should be screened for performance status, liver function, and extent of metastasis. Outcomes for TARE are improved with normal prothrombin time, albumin, and total bilirubin. The procedure provides a minimally invasive option for nonsurgical candidates with multifocal liver tumors. In early trials for TARE for metastatic colorectal cancer, SIR-Spheres in combination with systemic chemotherapy provided significantly longer median time to disease progression and significantly longer survival rate compared with systemic chemotherapy alone or TACE [38–40]. Subsequent prospective studies show no significant benefit, possibly due to patient selection bias and procedure technique [41].

The most common side effects of TARE are fatigue, nausea/vomiting, abdominal pain/discomfort, and cachexia, which are related to the radiation effects on the normal hepatic parenchyma [42–44]. A short course of tapering oral steroids may be administered in nondiabetic patients to minimize these transient sequelae. Complications can occur from nontarget embolization to the duodenum, stomach, pancreas, gallbladder, or diaphragm [45–47]. Biliary complications may also develop that include biloma, biliary necrosis, and abscess formation [48]. The arterial supply to these structures may be embolized with coils prior to injection of the radioembolic material. Shunting from the liver to the lung may result in radiation pneumonitis, with possible long-term sequela of pulmonary fibrosis [49], and is one of the main reasons for the initial evaluation with MAA as outlined above. Lastly, the rare complication of radiation-induced liver damage can occur in up to 4% of patients, with delayed presentation 4–8 weeks after treatment [50–51].

Percutaneous Thermal Ablation

Thermal ablation mediates cell death by the direct effects of thermal energy applied through the tip of a needle probe on surrounding tumor tissue. The two most common heat-based technologies are radiofrequency ablation (RFA) and microwave ablation (MA), while cryoablation is the alternative hypothermic technology. An important component of ablation is to ensure tumor-free margins, ideally with a 0.5–1 cm circumferential ablation margin [52]. To achieve these results, the tumor should be adequately visualized during placement of ablation needle probes, and the target diameter of the ablation should be larger than the tumor diameter, which might require multiple probes or overlapping ablation impacts. Real-time visualization of the tumor during needle placement is important and may be achieved with ultrasound, CT, MRI, or fusion imaging guidance [53].

Radiofrequency energy transmitted into the tissues surrounding the RFA probe converts to heat due to tissue resistance. Cellular death occurs from intolerable heat accumulation that causes coagulation necrosis over several days as the sequela of protein coagulation of cytosolic and mitochondrial enzymes and nucleic acid-histone protein complexes [54]. The degree of hyperthermic tissue damage depends on the achieved temperature, heating duration, and tissue specific factors [55]. In general, near-immediate coagulation occurs with temperatures of 60–100 °C [56, 57]. Complete tumor necrosis can be achieved in a greater percentage with tumors less than 3 cm and in locations without vasculature measuring greater than 2 mm [58].

RFA outcomes are reportedly decreased for tumors larger than 4 cm, due to challenges to achieve homogenous ablation temperatures in tumors that are larger than 4 cm, or in hypervascular tumors, or in locations prone to heat loss. Alternative ablation technologies have been advanced to overcome these challenges. The most common alternatives are microwave ablation (MWA) and cryoablation (CYA). Microwave ablation creates a hyperthermic zone by the application of electromagnetic energy through the needle probe, which causes rapid rotation of cellular water molecules in the adjacent tissues at equal to or greater than 900 kHz. The friction-induced heat is generated in a more uniform distribution than RFA. Cryoablation follows the Joule-Thomson effect, with conversion of a high-pressure argon gas to a low-pressure liquid at the tip of the probe. Temperatures reach as low as −150 °C at the needle tip and will form a therapeutic ellipsoid "ice ball" around the distal aspect of the needle that can be monitored with CT, MRI, or US. Irreversible cellular death occurs between −20 and −40 °C by the synergistic mechanisms of intracellular and extracellular ice crystal formation and ischemic necrosis from microvascular injury and vessel disruption [59, 60].

Regardless of the ablation technology, certain guiding principles exist to ensure a homogenous zone of ablation. Tumor factors that can adversely affect outcome include large tumor size and tumor hypervascularity. The technical factors that determine the size of the ablation zone include the type of ablation technology used, the duration of ablation, the number of ablation impacts, and the number of needles used. Overall, the degree of coagulation necrosis is governed by the amount of deposited energy, the local tissue interactions, and the temperature loss as outlined originally in the bio-heat equation [61]. Complications for all ablation procedures are generally similar and are secondary to collateral damage to the surrounding normal structures. Post-ablation syndrome is a combination of fever and flulike symptoms that is a self-limit immune-modulated response that occurs in approximately 5–10% of procedures [62, 63].

Hepatic Tumor Ablation

Hepatic ablation for primary tumors and metastases is predominantly performed with RFA or MWA, as cryoablation has shown a higher complication rate for bleeding (Fig. 5.3). Image guidance is usually performed with ultrasound, CT, or a combination of these two modalities. Again, ablation probe positioning within the tumor is important to ensure complete locoregional tumor control, and visualization of adjacent critical structures is necessary to avoid complications. Immediate evaluation of the ablation margins may be obtained with contrast-enhanced CT or contrast-enhanced US.

As RFA is a more established technology, longer-term outcome data is available. Survival depends on severity of underlying cirrhosis, performance status, tumor number, and tumor size. In patients with Child class A and solitary HCC, the 5-year

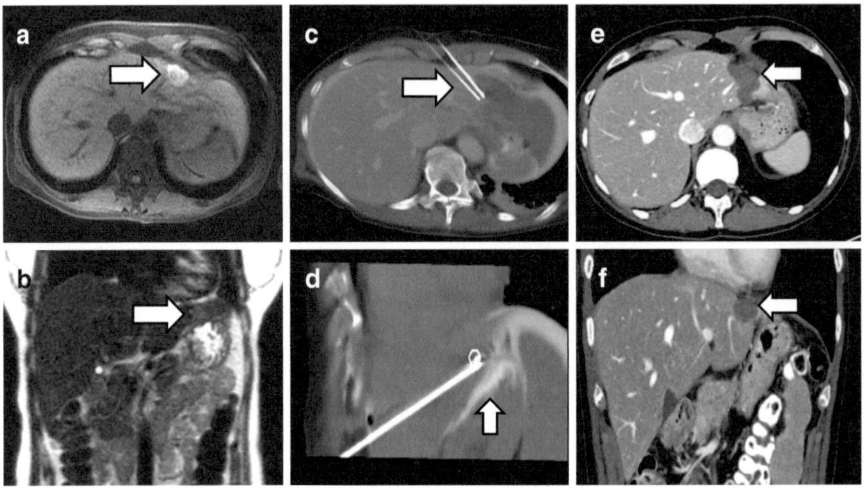

Fig. 5.3 A 56-year-old woman with metastatic leiomyosarcoma to the left liver. Axial MRI with contrast demonstrates enhancing nodule in the left liver segment 2 (**a**, arrow). Coronal MRI T2 without contrast demonstrates mildly hypointense lesion in the left liver between the heart and the stomach (**b**, arrow). Treatment with RFA using two electrodes (arrows in **c**, axial image, and **d**, sagittal image). Follow-up CT with contrast 16 months post-procedure with non-enhancing post-ablation scarring in the location of treatment indicative with local tumor control (arrows in **e**, axial image, and **f**, coronal image)

survival is between 40% and 65% [64–67]. An early randomized trial that compared RFA to surgical resection for small solitary hepatocellular carcinomas show similar overall survival rate and recurrence-free survival rates, although similar trials often have selection bias in favor of surgical resection as the gold standard therapy [68]. For metastatic colorectal cancer to the liver, RFA has results comparable to surgical resection with 5-year survival reported between 25% and 45% [69–74]. Locoregional outcomes for ablation of colorectal liver metastases are improvement in tumors less than 3 cm in size, low stage of primary tumor, small number of hepatic lesions, favorable tumor biology such as low carcinoembryonic antigen (CEA), and minimal tumor differentiation and cellular ploidy [75–77]. Recently tumors that exhibit wild-type KRAS mutation have been found to have a higher recurrence rate, requiring ablation margins to be extended due to increased infiltration into surrounding normal liver tissue [78]. In patients with liver recurrence after hepatectomy, RFA has been shown to increase possibility of curative treatment from 17% to 26% [79]. Incomplete ablation rates have been reported for metastatic colorectal cancer to the liver at 9%, 26.5%, and 45% for 290 metastases measuring 0–3 cm, 3–5 cm, and >5 cm, respectively [80]. Outcomes from MWA share the same dependent variables as RFA of underlying cirrhosis, performance status, tumor number, and tumor size. The 5-year survival of MWA for hepatocellular carcinoma has been reported between 50% and 60% [81, 82].

Complications from liver ablation are consistent with the minimally invasive nature of treatment. Minor complications are reported between 5% and 10%, major complications between 2% and 3%, and overall mortality rates ranging from 0.1% to 1.4% [83, 84]. Complications result from collateral damage to adjacent hepatic structures (bile duct injury, hepatic failure, portal vein thrombosis), extrahepatic structures (colon perforation), and infection (hepatic abscess, sepsis). Tumor seeding has been reported along the needle tract in approximately 0.5% of patients, with higher risk in poorly differentiated tumors and subcapsular locations [85, 86].

Renal Tumor Ablation

Treatment options for stage 1 renal cell carcinoma (RCC) have evolved to include percutaneous thermal ablation as a nephron-sparing procedure [87–89]. Percutaneous ablation is favorable in poor surgical candidates with multiple comorbidities or less than 10-year life expectancy and in patients with multiple bilateral renal tumors, solitary kidney, or poor renal function [90–92]. Optimal patient selection includes RCC stage T1a, with tumor measuring less than 4 cm in diameter [93–95]. Clinical outcomes between different ablation modalities for T1a RCC are similar and have reported 5-year cancer-specific survival outcomes that are within parameters observed in surgical total or partial nephrectomy, but with reduced periprocedural complications [96–100]. Locoregional control from T1b lesions that measure up to 7 cm is less likely however remains similar to results from partial surgical nephrectomy [101–103]. Peripheral tumor locations can improve safety and efficacy, due to decreased heat sink effect from the central vasculature and mitigated risk for collateral damage to the renal collecting system [104].

Major complications include perirenal hematoma, hematuria, ureteral injury, urinoma, abscess, and colon injury [105, 106]. Displacement of adjacent structures may be required with injection of liquid medium or carbon dioxide to minimize complications [107–110]. Again, high-quality image guidance during the ablation procedure is integral to achieve optimal locoregional control [111].

Pulmonary Tumor Ablation

Percutaneous thermal ablation may be used to treat either primary or oligometastatic lung cancers. The primary indication for pulmonary thermal ablation is locoregional curative treatment in patients who are not good surgical candidates (Fig. 5.4). This cohort may include patients with recurrence despite prior surgery or radiation therapy and those who refuse surgery or radiation. Ablation can also be performed as a palliative treatment for pain, cough, dyspnea, and hemoptysis [112, 113].

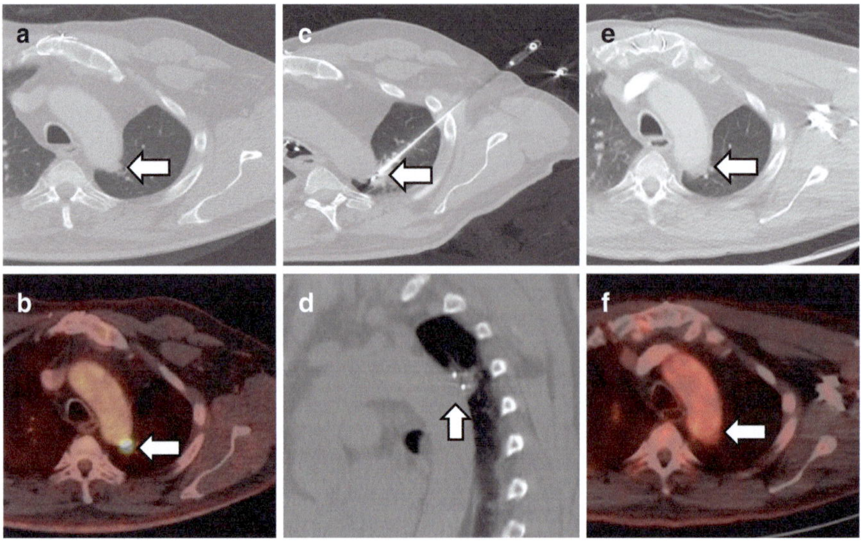

Fig. 5.4 A 59-year-old man with metastatic pleomorphic sarcoma presented for cryoablation of a 1 cm lung metastasis in the left upper lobe, located adjacent to the aorta (arrows in **a**, pre-procedure axial CT, and **b**, pre-procedure axial PET-CT). Cryoablation was performed using two probes, placed with an approach to minimize damage to the aortic wall (arrows in **c**, axial procedure CT, and **d**, oblique sagittal procedure CT). Post-procedure CT and PET-CT performed 3 months later with decreased nodule size and avidity, consistent with local control (arrows **e** and **f**, respectively)

For primary lung cancer, response rates have been reported as greater than 70% for lesions that measure less than 3 cm [114–116]. Care should be taken to evaluate for any hilar or mediastinal lymphadenopathy on pre-procedure imaging, which would preclude potential for locoregional control. Surgical resection is the gold standard treatment regardless of the technical ease of percutaneous ablation, as surgical intervention allows for palpation and visual inspection that can identify small pulmonary and mediastinal metastases. Hence thermal ablation should only be pursued in nonsurgical candidates or in patients who categorically refuse surgery.

Metastatic pulmonary tumors are more commonly treated with percutaneous ablation than primary lung disease. Patients that are most likely to respond to ablation include those with long disease-free interval, oligometastatic disease (<6 lesions), complete locoregional control of primary tumor location, metastases involving only the lung, and lesion size less than 3 cm [117]. For colorectal metastases to the lungs, overall median survival of 33 months (1-year, 85%; 2-year, 64%; and 3-year, 46%) has been reported after lung ablation using general exclusion guidelines of more than six lesions per hemithorax, maximal diameter greater than 5 cm, extrapulmonary metastases, and coagulopathy [118, 119]. A large retrospective review of 566 patients treated with RFA for 1037 lung metastases with median size of 1.5 cm reported a median overall survival of 62 months with a 4-year efficacy of 89% [120]. This outcome is comparable to 5-year overall survival reported between 27 and 68% for surgical resection of colon metastases [121–123].

Lung ablation is performed under CT guidance for real-time precision placement of ablation probes, assessment of ablation zone, and monitoring for immediate complications. As the surrounding air-filled lung can effectively act as insulation, the ablation energy required to achieve the same locoregional control may be decreased when compared to ablation of solid organ tumors [124–126]. Central lesions are more prone to major complications, which include bleeding, pneumothorax, and bronchopleural fistula [127]. With appropriate precautions, treatments in patients with emphysema or a solitary lung can be safely performed.

Musculoskeletal Tumor Ablation

Bone and soft tissue tumors can be treated by thermal ablation for both locoregional control and pain palliation (Fig. 5.5). Initial successes in the treatment of benign osteoid osteoma led to expansion of treatment to primary and metastatic tumors. Again, percutaneous ablation is reserved for patients that are not optimal surgical candidates or who refuse surgery and for lesions that recur or progress despite surgical resection, external radiation, and systemic chemotherapy. Outcomes for local tumor control are improved for tumors that measure less than 3 cm in greatest dimension [128]. Local control rates for both RFA and cryoablation have been reported between 67% and 97% with more than a 1-year follow-up [129–130].

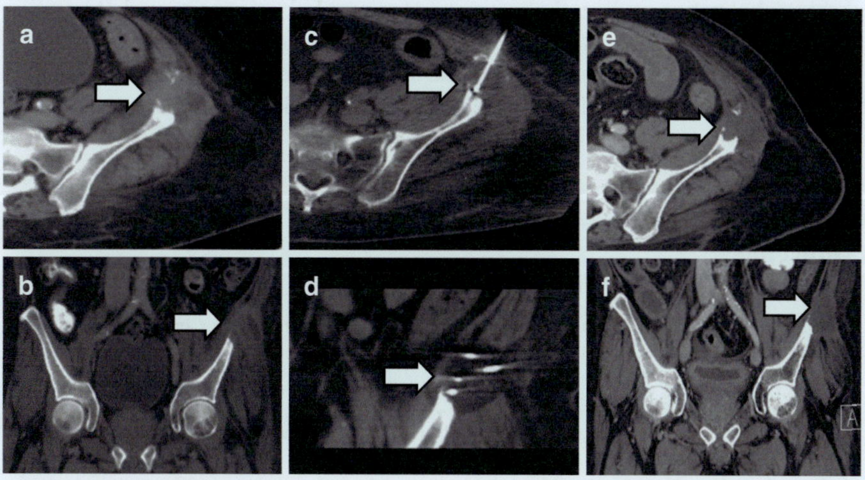

Fig. 5.5 A 58-year-old man with metastatic lung adenocarcinoma to the left iliac bone (arrows in **a**, pre-procedure axial CT with contrast, and **b**, pre-procedure coronal CT with contrast). Cryoablation performed with four cryoprobes (arrows in **c**, axial procedural CT, and **d**, coronal procedural CT). Post-procedure CT with contrast demonstrates decreased size of lesion and absence of enhancement, consistent with local tumor control (arrows in **e**, axial CT with contrast, and **f**, coronal CT with contrast)

Ablation of larger lesions can also confer local control if curative margins can be safely obtained; however, reports are limited to case reports or small case series.

Potential complications of musculoskeletal ablation include bleeding and damage to adjacent structures. Displacement techniques with fluid or carbon dioxide may decrease risk to adjacent large blood vessels, nerves, and hollow organs. Ablation may pose a risk to periarticular structures that can result in irreparable damage to the joint [131–132]. Furthermore, ablation of a weight-bearing bone such as a vertebral body may weaken the structural bone and subject the patient to post-procedure insufficiency fracture. Augmentation with a bone filler such as polymethyl methacrylate may prevent this painful complications [133]. If ablation is performed near the spinal cord or spinal and peripheral nerves, intra-procedural neurophysiologic monitoring may be arranged to minimize nerve damage. Nerve monitoring during ablation can be done with somatosensory evoked potentials (SSEPs), muscle motor evoked potentials (MEPs), and stimulated and spontaneous EMG activity [134].

Conclusion

Interventional oncology treatment options require the precise application of minimally invasive technology under real-time image guidance for curative or palliative effect. Locoregional therapy is performed to maximize tumor destruction and simultaneously minimize systemic and same-organ toxicity. Therapies for primary and metastatic liver tumors include hepatic intra-arterial chemotherapy infusion, chemoembolization, radioembolization, and thermal ablation. Thermal ablation is also commonly applied outside of the liver, to treat primary and metastatic disease in the kidneys, lungs, and musculoskeletal system. As for any locoregional therapy, a safe and effective treatment requires precise application of the most appropriate technology for the given tumor biology, tumor location, and patient comorbidities.

References

1. Ackerman NB. The blood supply of experimental liver metastases. IV. Changes in vascularity with increasing tumor growth. Surgery. 1974;75:589–96.
2. Sigurden ER, Ridge JA, Kemeny N, et al. Tumor and liver drug uptake following hepatic artery and portal vein infusion. J Clin Oncol. 1987;5:1836–40.
3. Chuang VP, Wallace S. Hepatic artery embolization in the treatment of hepatic neoplasms. Radiology. 1981;140:51–8.
4. Yamada R, Sato M, Kawabata M, et al. Hepatic artery embolization in 120 patients with unresectable hepatoma. Radiology. 1983;148:397–401.
5. Doyon D, Mouzon A, Jourde AM, et al. Hepatic arterial embolization in patients with malignant tumors. Ann Radiol (Paris). 1974;17:593–603.

6. Kemeny NE, Melendez FD, Capanu M, et al. Conversion to resectability using hepatic artery infusion plus systemic chemotherapy for the treatment of unresectable liver metastases from colorectal carcinoma. J Clin Oncol. 2009;27(21):3465–71.
7. Boige V, Malka D, Elias D, et al. Hepatic arterial infusion of oxaliplatin and intravenous LV5FU2 in unresectable liver metastases from colorectal cancer after systemic chemotherapy failure. Ann Surg Oncol. 2008;15(1):219–26.
8. Allard MA, Sebagh M, Baillie G, et al. Comparison of complete pathologic response and hepatic injuries between hepatic arterial infusion and systemic administration of oxaliplatin in patient with colorectal liver metastases. Ann Surg Oncol. 2015;22(6):1925–32.
9. Deschamps F, Rao P, Teriitehau C, et al. Percutaneous femoral implantation of an arterial port catheter for intraarterial chemotherapy: feasibility and predictive factors of long-term functionality. J Vasc Interv Radiol. 2010;21(11):1681–8.
10. Hildebrandt B, Pech M, Nicolaou A, et al. Interventionally implanted port catheter systems for hepatic arterial infusion of chemotherapy in patients with colorectal liver metastases: a phase II-study and historical comparison with the surgical approach. BMC Cancer. 2007;7:69.
11. Deschamps F, Elias D, Goere D, et al. Intra-arterial hepatic chemotherapy: a comparison of percutaneous versus surgical implantation of Port-Catheters. Cardiovasc Interv Radiol. 2011;34(5):973–9.
12. Sasaki Y, Imaoka S, Kasugai H, et al. A new approach to chemoembolization therapy for hepatoma using ethiodized oil, cisplatin, and gelatin sponge. Cancer. 1987;60:1194–203.
13. Sawada S. Transcatehter oily chemoembolization of hepatocellular carcinoma. Radiology. 1989;170:783–6.
14. Konno T. Tareting cancer chemotherapeutic agents by use of lipioidol contrast medium. Cancer. 1990;66:1897–903.
15. Ramsey DE, Kernagis LY, Soulen MC, et al. Chemoembolization of hepatocellular carcinoma. J Vasc Interv Radiol. 2002;13:S211–21.
16. Kruskal JB, Hlatky L, Hahnfeldt P, et al. In vivo and in vitro analysis of the effectiveness of docorubicin combined with temporary arterial occlusion in liver tumors. J Vasc Interv Radiol. 1993;4:741–7.
17. De Baere T, Arai Y, Lencioni R, et al. Treatment of liver tumors with lipiodol TACE: technical recommendations from expert opinion. Cardiovasc Intervent Radiol. 2016;39(3):334–43.
18. Nakajo M, Kobayashi H, Shimabukuro K, et al. Biodistribution and in vivo kinetics of iodine-131 lipiodol infused via the hepatic artery of patients with hepatic cancer. J Nucl Med. 1988;29:1066–77.
19. Nakamura H, Hashimoto T, Oi H, et al. Transcatheter oily chemoembolization of hepatocellular carcinoma. Radiology. 1989;170:793–86.
20. Clouse ME, Perry L, Stuart K, et al. Hepatic arterial chemoembolization for metastatic neuroendocrine tumors. Digestion. 1994;55(Suppl 3):92–7.
21. Raoul JL, Heresbach D, Bretagne JF, et al. Chemoembolization of hepatocellular carcinomas: a study of the biodistribution and pharmacokinetics of doxorubicin. Cancer. 1992;70:585–90.
22. Konno T, Maeda H, Iwai K, et al. Effect of arterial administration of high-molecular-weight anticancer agent SMANCS with lipid lymphagraphic agent on hepatoma. Eur J Cancer Clin Oncol. 1983;19:1053–65.
23. Nakamura H, Tanaka T, Jori S, et al. Transcatheter embolization of hepatocellular carcinoma: assessment of efficacy in case of resection following embolization. Radiology. 1983;147:401–5.
24. Bhattacharya S, Novell JR, Winslet MC, et al. Iodinized oil in the treatment of hepatocellular carcinoma. Br J Surg. 1994;81:1563–71.
25. Forner A, Reig M, Bruix J. Hepatocellular carcinoma. Lancet. 2018;391:1301–14.
26. Yau T, Tang VY, Yao TJ, et al. Development of Hong Kong Liver Cancer staging system with treatment stratification for patients with hepatocellular carcinoma. Gastroenterology. 2014;146:1691–700.

27. Llovet JM, Burroughs A, Bruix J. Hepatocellular carcinoma. Lancet. 2003;362(9399):1907–17.
28. Lencioni R, de Baere T. Soulen, et al. Lipiodol transarterial chemoembolization for hepatocellular carcinoma: a systematic review of efficacy and safety data. Hepatology. 2016;64:106–16.
29. Gupta S, Johnson MM, Murphy R, et al. Hepatic arterial embolization and chemoembolization for the treatment of patients with metastatic neuroendocrine tumors. Cancer. 2005;104(8):1590–602.
30. Lang EK, Brown CL. Colorectal metastases to the liver: selective chemoembolization. Radiology. 1993;189(2):417–22.
31. Rao PP, Pascale F, Seck A, et al. Irinotecan loaded in eluting bead: pre-clinical assessment in a rabbit VX2 liver tumor model. Cardiovasc Interv Radiol. 2012;35(6):1448–59.
32. Fiorentini G, Aliberti C, Tilli M, et al. Intra-arterial infusion of irnotecan-loaded drug-eluting beads (DEBIRI) versus intravenous therapy (FOLFIRI) for hepatic metastases from colorectal cancer: final results of a phase II study. Anticancer Res. 2012;32(4):1387–95.
33. Song SY, Chung JW, Han JK, et al. Liver abscess after transcatheter oily chemoembolization for hepatic tumors: incidence, predisposing factors and clinical outcome. J Vasc Interv Radiol. 2001;12:313–20.
34. Kim W, Clark TWI, Baym RA, et al. Risk factors for liver abscess formation after hepatic chemoembolization. J Vasc Interv Radiol. 2001;12:965–8.
35. Salem R, Gabr A, Riaz A, et al. Institutional decision to adopt Y90 as primary treatment for hepatocellular carcinoma informed by a 1,000-patient 15-year experience. Hepatology. 2018;68(4):1429–40.
36. Salem R, Gordon AC, Mouli S, et al. Y90 radioembolization significantly prolongs time to progression compared with chemoembolization in patients with hepatocellular carcinoma. Gastroenterology. 2016;151(6):1155–63.
37. Ho S, Lau WY, Leung TW, et al. Clinical evaluation of the partition model for estimating radiation doses from yttrium-90 microspheres in the treatment of hepatic cancer. Eur J Nucl Med. 1997;24(3):293–8.
38. Gray B, Van Hazel G, Hope M, et al. Randomised trial of SIR-Spheres plus chemotherapy vs chemotherapy alone for treating patients with liver metastases from primary large bowel cancer. Ann Oncol. 2001;12(12):1711–20.
39. Van Hazel G, Blackwell A, Anderson J, et al. Randomizedphase 2 trial of SIR-Spheres plus fluorouracil/leucovorin chemotherapy versus fluorouracil/leucovorin chemotherapy alone in advanced colorectal cancer. J Surg Oncol. 2004;88(2):78–85.
40. Lim LC, Gibbs YD, Shapiro J, et al. A prospective evaluation of treatment with selective internal radiation therapy (SIR-Spheres) in patients with unresectable liver metastases from colorectal cancer previously treated with 5-FU based chemotherapy. BMC Cancer. 2005;5(1):132.
41. Wasan H, Gibbs P, Sharma N, et al. First-line selective internal radiotherapy plus chemotherapy versus chemotherapy alone in patients with liver metastases from colorectal cancer (FOXFIRE, SIRFLOX, and FOXFIRE-Global): a combined analysis of three multicentre, randomized, phase 3 trials. Lancet. 2017;18(9):1159–71.
42. Lewandowski RJ, Thurston KG, Goin JE, et al. 90Y Microsphere (TheraSphere) treatment for unresectable colorectal cancer metastases of the liver: response to treatment at targeted doses of 135–150 Gy as measured by (18f) fluorodeoxyglucose positron emission tomography and computed tomographic imaging. J Vasc Interv Radiol. 2005;16(12):1641–51.
43. Murthy R, Nunez R, Szklaruk J, et al. Yttrium-90 microsphere therapy for hepatic malignancy: devices, indications, technical considerations, and potential complications. Radiographics. 2005;25(Suppl 1):S41–55.
44. Salem R, Lewandowski RJ, Atassi B, et al. Treatment of unresectable hepatocellular carcinoma with use of ^{90}Y microspheres (TheraSphere): safety, tumor response, and survival. J Vasc Interv Radiol. 2005;16(12):1627–39.
45. Liu DM, Salem R, Bui JT, et al. Angiographic considerations in patients undergoing liver-directed therapy. J Vasc Interv Radiol. 2005;16(7):911–35.

46. Salem R, Lewandowski RJ, Sato KT, et al. Technical aspects of radioembolization with 90Y microspheres. Tech Vasc Interv Radiol. 2007;10(1):12–29.
47. Yip D, Allen R, Ashton C, et al. Radiation-induced ulceration of the stomach secondary to hepatic embolization with radioactive yttrium microspheres in the treatment of metastatic colon cancer. J Gastroenterol Hepatol. 2004;19(3):347–9.
48. Lewandowski R, Salem R. Incidence of radiation cholecystitis in patients receiving Y-90 treatment for unresectable liver malignancies. J Vasc Interv Radio. 2004;15(2):S162.
49. Ho S, Lau WY, Leung TW, et al. Clinical evaluation of the partition model for estimating radiation doses from yttrium-90 microspheres in treating hepatic tumours. Eur J Nucl Med. 1996;23(8):947–52.
50. Kennedy AS, McNeillie P, Dezarn WA, et al. Treatment parameters and outcome in 680 treatments of internal radiation with resin 90-Y microspheres for unresectable hepatic tumors. Int J Radiat Oncol Biol Phys. 2009;74(5):1494–500.
51. Sangro B, Gil-Alzugaray B, Rodriguez J, et al. Liver disease induced by radioembolization of liver tumors: description and possible risk factors. Cancer. 2008;112(7):1598–46.
52. Dodd GD, Frank MS, Aribandi M, et al. Radiofrequency thermal ablation: computer analysis of the size of the thermal injury created by overlapping ablations. Am J Roentgenol. 2001;2001(177):777–82.
53. Sofocleous CT, Petre EN, Gonen M, et al. CT-guided radiofrequency ablation as a salvage treatment of colorectal cancer hepatic metastases developing after hepatectomy. J Vasc Interv Radiol. 2011;22(6):755–61.
54. Zevas N, Kuwayama A. Pathologic analysis of experimental thermal lesions: comparison of induction heating and radiofrequency electrocoagulation. J Neurosurg. 1972;37:418–22.
55. Mertyna P, Hines-Peralta A, Liu Z, et al. Radiofrequency ablation: variability in heat sensitivity in tumors and tissues. J Vasc Interv Radiol. 2007;18(5):647–54.
56. Trembley B, Ryan T, Strohbehn J. Interstitial hyperthermia: physics, biology, and clinical aspects. In: Hyperthermia and oncology, vol. 3. Utrecht: VSP; 1992. p. 11–98.
57. Goldberg SN, Gazelle GS, Compton CC, et al. Treatment of intrahepatic malignancy with radiofrequency ablation: radiologic-pathologic correlation. Cancer. 2000;88:2452–63.
58. Lu DS, Yu NC, Raman SS, et al. Radiofrequency ablation of hepatocellular carcinoma: treatment success as defined by histological examination of the explanted liver. Radiology. 2005;234:954–60.
59. Hoffmann NE, Bischof JC. The cryobiology of cryosurgical injury. Urology. 2002;60:40–9.
60. Rupp CC, Hoffmann NE, Schmidlin FR, et al. Cryosurgical changes in the porcine kidney: histologic analysis with thermal history correlation. Cryobiology. 2002;45:167–82.
61. Pennes H. Analysis of tissue and arterial blood temperatures in the resting human forearm. J Appl Physiol. 1948;1(2):93–122.
62. Kim KR, Thomas S. Complications of image-guided thermal ablation of liver and kidney neoplasms. Semin Intervent Radiol. 2014;31:138–48.
63. Zhong J, Bambrook J, Bhambra B, et al. Incidence of post-ablation syndrome following image-guided percutaneous cryoablation of renal cell carcinoma: a prospective study. Cardiovasc Intervent Radiol. 2018;41:270–6.
64. Lencioni R, Cioni D, Crocetti L, et al. Early-stage hepatocellular carcinoma in cirrhosis: long-term results of percutaneous image-guided radiofrequency ablation. Radiology. 2005;234:961–7.
65. Tateishi R, Shiina S, Teratani T, et al. Percutaneous radiofrequency ablation for hepatocellular carcinoma. Cancer. 2005;103:1201–9.
66. Cabassa P, Donato F, Simeone F, et al. Radiofrequency ablation of hepatocellular carcinoma: long-term experience with expandable needle electrodes. Am J Roentegnol. 2006;185:S316–21.
67. Choi D, Lim HK, Rhim H, et al. Percutaneous radiofrequency ablation for early-stage hepatocellular carcinoma as a first-line treatment: long-term results and prognostic factors in a large single-institution series. Eur Radiol. 2007;17:684–92.

68. Chen MD, Li JQ, Zheng Y, et al. A prospective randomized trial comparing percutaneous local ablative therapy and partial hepatectomy for small hepatocellular carcinoma. Ann Surg. 2006;243:321–8.
69. Elias D, Baton O, Sideris L, et al. Local recurrences after intraoperative radiofrequency ablation of liver metastases: a comparative study with anatomic and wedge resections. Ann Surg Oncol. 2004;11(5):500–5.
70. Berber E, Pelley r, Siperstein AE. Predictors of survival after radiofrequency thermal ablation of colorectal cancer metastases to the liver: a prospective study. J Clin Oncol. 2005;23:1358–64.
71. Gillams AR, Lees WR. Radio-frequency ablation of colorectal liver metastases in 167 patients. Eur Radiol. 2004;14:2261–7.
72. Jakobs TF, Hoffmann RT, Trumm C, et al. Radiofrequency ablation of colorectal liver metastases: mid-term results in 68 patients. Anticancer Res. 2006;26:671–80.
73. Lencioni R, Crocetti L, Cioni D, et al. Percutaneous radiofrequency ablation of hepatic colorectal metastases: technique, indications, results and new promises. Investig Radiol. 2004;39:689–97.
74. Sorensen SM, Mortensen FV, Nielsen DT. Radiofrequency alation of colorectal liver metastases: long-term survival. Acta Radiol. 2007;48:253–8.
75. Tanis E, Nordlinger B, Mauer M, et al. Local recurrence rates after radiofrequency ablation or resection of colorectal liver metastases. Analysis of the European Organisation for Research and Treatment of Cancer #40004 and #40983. Eur J Cancer. 2014;50(5):912–9.
76. Nishiwada S, Ko S, Mukogawa T, et al. Comparison between percutaneous radiofrequency ablation and surgical hepatectomy focusing on local disease control rate for colorectal liver metastases. Hepato-Gastroenterology. 2014;61(130):436–41.
77. Vigano L, Capussotti L, Lapointe R, et al. Early recurrence after liver resection for colorectal metastases: risk factors, prognosis, and treatment. A LiverMetSurvey-based study of 6025 patients. Ann Surg Oncol. 2014;21(4):1276–86.
78. Calandri M, Yamashita S, Gazzera C, Fonio P, Veltri A, Bustreo S, Sheth RA, Yevich SM, Vauthey JN, Odisio BC. Ablation of colorectal liver metastasis: interaction of ablation margins and RAS mutation profiling on local tumour progression-free survival. Eur Radiol. 2018;28(7):2727–34.
79. Elias D, DeBaere T, Smayra T, et al. Percutaneous radiofrequency thermoablation as an alternative to surgery for treatment of liver tumour recurrence after hepatectomy. Br J Surg. 2002;89:752–6.
80. Nielsen K, van Tilborg AA, Meijerink MR, et al. Incidence and treatment of local site recurrences following RFA of colorectal liver metastases. World J Surg. 2013;37(6):1340–7.
81. Dong B, Liang P, Yu X, et al. Percutaneous sonographically guided microwave coagulation therapy for hepatocellular carcinoma: results in 234 patietns. Am J Roentgenol. 2003;180:1547–1.
82. Liang P, Dong B, Yu X, et al. Prognostic factors for survival in patients with hepatocellular carcinoma after percutaneous microwave ablation. Radiology. 2005;235:299–307.
83. Rhim H. Complications of radiofrequency ablation in hepatocellular carcinoma. Abdom Imaging. 2005;30:409–18.
84. DeBaere T, Risse O, Kuoch V, et al. Adverse events during radiofrequency treatment of 582 hepatic tumors. Am J Roentenol. 2003;181:695–700.
85. Livraghi T, Solbiati L, Meloni MF, et al. Treatment of focal liver tumors with percutaneous radiofrequency ablation: complications encountered in a multicenter study. Radiology. 2003;226:441–51.
86. Llovet JM, Vilana R, Bru C, Barcelona Clinic Liver Cancer (BCLC) Group, et al. Increased risk of tumor seeding after percutaneous radiofrequency ablation for single hepatocellular carcinoma. Hepatology. 2001;33:1124–9.
87. Chiou YY, Hwang JI, Chou YH, et al. Percutaneous radiofrequency ablation of renal cell carcinoma. J Chin Med Assoc. 2005;68:221–5.
88. Silverman SG, Tuncali K, vanSonnenberg E, et al. Renal tumors: MR imaging-guided percutaneous cryotherapy – initial experience in 23 patients. Radiology. 2005;236:716–24.

89. Higgins LJ, Hong K. Renal ablation techniques: state of the art. Am J Roentgenol. 2015;205:735–41.
90. Ljungberg B, Bensalah K, Canfield S, et al. EAU guidelines on renal cell carcinoma: 2014 update. Eur Urol. 2015;67:913–24.
91. Finelli A, Ismaila N, Bro B, et al. Management of small renal masses: American society of clinical oncology clinical practice guideline. J Oncol Pract. 2017;35:668–80.
92. Escudier B, Porta C, Schmidinger M. et la. ESMO Clinical Practice Guidelines for diagnosis, treatment, and follow-up. Ann Oncol. 2019;30:706–20.
93. Gervais DA, McGovern FJ, Arellano RS, et al. Radiofrequency ablation of renal cell carcinoma: part 1, indications, results, and role in patient management over a 6-year period and ablation of 100 tumors. AJR Am J Roentgenol. 2005;185:64–71.
94. Mayo-Smith WW, Dupuy DE, Parikh PM, et al. Imaging-guided percutaneous radiofrequency ablation of solid renal masses: techniques and outcomes of 38 treatment sessions in 32 consecutive patients. AJR Am J Roentgenol. 2003;180:1503–8.
95. Ahrar K, Matin S, Wood CG, et al. Percutaneous radiofrequency ablation of renal tumors: technique, complications, and outcomes. J Vasc Interv Radiol. 2005;16:679–88.
96. Talengeld AD, Gennarelli RL, Elkin EB, et al. Percutaneous ablation versus partial and radical nephrectomy for T1a renal cancer: a population-based analysis. Ann Intern Med. 2018;169:69.
97. Xing M, Kokabi N, Zhang D, et al. Comparative effectiveness of thermal ablation, surgical resection, and active surveillance for T1a renal cell carcinoma: a Surveillance, Epidemiology, and End Results (SEER)-Medicare-linked Population Study. Radiology. 2018;288:81–90.
98. Katsanos K, Mailli L, Krokidis M, et al. Systematic review and meta-analysis of thermal ablation versus surgical nephrectomy for small renal tumours. Cardiovasc Intervent Radiol. 2014;37:427–37.
99. Yin X, Cui L, Li F, et al. Radiofrequency ablation versus partial nephrectomy in treating small renal tumors: a systematic review and meta-analysis. Medicine. 2015;94:e2255.
100. Wang S, Qin C, Peng Z, et al. Radiofrequency ablation versus partial nephrectomy for the treatment of clinical stage 1 renal masses: a systematic review and meta-analysis. Chin Med J. 2014;127:2497–503.
101. Hasegawa T, Yamanaka T, Gobara H, et al. Radiofrequency ablation versus cryoablation for T1b renal cell carcinoma: a multicenter study. Jpn J Radiol. 2018;36:551–8.
102. Chang X, Zhang F, Liu T, et al. Radio frequency ablation versus nephrectomy for clinical T1b renal cell carcinoma: long-term clinical and oncologic outcomes. J Urol. 2015;193:430–5.
103. Wells SA, Wheeler KM, Mithqal A, et al. Percutaneous microwave ablation of T1a and T1b renal cell carcinoma: short-term efficacy and complications with emphasis on tumor complexity and single session treatment. Abdom Radiol. 2016;41:1203–11.
104. Gervais DA, McGover FJ, Arellano RS, et al. Renal cell carcinoma: clinical experience and technical success with radio-frequency ablation of 42 tumors. Radiology. 2003;226:417–24.
105. Krokidis ME, Orsi F, Katsanos K, et al. CIRSE guidelines on percutaneous ablation of small renal cell carcinoma. Cardiovasc Intervent Radiol. 2017;40:177–91.
106. Choi SH, Kim JW, Kim JH, et al. Efficacy and safety of microwave ablation for malignant renal tumors: an updated systematic review and meta-analysis of the literature since 2012. Korean J Radiol. 2018;19:938–49.
107. Farrell MA, Charboneau JW, Callstrom MR, et al. Paranephric water instillation: a technique to prevent bowel injury during percutaneous renal radiofrequency ablation. Am J Roentgenol. 2003;181:1315–7.
108. Kariya Z, Yamakado K, Nakatuka A, et al. Radiofrequency ablation with and without balloon occlusion of the renal artery: an experimental study in porcine kidneys. J Vasc Interv Radiol. 2003;14:241–5.
109. Raman SS, Aziz D, Chang X, et al. Minimizing diaphragmatic injury during radiofrequency ablation: efficacy of intraabdominal carbon dioxide insufflation. Am J Roentgenol. 2004;183:197–200.

110. Lee SJ, Choyke LT, Locklin JK, et al. Use of hydrodissection to prevent nerve and muscular damage during radiofrequency ablation of kidney tumors. J Vasc Interv Radiol. 2006;17:1967–9.
111. Mauri G, Sconfienza LM. Is operators' experience more important that the ablation technique in image-guided thermal ablations? Int J Hyperth. 2017;33:955–6.
112. VanSonnenberg E, Shankar S, Morrison PR, et al. Radiofrequency ablation of thoracic lesions: part 2, initial clinical experience – technical and multidisciplinary considerations in 30 patients. Am J Roentgenol. 2005;184(2):381–90.
113. Wang H, Littrup PJ, Duan Y, et al. Thoracic masses treated with percutaneous cryoablation: initial experience with more than 200 procedures. Radiology. 2005;235(1):289–98.
114. Belfiore G, Moggio G, Tedeschi E, et al. CT-guided radiofrequency ablation: a potential complementary thgerapy for patients with unresectable primary lung cancer – a preliminary report of 33 patients. Am J Roentgenol. 2004;183(4):1003–11.
115. Ambriogi MC, Lucchi M, Dini P, et al. Percutaneous radiofrequency ablation of lung tumours: results in the mid-term. Eur J Cardiothorac Surg. 2006;30(1):177–83.
116. Simon CJ, Dupuy D, Safran H, et al. Pulmonary radiofrequency ablation: long-term safety and efficacy in 153 patients. Radiology. 2006;243(1):268–75.
117. Pastorino U, Buyse M, Friedel G, et al. International registry of lung metastases, long-term results of lun metastasectomy: prognostic analysis based on 5206 cases. J Thorac Cardiovasc Surg. 1997;113:37–49.
118. Yan T, King J, Sjarif A, et al. Percutaneous radiofrequency ablation of pulmonary metastases from colorectal carcinoma: prognostic determinants for survival. Ann Surg Oncol. 2006;13(11):1529–37.
119. Yan TD, King J, Sjarif A, et al. Learning curve for percutaneous radiofrequency ablation of pulmonary metastases from colorectal carcinoma: a prospective study of 70 consecutive cases. Ann Surg Oncol. 2006;13(12):1588–95.
120. De Baere T, Auperin A, Deschamps F, et al. Radiofrequency ablation is a valid treatment option for lung metastases: experience in 566 patients with 1037 metastases. Ann Oncol. 2015;26(5):987–91.
121. Iida T, Nomori H, Shiba M, et al. Prognotic factors after pulmonary metastasectomy for colorectal cancer and rationale for determining surgical indications: a retrospective analysis. Ann Surg. 2013;257(6):1059–64.
122. Gonzalez M, Poncet A, Combescure C, et al. Risk factors for survival after lung metastasectomy in colorectal cancer patients: a systematic review and meta-analysis. Ann Surg Oncol. 2013;20(2):572–9.
123. Pfannschmidt J, Hoffmann H, Dienemann H. Reported outcome factors for pulmonary resection in metastatic colorectal cancer. J Thorac Oncol. 2010;5(6 Suppl 2):S172–8.
124. Goldberg NS, Dupuy DE. Image-guided radiofrequency tumor ablation: challenges and opportunities part I. J Vasc Interv Radiol. 2001;12(9):1021–32.
125. Dupuy DR, Goldberg SN. Image-guided radiofrequency tumor ablation: challenges and opportunities part II. J Vasc Interv Radiol. 2001;12(10):1135–48.
126. Ahmed M, Liu Z, Afzal KS, et al. Radiofrequency ablation: effect of surrounding tissue composition on coagulation necrosis in a canine tumor model. Radiology. 2004;230(3):761–7.
127. Hiraki T, Tajiri N, Mimura H, et al. Pneumothorax, pleural effusion, and chest tube placement after radiofrequency ablation of lung tumors: incidence and risk factors. Radiology. 2006;241:275–83.
128. McMenomy B, Kurup N, Johnson G, et al. Percutaneous cryoablation of musculoskeletal oligometastatic disease for complete remission. J Vasc Interv Radiol. 2013;24:207–13.
129. Kurup N, Morris J, Callstrom M. Ablation of musculoskeletal metastases. Am J Roentgenol. 2017;209:713–21.
130. Deschamps F, Farouil G, de Baere T. Percutaneous ablation of bone tumors. Diagn Interv Imaging. 2014;95(7–8):659–63.

131. Friedman MV, Hillen TJ, Wessell DE, et al. Hip chondrolysis and femoral head osteonecrosis: a complication of periacetabular cryoablation. J Vasc Interv Radiol. 2014;25:1580–8.
132. Prologo JD, Patel I, Buethe J, et al. Ablation zones and weight-bearing bones: points of caution for the palliative interventionalist. J Vasc Interv Radiol. 2014;25:769–75.
133. Wallace AN, Greenwood TJ, Jennings JW. Radiofrequency ablation and vertebral augmentation for palliation of painful spinal metastases. J Neuro-Oncol. 2015;124:111–8.
134. Kurup AN, Morris JM, Boon AJ, et al. Motor evoked potential monitoring during cryoablation of musculoskeletal tumors. J Vasc Interv Radiol. 2014;25(11):1657–64.

Chapter 6
Radiation Dosimetry Considerations of Locoregional Radionuclide Cancer Therapy

Franklin C. L. Wong and Richard B. Sparks

Introduction

Locoregional radionuclide cancer therapy (LRCT) is a feasible modality to treat human cancer with the intended goal of maximizing radiation-absorbed dose (RAD) to tumor and minimizing potential toxicity to critical organs. There have been increasing LRCT clinical applications as illustrated by approved cancer therapies using Y-90 microspheres [1] and clinical trials such as P-32 silicon particles [4]. The use of radionuclides in therapy allows direct monitoring (via imaging) of the spatial and temporal distribution of the treating agent and hence estimation of actual RAD delivered to the tumor target (target dosimetry, or TD) and surrounding tissues (depth dosimetry, or, DD). Upon integration with biodistribution and pharmacokinetic information based on anthropomorphic models and imaging, it is possible to estimate RAD to vital organs and the rest of the body (whole-body dosimetry, WBD).

Dosimetric models have been published to estimate radiation self-dose per unit cumulated activity to spheres representing tumors from various individual radionuclides. However, such estimates (1) require the user to derive their own nonlinear interpolation for specific tumor sizes, (2) only allow for uniform distribution of activity in the source representing tumor, and (3) do not provide depth-dose estimates of radiation exposure to the surrounding tissues. It is thus desirable to have more complete radiation dosimetry models to estimate TD and DD across a clinically relevant volume (e.g., 0.5–250 mL) of tumor sizes.

F. C. L. Wong (✉)
Department of Nuclear Medicine, University of Texas, M. D. Anderson Cancer Center, Houston, TX, USA
e-mail: fwong@mdanderson.org

R. B. Sparks
CDE Dosimetry Services, Inc., Knoxville, TN, USA
e-mail: rsparks@creativedevelopment.com

F. C. L. Wong (ed.), *Locoregional Radionuclide Cancer Therapy*,
https://doi.org/10.1007/978-3-030-56267-0_6

This chapter reports on the construction of radiation transport models from a set of five spheres of increasing fixed volumes with 23 different commercially available radionuclides that allow for both uniform and peripheral distributions in the source and provides estimates not only of self-dose (TD) per unit cumulated activity, but also dose to surrounding tissues as a function of depth (DD). The uniform distribution (or, spheres) model simulates homogeneous distribution of activity in the tumor. The peripheral distribution (or, shells) model simulates uneven distribution after intratumoral injection such as into a cavitary tumor where the tumorous tissues are on the surface of the cavity and will concentrate the radiopharmaceuticals before diffusion and eventual absorption into the capillaries and return to the circulation. The uniform and peripheral distribution models together cover the extremes of homogeneous to heterogeneous distribution that might be expected and thus estimate upper and lower bounds of potential radiation exposure.

Dosimetry estimates to the tumor and surrounding tissues using the dose per unit cumulated activity determined by the models described herein also require the determination of the cumulated activity (residence time). Cumulated activity (residence time) in the tumor source is dependent on the rate of clearance of activity from the tumor. The routes of clearance of interstitially deposited medication including radiopharmaceuticals depend on the physical form of the pharmaceutical preparation. Particles including colloids (>0.2 micron) [3] and solutes of higher molecular weights (greater than 20 kD) [12] are predominantly processed through the lymphatics and typically have slower clearance rates. Solutes of lower molecular rate (less than 5 kD) are typically cleared promptly back to general circulation via the neighboring capillaries to the venous system [2]. Injection of radiopharmaceuticals into a cavitary lesion may result in layering to the wall of the cavity before absorption via the capillaries or lymphatics, again depending on form of the pharmaceutical preparation. Sequential imaging or clearance models can be used to determine cumulated activities using the standard methodology, and these results can be combined with the model results herein to produce the TD and DD estimates.

In order to increase the usefulness of this work, the results were normalized by the tumor volumes to produce volume normalized S-values, and empirical logarithmic or power models were produced to simplify the process of determining the dose estimates.

Methodology

Uniform Distribution (or, Spheres) Models

Uniform distributions in the tumors are modeled by assuming each tumor source is spherical as shown in Eq. (6.1), with radii of 0.457, 0.782, 1.336, 2.285, and 3.908 cm for the 0.4, 2.0, 10, 50, and 250 cc tumor/sphere sources, respectively. The surrounding tissues are modeled as a series of concentric spherical shells starting at the outer edge of the source sphere using Eqs. (6.2) and (6.3) where i is the shell number and t is the shell thickness.

$$\left(\frac{x}{r}\right)^2+\left(\frac{y}{r}\right)^2+\left(\frac{z}{r}\right)^2\leq 1 \tag{6.1}$$

$$\left(\frac{x}{r+(i-1)t}\right)^2+\left(\frac{y}{r+(i-1)t}\right)^2+\left(\frac{z}{r+(i-1)t}\right)^2>1 \tag{6.2}$$

$$\left(\frac{x}{r+it}\right)^2+\left(\frac{y}{r+it}\right)^2+\left(\frac{z}{r+it}\right)^2\leq 1 \tag{6.3}$$

Peripheral Distribution (or, Shells) Models

Peripheral distributions in the tumors are modeled assuming each tumor source is a thin spherical shell (using Eqs. (6.2) and (6.3)) starting on the outside edge of the source spheres described in the uniform distribution model. The surrounding tissues are modeled as a series of concentric spherical shells exactly as was done for the uniform distribution model. For the tumor sources and surrounding tissues in both the uniform and peripheral distribution models, the soft tissue elemental composition as defined in the Cristy-Eckerman phantom [6] is assumed. The dimensions of these models are described in Table 6.1.

MCNP Radiation Transport Simulations

Monte Carlo radiation transport simulation [7] is used to estimate the fraction of energy emitted from the radioactive decays in the tumor source that is absorbed in the tumor itself and in the surrounding tissues as a function of depth (absorbed fractions). Every emission of each radionuclide is modeled in the simulation, accounting for both the abundance of discrete emissions and the full spectrum of beta as well as gamma emissions. Table 6.2 shows an example of the emissions, as used for Zr-89 [11].

The radiation transport code MCNP 4b [5] is used in this study to run the simulations. For each of the models, between 2 million and 10 million particle histories are simulated. Emission energies and yields for each nuclide are taken from the RADAR

Table 6.1 Radius and thickness values for 0.4 cc, 2 cc, 10 cc, 50 cc, 250 cc models

Model	r (cm)	t (cm)
0.4 cc	0.457	0.05
2 cc	0.782	0.1
10 cc	1.336	0.1
50 cc	2.285	0.1
250 cc	3.908	0.1

Table 6.2 Radioactive emissions of Zr-89

Emission	Mean energy (MeV)	Frequency
β+	0.3955	0.2274
Auger-L e–	0.0019	0.79
Auger-K e–	0.0127	0.1947
L X-ray	0.0019	0.018
Kα2 X-ray	0.0149	0.1388
Kα1 X-ray	0.015	0.2674
Kβ X-ray	0.0167	0.0735
γ +/–	0.511	0.4548
γ	0.9092	0.9904
γ	1.6208	0.0007
γ	1.6573	0.0011
γ	1.713	0.0075
γ	1.7445	0.0012

Note: For beta emission, the full beta spectrum was utilized

emissions database [11]. For the photon simulations, sufficient numbers of histories are run such that the relative errors are less than 1%. For the electron simulations sufficient numbers of histories are run such that the relative errors are less than 7%. The MCNP relative error criteria for generally reliable results are 10% or less.

The resultant absorbed fractions are used with calculated masses of the target shells and the mean energy emitted per nuclear transition, to determine S-values using the standard MIRD methodology [8]. Dose tables are produced by multiplying the residence times in the source regions by the calculated S-values. Residence times for the purposes of table construction in this chapter are determined by assuming physical decay only (no biologic loss) of the activity in the tumor.

Results

Target Dose (TD) and Depth Dose (DD) of the Uniform Distribution Models

The TD and DD of the uniform distribution models are listed in Appendices I (target dose) and II (fractional depth dose as fraction of source dose), respectively. Division by the residence times yields the S-value and allows for comparison of radiation-absorbed doses from various radiopharmaceuticals. In the current models, complete decay is assumed, i.e., there is no biologic loss of activity from the tumor, and residence times can be determined by multiplying 1.44 times the physical half-lives (in hours). When biologic loss is considered and accurately determined using imaging or known pharmacokinetic models, the residence time can be determined by multiplying 1.44 times the effective half-lives. The S-values with units of cGy/(mCi hr.) of the 23 radionuclides in sphere models are illustrated in Fig. 6.1. Further normalization can be made to account for the volume of the radionuclides in the source spheres to create a volume-normalized S-value in units of cGy/ (mCi hr. ml) as illustrated in Fig. 6.2 to compare the effects of the source volume on the S-values for different radionuclides. Based on the five chosen volumes of clinical significance, as source volume increases, steadily rising trends of volume-normalized S-values toward plateaus are noted for most of the radionuclides examined.

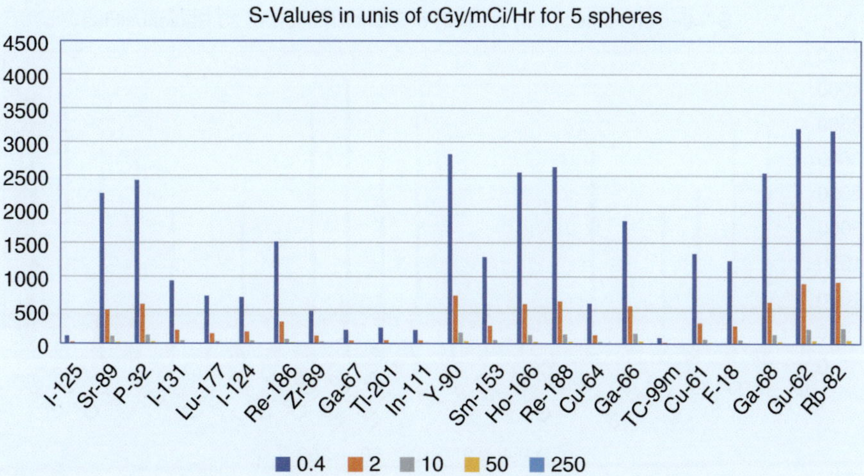

Fig. 6.1 S-values (in units of cGy/mCi/Hr) of five-sphere models of 23 radionuclides

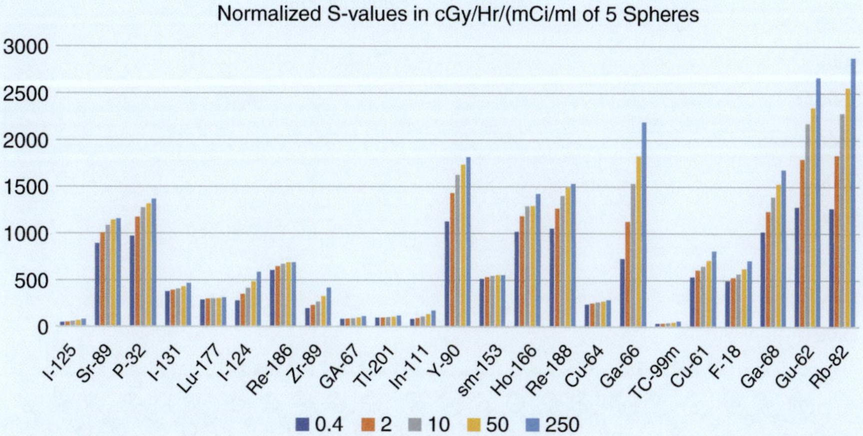

Fig. 6.2 Volume-normalized S-values in cGy/Hr/ (mCi/ml) of five sphere models of 23 radionuclides

TD and DD of the Peripheral Distribution Models

The TD and DD of the peripheral distribution models are listed in Appendices III (target dose) and IV (fractional depth dose), respectively. The S-values and volume-normalized S-values of the peripheral distribution models are illustrated in Figs. 6.3 and 6.4 to compare the volume effects. Steadily rising trends are again noted with respect to increasing volumes.

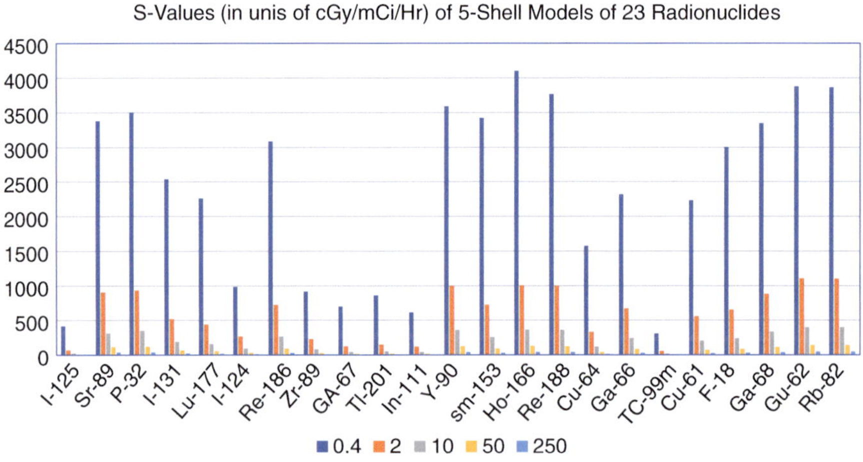

Fig. 6.3 S-Values (in unis of cGy/mCi/Hr) of 5-Shell Models of 23 Radionuclides

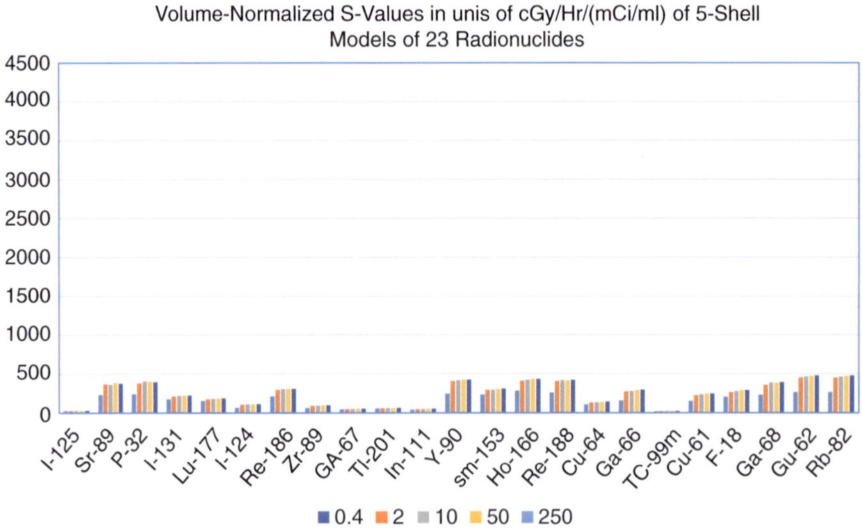

Fig. 6.4 Volume-Normalized S-Values in unis of cGy/Hr/(mCi/ml) of 5-Shell Models of 23 Radionuclides

Ranges of Depth Doses

Depth dosimetry (DD) – Radiation exposure in the surrounding tissues declines drastically with increasing distance from the radionuclide sources. In general, beyond 0.25 cm there is less than 50% of radiation-absorbed doses of the target sources in the uniform distribution models (Appendix V) and peripheral models (Appendix VI). Other measures of interest are the distance of the layer that received less than 10% of radiation dose rate, as well as distance of the layer at which more than 90% of total cumulative radiation-absorbed dose has been deposited (i.e., less than 10% cumulative dose on or beyond that layer). These latter measures show greater differences than the 50% depth dose layer for the 23 radionuclides.

Interpolation and Analytic Solutions for Predicting TD and DD

Steadily rising trends with decreasing slope of the volume normalized S-values allow for accurate regression analysis to provide empirical interpolation and extrapolation to predict volume-normalized-S values of TD and DD. As demonstrated by the look-up tables for TD and DD, respectively, in Appendices VII and VIII, the volume-normalized S-values for spheres between 0.4 and 250 ml can be reliably derived from simple logarithmic or power equations with three parameters (for TD) and four parameters (for DD).

Comparison of TD and DD of Uniform and Peripheral Models

TD of the uniform and the peripheral distribution models likely bracket the extremes of radionuclide distributions within the target volumes. Variations of DD between corresponding depths (layers) of the uniform vs the peripheral models were significant only in the innermost few layers (up to 0.3 cm from the outer edge of the tumor source).

TD and DD can also be derived and compared for uniform distribution model spherical tumors filled with any or all the above 23 commercially available radionuclides. Similarly, the peripheral models will allow dosimetry estimation of radionuclides that distribute in a shell (as in a post-surgical cavity) or in extremely heterogeneous patterns within the spherical tumor source.

An Example for Calculation of TD from Ga-68 GIMA for IRCT

Based on experiments of canine transmissible tumor (cTVT) model (further described in Fig. 8.9a–c of Chap. 8), the radiation-absorbed dose or the target dose (TD) of intratumoral injection can be estimated. Requirements of this exercise are the volume of the injectate, the residence time of the radionuclide (based on serial scintigraphy imaging, known pharmacokinetic models, or based on assumption of complete decay from physical half-life), and the S-value or volume-normalized S-value.

Upon an MRI-guided intratumoral injection of 0.27 mCi of Ga-68 gallium iron macroaggregates (GIMA) cTVT tumor graft of 2 × 2 × 2 cm implanted into the right lung, prolonged aggregation of GIMA more than 3 h (more than three half-lives) was confirmed by serial PET imaging findings of persistent SUV greater than 1600. This finding justified the assumption of complete decay inside the tumor allowing derivation of residence time based on the physical half-life of 1.13 h, yielding a residence time of 1.63 h The final injectate volume after injection was determined by paramagnetic signals on MRI over 4 days to be 0.5 ml. The volume-normalized S-value is estimated for Ga-68 from Appendix VII: y = 1139 + 100.5 * ln (0.5) = 1069.3 cGy/(mCi hr. ml). The S-value for the injectate volume inside the tumor based on the interpolation formula is 1069.3 × 0.5 ml = 534.7 cGy/(mCi hr.). The TD is therefore the product of S-value, residence time, and injected radioactivity (=534.7 cGy/(mCi hr.) × 1.63 h × 0.27 mCi = 235.3 cGy). This radiation dose was in the range to suppress tumor growth over 5 days, as illustrated by a follow-up F-18 FDG PET-CT scan showing a stable tumoral SUV of 6.6 versus 6.5 (baseline before injection of GIMA). Another cTVT tumor implanted in the left lung of the same animal had an increased SUV of 8.8 scan from baseline value of 6.2 before GIMA injection.

Depth dosimetry (DD) can be derived from Appendix VIII to obtain parameters including distance within which 90% of radiation-absorbed dose have been deposited. For example, the radiation-absorbed dose of the above sphere at 0.3 cm from the edge of the sphere (of 0.5 ml) can be derived from Appendix VIII using the following formula: z = 0.041 + 0.004 * ln(0.5) – 0.041 * ln(0.3) – 0.00006 * ln(0.3) * ln(0.3) = 0.0875, and the radiation absorbed dose at 0.3 cm is: 0.875 × 235.3 = 20.6 cGy.

Conclusion

Using uniform and peripheral distribution models of clinically relevant sized spheres, radiation absorbed doses inside a target (i.e., TD) and outside of a target (i.e., DD) filled with individual radionuclides can be estimated. Furthermore, after normalization of the radiation absorbed doses by residence time and target volumes, the resultant volume normalized S-values can be reliably interpolated by routine regression analyses. These findings allow ready and reliable comparison of radiopharmaceuticals of the 23 commercially available radionuclides, as long as residence times and target volumes can be determined, perhaps with the aid of advanced hybrid imaging.

Discussion

Radiation-Absorbed Dose Versus S-Values Versus Normalized S-Values Versus Half-Lives

The control of tumors certainly depends on TD which ablates the body of malignant tissues; it also depends on the DD which ablates micrometastases surrounding the tumor that are beyond detection limits by physical exam or even the most advanced imaging modality. The degree of micrometastasis depends on tumor types and other tumor biologic factors that may or may not be readily determined. These issues are empirically dealt with by different types of target tumor volumes such as gross tumor volumes (GTV), clinical tumor volumes (CTV), internal tumor volume (ITP), and planned tumor volumes (ITP) in the practice of clinical radiation oncology as further described in Chap. 3. Since DD have limited ranges (50% dose range below 0.25 cm), empirical radiation oncology guidelines for tumors may be followed in the initial planning of IRCT for TD until there are practice-validated quantifications of micrometastasis. The short ranges of DD, on the other hand, may assist treatment planning by providing estimates of safety to adjacent vital organs as illustrated with Y-90 and I-131 radiopharmaceuticals in the abdomen [10].

Modeling of Tumor Masses that Are Not Spherical-Additive Dosimetry

Because of the additive properties of dosimetric values, radiation-absorbed doses (TD or DD) of nonspherical masses may be approximated by adding TD or DD from fitted spheres of known spherical sizes. Additionally, injection of mixture or compounds with more than one radionuclide may be additive also, assuming that the volume and residence time (area under time-activity curve) can be independently and accurately determined.

Derivation of Tumor TD and DD from Integration of Dosimetry Models with Biodistribution from Advanced and Hybrid Imaging

While the current models assume complete decay of study radiopharmaceuticals, in most clinical situations, biologic removal will occur, and the pharmacokinetics and pharmacodynamics will determine the residence times in the tumor sources which are required to calculate TD and DD. Serial scintigraphy measurements will allow determination of the area under the time-activity curve for calculating the residence times. Recent advances in SPECT and PET have allowed refined and accurate measurement of radioactivity inside the human body. Advanced imaging including hybrid imaging modalities with fusion between SPECT and PET with CT, MRI, and/or sonography also allows reliable determination of location and volume of tumors. These recent advances in imaging technology have made possible integration of dosimetry models with anatomic and function imaging to derive TD and DD. Nevertheless, the translation of such possibilities still needs to be validated for each modality of combinations until LRCT becomes routine practice and standard of care.

Important Issues to Be Further Explored

Determination of Injectate Volume

The example of calculation of radiation dosimetry of GIMA above in a canine model had an independent measurement of injectate volume using MRI on the paramagnetic radiopharmaceutical based on paramagnetic property that is independent of the radioactivity (of Ga-68). Otherwise, the determination of injectate volume of radiopharmaceuticals inside an organ or a tumor is difficult because the movement of the admixture often renders an appearance of a sphere of which the measured size from scintigraphy is arbitrary and depends on sensitivity and settings of imaging parameters. An alternative will be empirically including internal standards of multiple relevant sizes and relevant radioactivities before or during imaging to derive a look-up table for interpolation for sizes of the spheres. The construction of such look-up table may be augmented by artificial intelligence.

The determination of injectate volume may have to assume that the volume does not vary too rapidly over time, so that fewer repeated measurements are needed. Such assumption may be justified for the use of particulate injectate (as in the example of cTVT tumor injection with GIMA) because of the scanty and slow lymphatic transport compared with the relatively short half-life. For soluble radiopharmaceuticals that bind tightly to the interstitium, a steady injectate volume may also be justified for radionuclides with relatively short half-lives. The assumption of steady injectate volume for soluble small molecules may require additional consideration and adjustment for clearance by the systemic circulation.

High-Dose Rate (HDR) Versus Low-Dose Rate (LDR) Considerations in LRCT

With biologic clearance and physical decay, an effective LRCT would invariably involve initial high-dose-rate (HDR) and subsequent low-dose-rate (LD) irradiation which have been described in Chap. 3 as >12 Gy/ Hr. and between 0.4 and 2.0 Gy/

Hr., respectively. Each of these dose rates of irradiation has advantages and disadvantages and has been utilized individually or in combination in conventional brachytherapy. A typical example is seen in patients with prostate cancer receiving 25 sessions of 100 cGy at HDR (of brief duration of 1–2 min) every other day (totaling 2500 cGy) followed by permanent implantation of I-125 seeds for brachytherapy to achieve LDR over several months [9, 13, 14]. In conventional radiotherapy, the HDR and LDR can be precisely selected because of steady output of the radiation source. The HDR source can be readily turned on or off, applied, or discontinued at will. With LRCT the injectate stays inside the tumor, and the radiation-absorbed dose is often from a combination of HDR and LDR, while the transition occurs along the course of radiation decay and biologic clearance. Individual HDR and LDR contribution may be determined by time-activity curves from serial scintigraphy or from simulation with reasonable measurement or assumptions of biologic half-lives.

The combination of HDR and LDR in LRCT can be illustrated with the canine cTVT tumor model in lungs further described in Chap. 8 Fig. 8.9b. With an injected activity of 0.27 mCi of Ga-68 GIMA and fair assumption of no biologic clearance during decay, a sublethal dose of 235.3 cGy was deposited into the tumor, and only LDR contribution (171 cGy or 72.8%) was realized as illustrated in Fig. 6.5a. If the radioactivity is increased 20-fold to 5.4 mCi to deliver a total of 4706 cGy, a larger portion of dose contribution (2718 cGy or 57.3%) will be from HDR, while LDR (258.4 cGy) only contributes 5.4% as in Fig. 6.5b. That also leaves questions open about the theoretical and clinical significance in LRCT of the radiation dose deposited at rates between HDR and LDR (<12 Gy/Hr. but >2Gy/Hr.) which consists of 1695.2 cGy or 35.7% in Fig. 6.5b. Perhaps, it should be coined a term mid-dose range or MDR which should be considered in future LRCT studies. Furthermore, the significance or non-significance of radiation-absorbed dose from dose rate below LDR (171 cGy in Fig. 6.5a and 70 cGy in Fig. 6.5b) also needs to be further investigated.

The determination of individual contribution of HDR and LDR in LRCT to conform to conventional radiation oncology practice could be important for successful adoption of LRCT in clinical practice. With more development of LRCT into clinical practice and the ability to assess TD and DD of LRCT, it will be important to derive other parameters such as the contributions and ratios of radiation-absorbed doses in HDR versus LDR and MDR. These parameters in LRCT are likely affected by S-values, injected radioactivities, and distributed volumes of the injectate and may allow optimization during treatment planning. With more in vivo experiments and correlation with conventional radiotherapy, HDR versus LDR and MDR ratios may be constructed to further correlate with treatment outcomes and to optimize designs of LRCT.

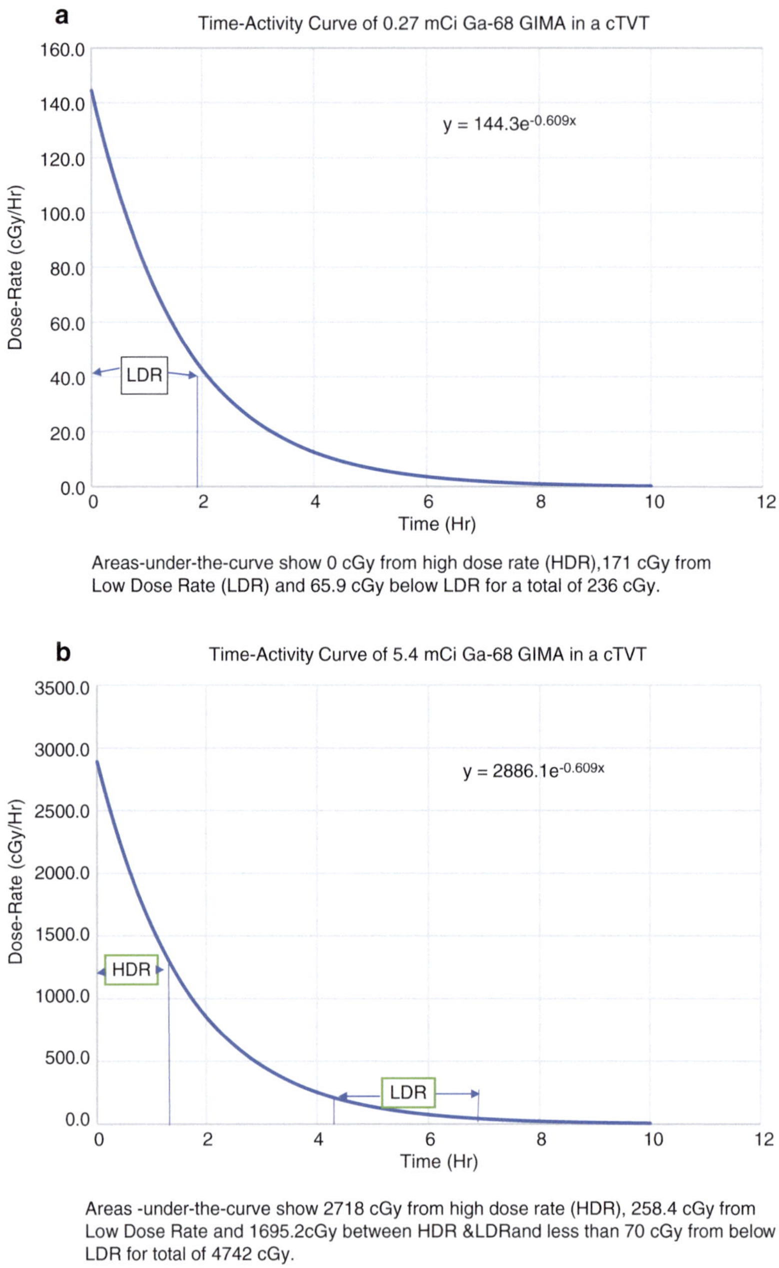

Fig. 6.5 (**a**) Time-Activity Curve of 0.27 mCi Ga-68 GIMA in a cTVT. Areas under the curve show 0 cGy from high-dose rate (HDR), 171 cGy from low-dose rate (LDR) and 65.9 cGy below LDR for a total of 236 cGy. (**b**) Time-Activity Curve of 5.4 mCi Ga-68 GIMA in a cTVT. Areas under the curve show 2718 cGy from high-dose rate (HDR), 258.4 cGy from low-dose rate and 1695.2 cGy between HDR and LDR and less than 70 cGy from below LDR for total of 4742 cGy

Appendix I Target dose (cGy/mCi) of Five-Sphere (0.4–250 ml) Model of 23 Radionuclides

Sph Vol in ml.	I-125	Sr-89	P-32	I-131	Lu-177	I-124	Re-186	Zr-89	6a-67	Tl-201	In-111	Y-90	Sm-153	Ho-156	Re-188	Cu-64	Ga-66	Tc-99m	Cu-61	F-18	Ga68	Cu-62	Rb-82
0.40	240000.0	3900000.0	12000000.0	260000.0	165000.0	100000.0	198000.0	55000.0	22700.0	24900.0	19900.0	260000.0	86700.0	98500.0	64400.0	11000.0	25000.0	768.0	6600.0	3260.0	4160.0	750.0	99.1
2.00	51000.0	880000.0	290000.0	54291.8	34400.0	25000.0	42282.5	13000.0	4756.0	5100.0	4460.5	66000.0	17977.0	22903.9	15499.8	2300.0	7700.0	164.0	1500.0	697.2	1012.1	210.0	28.7
10.00	12000.0	190000.0	63000.0	11350.7	699.0	6000.0	8794.7	3000.0	1006.3	1060.0	1044.6	15000.0	3684.9	4995.4	3434.6	480.0	2100.0	36.2	320.0	150.0	227.9	51.0	7.2
50.00	2700.0	40000.0	13000.0	2400.0	14100	1400.0	1800.0	730.0	220.0	220.0	260.0	3200.0	750.0	1000.0	730.0	99.0	500.0	8.3	70.0	33.0	50.0	11.0	1.6
250.00	640.0	8100.0	2700.0	520.0	287.0	340.0	360.0	190.0	50.0	49.0	67.0	670.0	150.0	220.0	150.0	21.0	120.0	2.1	16.0	7.5	11.0	25	0.4

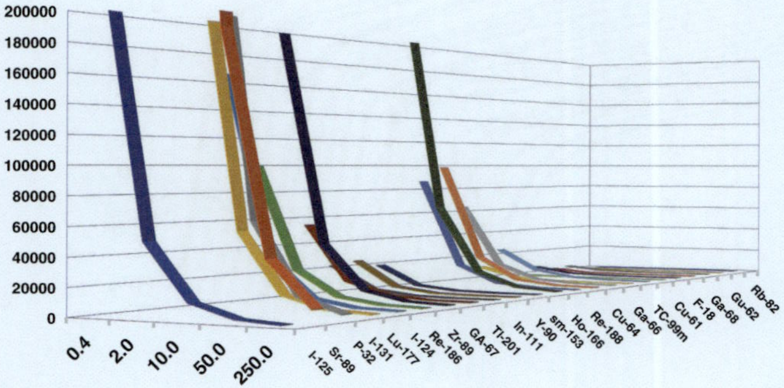

Appendix II Fractional Depth dose of 23 Radionuclides in the 2 ml Sphere Model

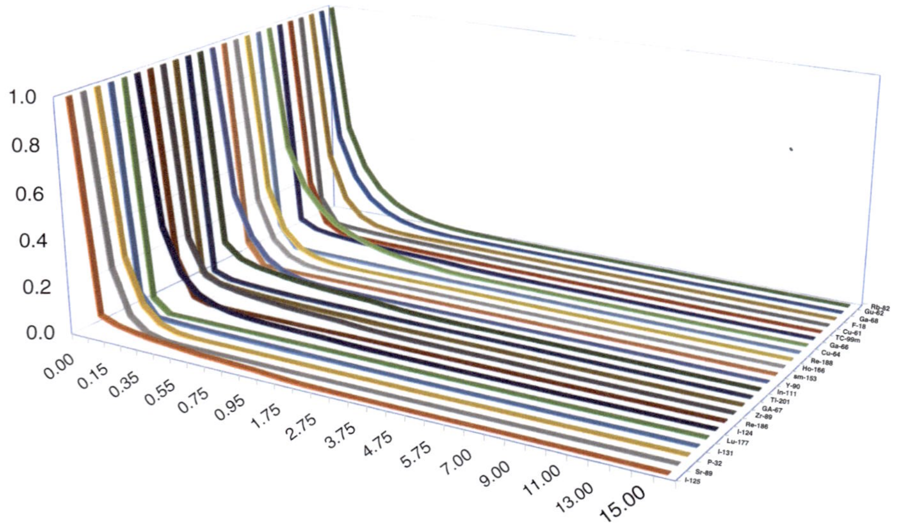

Appendix III Target dose (cGy/mCi) of Five-Shell Model (Core of 0.4–250 ml) of 23 Radionuclides

Shell Model	core vol mL	Dist. (cm)	Rb-82	I-125	Sr-89	P-32	I-131	Lu-177	I-124	Re-186	Zr-89	Ga-67	Tl-201	In-111	Y-90	Sm-153	Ho-166	Re-188	Cu-64	Ga-66	Tc-99m	Cu-61	F-18	Ga-68	Cu-62
Core(0.457 cm)	0.4	0	51	15000	1400000	490000	45000	19400	42000	53000	17000	1700	1200	2900	110000	15000	36000	26000	2100	13000	62	2200	710	1800	370
Source Shell	0.4	0.025	84	600000	4100000	1200000	490000	364000	99000	280000	72000	55000	63000	42000	230000	160000	110000	64000	20000	22000	1850	7600	5500	3800	630
Core(0.782 cm)	2	0	12	4900	240000	86000	5800	2070	8600	7500	3200	330	230	680	23000	1800	6400	4800	260	3500	15	360	100	330	84
Source Shell	2	0.05	24	100000	1100000	320000	100000	70600	27000	66000	18000	9900	11000	8200	64000	34000	27000	17000	4200	6400	333	1900	1200	1000	180
Core(1.336 cm)	10	0	3	1800	52000	19000	1400	450	2100	1600	900	99	67	230	5200	400	1400	1100	61	920	5	84	26	76	20
Source Shell	10	0.05	9	38000	380000	120000	37000	25400	9700	24000	6500	3600	4000	3000	23000	12000	9800	6100	1500	2300	121	700	440	380	65
Core(1.8128 cm)	50	0	1	580	11000	3900	360	98	540	330	260	31	21	76	1100	86	300	230	15	220	2	20	7	17	5
Source Shell	50	0.05	3	13000	140000	41000	13000	8970	3400	8400	2300	1300	1400	1100	8100	4300	3500	2100	540	830	43	250	160	130	23
Core(3.908 cm)	250	0	0	180	2200	810	96	22	140	69	80	10	7	26	230	19	62	47	4	53	1	5	2	4	1
Source Shell	250	0.05	1	4700	47000	14000	4500	3120	1200	2900	820	440	490	380	2800	1500	1200	740	190	290	15	87	55	46	8

Appendix IV Fractional Depth dose of 23 Radionuclides in the 2 ml Shell Model to 15 cm

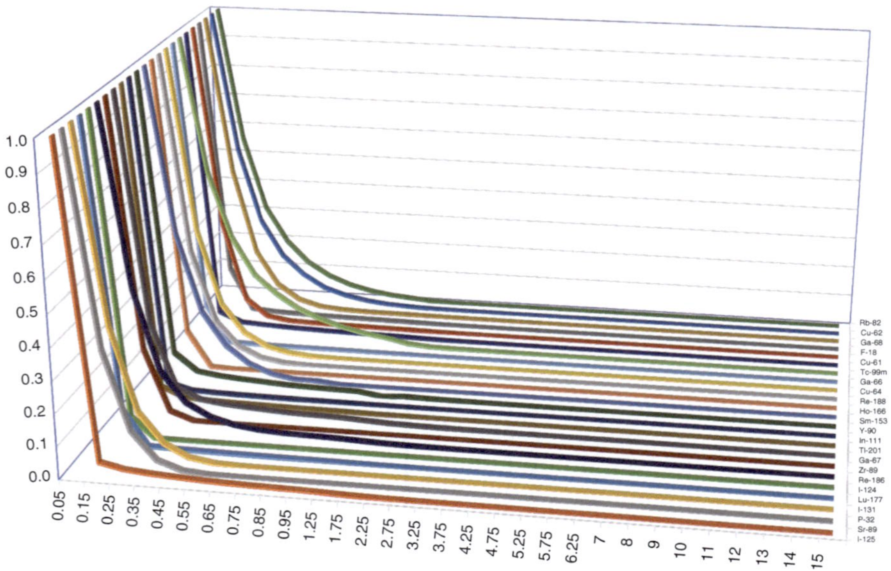

Appendix V Ranges (cm) of for Five-Sphere Models, at <50% and 10% Residual Dose Rate and 10% Cumulative Dose

Vol (ml)	I-125	Sr-89	P-32	I-131	Lu-177	I-124	Re-186	Zr-89	Ga-67	Tl-201	In-111	Y-90	Sm-153	Ho-166	Re-188	Cu-64	Ga-66	Tc-99m	Cu-61	F-18	Ga-68	Cu-62	Rb-82
	range (cm) <50% dose rate																						
0.4	0.025	0.025	0.025	0.025	0.025	0.025	0.025	0.025	0.025	0.025	0.025	0.025	0.025	0.025	0.025	0.025	0.075	0.025	0.025	0.025	0.025	0.025	0.075
2	0.05	0.05	0.05	0.05	0.05	0.05	0.05	0.05	0.05	0.05	0.05	0.05	0.05	0.05	0.05	0.05	0.05	0.05	0.05	0.05	0.05	0.05	0.05
10	0.05	0.05	0.05	0.05	0.05	0.05	0.05	0.05	0.05	0.05	0.05	0.05	0.05	0.05	0.05	0.05	0.05	0.05	0.05	0.05	0.05	0.05	0.05
50	0.05	0.05	0.05	0.05	0.05	0.05	0.05	0.05	0.05	0.05	0.05	0.05	0.05	0.05	0.05	0.05	0.05	0.05	0.5	0.05	0.05	0.05	0.05
250	0.05	0.05	0.05	0.05	0.05	0.05	0.05	0.05	0.05	0.05	0.05	0.05	0.05	0.05	0.05	0.05	0.05	0.05	0.05	0.05	0.05	0.05	0.05
	range (cm) <10% dose rate																						
0.4	0.025	0.125	0.175	0.075	0.075	0.225	0.075	0.1	0.025	0.025	0.075	0.225	0.075	0.175	0.175	0.075	0.4	0.025	0.125	0.075	0.175	0.3	0.3
2	0.05	0.15	0.15	0.15	0.05	0.25	0.15	0.14	0.05	0.05	0.15	0.25	0.05	0.15	0.25	0.15	0.45	0.05	0.15	0.15	0.25	0.35	0.35
10	0.25	0.15	0.15	0.15	0.05	0.35	0.15	0.35	0.05	0.05	0.45	0.25	0.15	0.25	0.25	0.15	0.45	0.15	0.15	0.15	0.25	0.35	0.35
50	0.65	0.15	0.25	0.15	0.05	0.45	0.15	0.95	0.15	0.05	1.25	0.25	0.15	0.25	0.25	0.15	0.55	0.75	0.25	0.25	0.25	0.35	0.45
250	1.25	0.15	0.25	0.15	0.05	1.25	0.15	2.25	0.95	0.35	2.75	0.25	0.15	0.25	0.25	0.15	0.75	2.25	0.35	0.95	0.35	0.45	0.45
	range (cm) <10% culmulative RAD																						
0.4	0.175	0.125	0.125	0.025	0.025	0.175	0.025	0.175	0.025	0.025	0.225	0.175	0.025	0.125	0.125	0.025	0.3	0.125	0.075	0.025	0.125	0.225	0.225
2	0.45	0.05	0.05	0.05	0	0.35	0.05	0.46	0.15	0.05	0.55	0.15	0.05	0.15	0.15	0.05	0.45	0.45	0.15	0.24	0.15	0.25	0.35
10	0.75	0.05	0.05	0.35	0	0.65	0.05	0.8	0.65	0.35	0.85	0.15	0.05	0.15	0.15	0.15	0.55	0.85	0.35	0.55	0.25	0.35	0.35
50	0.95	0.05	0.15	0.75	0.05	0.95	0.05	1.25	0.95	0.85	1.75	0.15	0.05	0.15	0.15	0.65	0.65	1.75	0.85	0.95	0.45	0.45	0.45
250	1.25	0.05	0.15	1.75	0.25	2.25	0.05	2.75	2.75	2.25	2.75	0.15	0.45	0.15	0.15	1.25	0.95	3.25	1.75	2.25	0.95	0.65	0.65

Appendix VI Ranges (cm) of for Five-Shell Models, at <50% and 10% Residual Dose Rate and 10% Cumulative Dose

Core Vol (ml)	I-125	Sr-89	P-32	I-131	Lu-177	I-124	Re-186	Zr-89	Ga-67	Tl-201	In-111	Y-90	Sm-153	Ho-166	Re-188	Cu-64	Ga-66	Tc-99m	Cu-61	F-18	Ga-68	Cu-62	Rb-82
	range(cm) <50% dose rate																						
0.4	0.075	0.075	0.125	0.075	0.075	0.125	0.075	0.075	0.075	0.075	0.075	0.075	0.075	0.075	0.075	0.075	0.125	0.075	0.075	0.075	0.075	0.125	0.125
2	0.15	0.15	0.15	0.15	0.15	0.15	0.15	0.15	0.15	0.15	0.15	0.15	0.15	0.15	0.15	0.15	0.25	0.15	0.15	0.15	0.15	0.25	0.15
10	0.15	0.15	0.15	0.15	0.15	0.15	0.15	0.15	0.15	0.15	0.15	0.15	0.15	0.15	0.15	0.15	0.25	0.15	0.15	0.15	0.15	0.25	0.25
50	0.15	0.15	0.15	0.15	0.15	0.15	0.15	0.15	0.15	0.15	0.15	0.25	0.15	0.15	0.15	0.15	0.25	0.15	0.15	0.15	0.25	0.25	0.25
250	0.15	0.15	0.15	0.15	0.15	0.25	0.15	0.15	0.15	0.15	0.15	0.25	0.15	0.15	0.15	0.15	0.25	0.15	0.15	0.15	0.25	0.25	0.25
	range(cm) <10% dose rate																						
0.4	0.075	0.225	0.225	0.125	0.125	0.3	0.175	0.175	0.075	0.075	0.125	0.3	0.125	0.225	0.3	0.125	0.5	0.075	0.175	0.125	0.3	0.4	0.4
2	0.25	0.35	0.35	0.25	0.15	0.35	0.25	0.25	0.15	0.15	0.15	0.45	0.25	0.35	0.35	0.25	0.65	0.15	0.25	0.25	0.35	0.45	0.55
10	0.15	0.35	0.35	0.25	0.15	0.45	0.25	0.25	0.15	0.15	0.25	0.45	0.25	0.35	0.45	0.25	0.75	0.15	0.25	0.25	0.35	0.55	0.55
50	0.15	0.35	0.35	0.25	0.15	0.45	0.25	0.35	0.15	0.15	0.25	0.45	0.25	0.35	0.35	0.25	0.75	0.15	0.35	0.25	0.45	0.55	0.65
250	0.15	0.35	0.35	0.25	0.15	0.45	0.25	0.35	0.15	0.15	0.25	0.45	0.25	0.35	0.35	0.15	0.75	0.15	0.15	0.25	0.45	0.55	0.65
	range (cm) <10% culuminative RAD																						
0.4	0.025	0.175	0.175	0.075	0.075	0.225	0.125	0.175	0.025	0.025	0.075	0.225	0.96	0.175	0.175	0.075	0.3	0.075	0.125	0.075	0.175	0.225	0.3
2	0.25	0.15	0.25	0.15	0.05	0.35	0.15	0.35	0.05	0.05	0.35	0.25	0.15	0.25	0.25	0.15	0.55	0.15	0.15	0.15	0.25	0.35	0.35
10	0.35	0.15	0.25	0.15	0.05	0.45	0.15	0.55	0.15	0.05	0.55	0.25	0.15	0.25	0.25	0.15	0.55	0.35	0.25	0.15	0.25	0.45	0.45
50	0.55	0.25	0.25	0.15	0.05	0.55	0.15	0.75	0.25	0.15	0.75	0.35	0.15	0.25	0.25	0.15	0.65	0.65	0.25	0.35	0.35	0.45	0.45
250	0.65	0.25	0.25	0.15	0.05	0.75	0.15	0.95	0.55	0.25	0.95	0.35	0.15	0.25	0.25	0.15	0.75	0.85	0.35	0.55	0.35	0.45	0.55

Appendix VII Statistically Significant Regression of Volume-Normalized S-Values of the Five-Sphere Model

A common two-parameter equation: y = a + b* lnx with valid statistics was found by SigmaPlot Table Curve 2D. The volume-normalized S-values can be reliably predicted based on the volume (X) of the sphere for each radionuclide

TC2D Fit	I-125	Sr-89	P-32	I-131	Lu-177	I-124	Re-186	Zr-89	Ga-67	Tl-201	In-111	Y-90	Sm-153	Ho-166	Re-188	Cu-64	Ga-66	Tc-99m	Cu-61	F-18	Ga-68	Cu-62	Rb-82
a	**47.8**	**961.5**	**1087.8**	**381.2**	**290.5**	**312.7**	**630.6**	**208.4**	**81.8**	**36.1**	**84.9**	**1305.1**	**526.3**	**1111.1**	**1178.5**	**245.9**	**962.7**	**36.1**	**570.9**	**509.4**	**1139.2**	**1577.0**	**1600.9**
Pa	*0.00*	*0.00*	*0.00*	*0.00*	*0.00*	*0.00*	*0.00*	*0.00*	*0.00*	*0.00*	*0.00*	*0.00*	*0.00*	*0.00*	*0.00*	*0.00*	*0.00*	*0.00*	*0.00*	*0.00*	*0.00*	*0.00*	*0.00*
b	**4.8**	**41.6**	**57.9**	**14.2**	**3.5**	**47.2**	**12.8**	**33.7**	**4.6**	**3.7**	**13.7**	**104.3**	**6.6**	**56.9**	**73.5**	**6.9**	**225.0**	**3.7**	**40.7**	**32.9**	**100.5**	**206.9**	**245.2**
Pb	*0.00*	*0.01*	*0.02*	*0.00*	*0.01*	*0.00*	*0.02*	*0.01*	*0.01*	*0.01*	*0.01*	*0.01*	*0.01*	*0.01*	*0.01*	*0.00*	*0.00*	*0.01*	*0.00*	*0.00*	*0.00*	*0.00*	*0.00*
rSq Coef	*0.96*	*0.93*	*0.89*	*0.97*	*0.92*	*0.99*	*0.88*	*0.95*	*0.94*	*0.90*	*0.94*	*0.93*	*0.90*	*0.92*	*0.93*	*0.99*	*1.00*	*0.90*	*0.98*	*0.96*	*0.99*	*0.97*	*0.98*
F value	78.57	37.57	24.23	100.57	35.34	362.87	21.06	52.84	43.86	27.39	44.53	40.65	27.25	36.42	37.37	266.12	981.46	27.39	131.56	79.77	326.76	92.18	127.54

Appendix VIII Statistically Significant Regression of Depth Dose fraction of the Five-Sphere Model

Empirical curve fitting with SigmaPlot Table Curve 3D found three sets of equations that could reliably predict the normalized S-values of the five-sphere model of the 23 radionuclides, based on the distance from the sphere (X) and the volume of the sphere (y)

T1/2P (hr)	1443.36	1212	342.24	192.96	161.04	100.32	90.64	78.48	78.26	73.1	67.92	64	46.7	26.8	16.98	12.7	9.49	6.01	3.41	1.83	1.13	0.16	0.02
TC3D Fit	I-125	Sr-89	P-32	I-131	Lu-177	I-124	Re-186	Zr-89	Ga-67	Tl-201	In-111	Y-90	Sm-153	Ho-166	Re-188	Cu-64	Ga-66	Tc-99m	Cu-61	F-18	Ga-68	Cu-62	Rb-82
TC3D Eq#	82	2160	2160	82	82	82	2160	82	82	82	82	2160	83	2160	2160	82	82	82	82	82	82	83	83
A	0.024	−0.203	−0.227	0.013	0.005	0.012	−0.155	0.040	0.013	0.008	0.033	−0.293	−0.006	−0.214	−0.239	0.012	0.083	0.020	0.028	0.019	0.041	0.008	0.013
P	*0.00*	*0.00*	*0.00*	*0.00*	*0.00*	*0.00*	*0.00*	*0.00*	*0.00*	*0.00*	*0.00*	*0.01*	*0.00*	*0.00*	*0.00*	*0.00*	*0.00*	*0.00*	*0.00*	*0.00*	*0.00*	*0.00*	*0.00*
b	0.013	0.256	0.285	0.006	0.001	0.005	0.196	0.019	0.011	0.007	0.020	0.366	0.001	0.272	0.302	0.005	0.006	0.017	0.007	0.011	0.004	0.003	0.003
P	*0.00*	*0.00*	*0.00*	*0.00*	*0.04*	*0.00*	*0.00*	*0.00*	*0.00*	*0.00*	*0.00*	*0.00*	*0.00*	*0.00*	*0.00*	*0.00*	*0.00*	*0.00*	*0.00*	*0.00*	*0.05*	*0.00*	*0.00*
c	−0.031	−0.059	−0.056	−0.017	−0.006	−0.016	−0.068	−0.048	−0.019	−0.013	−0.042	−0.049	−0.010	−0.058	−0.054	−0.016	−0.071	−0.029	−0.032	−0.026	−0.041	−0.053	−0.057
P	*0.00*	*0.00*	*0.00*	*0.00*	*0.00*	*0.00*	*0.00*	*0.00*	*0.00*	*0.00*	*0.00*	*0.00*	*0.00*	*0.00*	*0.00*	*0.00*	*0.00*	*0.00*	*0.00*	*0.00*	*0.00*	*0.00*	*0.00*
d	−0.00004			−0.00002	−0.00001	−0.00002		−0.00007	−0.00003	−0.00002	−0.00006		0.00678			−0.00002	−0.00010	−0.00004	−0.00004	−0.00004	−0.00006	0.02452	0.02502
P	*0.00*			*0.00*	*0.00*	*0.00*		*0.00*	*0.00*	*0.00*	*0.00*		*0.00*			*0.00*	*0.00*	*0.00*	*0.00*	*0.00*	*0.00*	*0.00*	*0.00*
e													0.00001									0.00004	0.00004
P													*0.00*									*0.00*	*0.00*
rSq	*0.98*	*0.89*	*0.88*	*0.99*	*1.00*	*0.99*	*0.92*	*0.96*	*0.99*	*0.99*	*0.97*	*0.85*	*1.00*	*0.89*	*0.87*	*0.99*	*0.93*	*0.98*	*0.96*	*0.98*	*0.94*	*0.99*	*0.99*
F Value	*1812*	*538*	*474*	*3772*	*10275*	*3492*	*770*	*1039*	*3829*	*7826*	*1217*	*369*	*8347*	*511*	*441*	*3492*	*583*	*1710*	*1093*	*2132*	*652*	*4934*	*5196*
Eqn 83 z=a+blnx+clny+d(lny)2+e(lny)3				*rSq >0.99*																			
Eqn 82 z=a+blnx+clny+d(lny)2				*rSq >0.93*																			
Eqn 2160 z=a+POWX(b,c)*POWY(1,c)				*rSq>0.85*																			

References

1. Arnold CA, Pezhouh MK, Lam-Himlin D, Pittman ME, VandenBussche C, Voltaggio L. 90Y-TheraSpheres: the new look of Yttrium-90. Am J Surg Pathol. 2019;43(5):688–94. https://doi.org/10.1097/PAS.0000000000001223.
2. Ballard BE. Biopharmaceutical considerations in subcutaneous and intramuscular drug administration. J Pharm Sci. 1968;57(3):357–78. https://doi.org/10.1002/jps.2600570301.
3. Bergqvist L, Strand SE, Persson BR. Particle sizing and biokinetics of interstitial lymphoscintigraphic agents. Semin Nucl Med. 1983;13(1):9–19. https://doi.org/10.1016/s0001-2998(83)80031-2.
4. Bhutani MS, Klapman JB, Tuli R, El-Haddad G, Hoffe S, Wong FCL, Herman JM. An open-label, single-arm pilot study of EUS-guided brachytherapy with phosphorus-32 microparticles in combination with gemcitabine +/− nab-paclitaxel in unresectable locally advanced pancreatic cancer (OncoPaC-1): technical details and study protocol. Endosc Ultrasound. 2020;9(1):24. https://doi.org/10.4103/eus.eus_44_19.
5. Briesmeister JF. MCNP – a general Monte Carlo N-particle transport code, version 4A LA-12625-M. 1993.
6. Cristy M, Eckerman K. Specific absorbed fractions of energy at various ages from internal photons sources. ORNL/TM-8381 V1-V7. Oak Ridge: Oak Ridge National Laboratory; 1987.
7. Hendricks JS, Adam KJ, Booth TE, Briesmeister JF, Carter LL, Cox LJ, Prael RE. Present and future capabilities of MCNP. Appl Radiat Isot. 2000;53(4–5):857–61. https://doi.org/10.1016/s0969-8043(00)00231-1.
8. Loevinger R, Budinger TF, Watson EE. MIRD primer. Society of nuclear medicine. 1991.
9. Sandler KA, Cook RR, Ciezki JP, Ross AE, Pomerantz MM, Nguyen PL, Kishan AU. Prostate-only versus whole-pelvis radiation with or without a brachytherapy boost for gleason grade group 5 prostate cancer: a retrospective analysis. Eur Urol. 2020;77(1):3–10. https://doi.org/10.1016/j.eururo.2019.03.022.
10. Sparks RB, Crowe EA, Wong FC, Toohey RE, Siegel JA. Radiation dose distributions in normal tissue adjacent to tumors containing (131)I or (90)Y: the potential for toxicity. J Nucl Med. 2002;43(8):1110–4.
11. Stabin MG, da Luz LC. Decay data for internal and external dose assessment. Health Phys. 2002;83(4):471–5. https://doi.org/10.1097/00004032-200210000-00004.
12. Supersaxo A, Hein WR, Steffen H. Effect of molecular weight on the lymphatic absorption of water-soluble compounds following subcutaneous administration. Pharm Res. 1990;7(2):167–9. https://doi.org/10.1023/a:1015880819328.
13. Tanaka N, Asakawa I, Hasegawa M, Fujimoto K. Low-dose-rate brachytherapy for prostate cancer: a 15-year experience in Japan. Int J Urol. 2020;27(1):17–23. https://doi.org/10.1111/iju.14098.
14. Tharmalingam H, Tsang Y, Choudhury A, Alonzi R, Wylie J, Ahmed I, Hoskin PJ. External beam radiation therapy (EBRT) and high-dose-rate (HDR) brachytherapy for intermediate and high-risk prostate cancer: the impact of EBRT volume. Int J Radiat Oncol Biol Phys. 2020;106(3):525–33. https://doi.org/10.1016/j.ijrobp.2019.09.044.

Chapter 7
Voxel-Based Targeted Radionuclide Therapy Dosimetry

Greta S. P. Mok

Introduction

Along with the development of novel theranostic radionuclide tracers [1], the effectiveness of targeted radionuclide therapy (TRT) is well-recognized for a range of primary and metastatic cancers [2]. The goal of TRT is to deliver a lethal dose of radiation to tumors from internal radioactive sources by targeting the tumors' specific molecular or functional receptors with a specific agent, which is administered to the patients via intravenous injection [3–5], oral uptake [6], and locoregional, arterial [7], or direct intratumoral injection. The local absorbed dose is mainly delivered directly by beta, Auger, or alpha particles [8] with short travelling distance or indirectly via the "bystander" effect [9]. Therefore, compared to conventional external radiotherapy or chemotherapy, it could possibly deliver therapeutic radiation more specifically to radiosensitive cancer cells without causing toxicity to adjacent normal tissues [10].

Iodine-based thyroid therapy is a classic example of TRT. More recently, the clinical applications with promising treatment effects include the Y-90 microsphere treatment for hepatic tumors [11], Lu-177-DOTA octreotide for neuroendocrine tumors [12], and Lu-177 prostate-specific membrane antigen (PSMA) for prostate cancers [13]. While the "one-dose-fits-all" or activity per unit body weight approach is still a preferred TRT practice especially for I-131 therapy, more sophisticated and personalized TRT dosimetry is recognized and in demand for precision medicine. Strigari et al. showed that personalized treatment planning would increase the survival rate and improve clinical efficacy based on a review of 79 studies [14].

The spatial distribution of the radionuclides varies among patients. Thus, a priori knowledge of the TRT agent's biokinetics before actual treatment would be desired,

G. S. P. Mok (✉)
Biomedical Imaging Laboratory, Department of Electrical and Computer Engineering, Faculty of Science and Technology, University of Macau, Macau SAR, China
e-mail: gretamok@umac.mo

F. C. L. Wong (ed.), *Locoregional Radionuclide Cancer Therapy*,
https://doi.org/10.1007/978-3-030-56267-0_7

with preliminary estimates of the cumulative activity and absorbed dose of tumors and critical organs for each patient. This information can be obtained noninvasively from single or sequential nuclear medicine scans and combined with optional blood sampling. Conventional internal dosimetry is organ-based and provides 2D dose information. Thus, planar imaging is a common imaging choice, with limited quantitative accuracy due to organs overlapping and background activity. Pursuing 3D dose information at voxel level is the new trend which considers patient-specific anatomy, activity, and tissue heterogeneity. For this purpose, emission computed tomography (ECT) with improved quantitative accuracy is necessary. With proper dose calibration, quantitative 3D reconstructed images at different time points allow fitting of time activity curves (TAC) for the critical organs and tumors. From the integration of area under these time activity curves, one can obtain the cumulative activity and further convert it to the 3D absorbed dose indices, e.g., dose volume histogram, 3D dose maps, or isodose contours, with conventional 2D absorbed dose information still available. This information can be used to (i) better assess the treatment response; (ii) adjust the administered dose to each individual patient to improve the therapeutic efficacy; and (iii) verify the post-therapy absorbed dose distribution. The whole dosimetry workflow is shown in Fig. 7.1. A general description on the Medical Internal Radiation Dose (MIRD) scheme for radiopharmaceutical dosimetry can be found from a recent review of Ljungberg et al. [15].

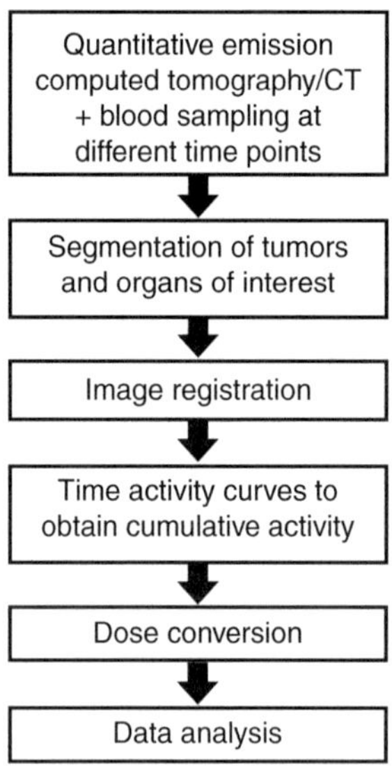

Fig. 7.1 Flowchart for voxel-based TRT dosimetry

Radiopharmaceuticals for Radionuclide Therapy

Imaging for the therapeutic agents in TRT is a more challenging task as compared to the conventional diagnostic radionuclide. Many TRT radionuclides are not suitable for imaging as either they do not have simultaneous gamma/positron emission, the photon energy is too high, or the abundance of gamma photons/positrons is too low.

Although direct imaging of these radionuclides is still possible using PET or a conventional gamma camera with suitable combinations of energy window, collimator, and detectors, the image quality of TRT agents is usually inferior to the current Tc-99m-based SPECT and F-18-based PET studies. Therefore, quantitation is even more challenging. On the other hand, the activity distribution of these TRT tracers can be obtained indirectly with the use of their theranostic imaging "surrogate". This refers to the same biomolecule labeled with another radioisotope with similar biological and chemical characteristics. This imaging "surrogate" should have better characteristics, e.g., single photon emissions with suitable energy range for SPECT imaging or positron emission for PET imaging. Since surrogate imaging isotopes may have different half-lives as compared to their therapeutic partners, decay corrections are warranted [16]. Common TRT radiopharmaceuticals, their imaging surrogates, and targeting mechanisms are listed in Table 7.1.

Table 7.1 Common radiopharmaceuticals and their imaging surrogates for TRT

Therapeutic radionuclide/ imaging surrogate	Half-lives	Emission type (keV)	Radiopharmaceutical	Targeting mechanism	Indication
I-131/I-123, I-124	8.04 d	β^- (max 606) and γ (364)/ γ (159), β^+ (2095)	Iodide	Thyroid hormone synthesis	Thyroid carcinoma
			Tositumomab	CD20 antigen binding	NHL
			MIBG	Active transport into the neuroendocrine cells and intracellular storage	Neuroblastoma, pheochromocytoma, carcinoid, paraganglioma, medullary thyroid carcinoma
Y-90/In-111, Y-86, Zr-89	64 h	β^- (max 2280)/γ (245, 171), β^+ (2010.4, 902)	Ibritumomab tiuxetan	CD20 antigen binding	NHL
			Microspheres	Intravascular trapping	Liver metastasis, hepatocellular carcinoma
			Octreotide	Somatostatin receptor binding	Neuroendocrine tumor

(continued)

Table 7.1 (continued)

Therapeutic radionuclide/ imaging surrogate	Half-lives	Emission type (keV)	Radiopharmaceutical	Targeting mechanism	Indication
Lu-177/ Ga-68	6.65 d	β^- (max 498.3) and γ (208 and 113)/β^+ (1899)	Octreotide	Somatostatin receptor binding	Neuroendocrine tumor, endocrine pancreatic tumor
			Prostate	PSMA	Prostate cancer
Ho-166	26 h	β^- (max 1770 and 1850) and γ (81)	Microspheres	Intravascular trapping	Liver metastasis, hepatocellular carcinoma
Sm-153	46.3 h	β^- (max 807) and γ (103)	EDTMP	Chemo-adsorption	Bone pain palliation
Sr-89	50.5 d	β^- (max 1463)	Chloride	Calcium analog	Bone pain palliation
Re-186	89.3 h	β^- (max 1070) and γ (137)	HEDP	Pyrophosphate analog	Bone pain palliation
Sc-47/Sc-44	3.34 d	β^- (max 441.1) and γ (159.38)/ β^+ (1474.3)	cm10 (DOTA-folate conjugate)	Small-molecular-weight albumin-binding	Epithelial ovarian cancers

MIBG metaiodobenzylguanidine, *NHL* non-Hodgkin lymphoma, *EDTMP* ethylenediamine tetramethylene phosphonate, *HEDP* hydroxyethylidene diphosphonate, *PSMA* prostate-specific membrane antigen

Quantitative Imaging for Voxel-Based Dosimetry

The accuracy and precision of voxel-based TRT dosimetry highly depend on the quantitative accuracy of the 3D imaging techniques. There are two main imaging systems for ECT: SPECT which consists of two- or three-head gamma cameras for single gamma emitters and PET which consists of a full ring of pixelated detector blocks for positron emitters.

A typical general purpose gamma camera for SPECT has an axial dimension of 40–45 cm and a transverse length of 50–55 cm. Typically, the collimator septa thickness is 0.2 mm for photon energies up to 150 keV and 1.05 mm for 150–250 keV. Higher-energy collimators with thicker septa (~1.8 mm) are also available but suffer from poor spatial resolution and low sensitivity. It is important to mention that mechanical collimation is a highly inefficient step, severely limiting the sensitivity of a gamma camera: only about 1 of 10,000 photons will be passing through the collimator. The standard detector in a gamma camera is a 3/8″-thick NaI detector, which is optimized for imaging low-energy photons. For SPECT and bremsstrahlung imaging, projections are acquired at different angles, and a three-dimensional image of the activity distribution is obtained from these data by an image reconstruction algorithm. A PET system always generates tomographic images with no gantry rotation required due to the full ring design. Current PET systems operate in fully 3D mode without septa which leads to a higher sensitivity than SPECT, in the range of 1–2.5%, and their axial length varies from 16 to 25 cm, and can reach >190 cm for state-of-the-art total body scanner. Common scintillators for PET are Lu-based such as L(Y)SO and LSO. Nowadays clinical SPECT is usually combined with a CT scanner, and PET is always combined with either a CT or MRI.

Statistical 3D iterative image reconstruction methods, e.g., maximum likelihood expectation maximization (ML-EM), its accelerated alternate of ordered subset expectation maximization (OS-EM), and maximum a posteriori (MAP), are the common image reconstruction methods for ECT in this era. As compared to the conventional filtered back projection (FBP) method, the statistical methods can incorporate the noise modeling and provide improved quantitative accuracy. The effects of physical image degradation factors such as attenuation, scatter, collimator-detector response (CDR), and partial volume effect can be modeled and compensated in the system matrix during the projector/back projector process. The three main 3D quantitative imaging techniques are described in details below.

Quantitative SPECT/CT

The use of SPECT improves image contrast caused by background activity and organ overlap in planar scintigraphy. It provides 3D spatial information with improved quantitation accuracy for 3D voxel-based dosimetry. The tracers of SPECT usually possess longer half-lives and are more suitable for sequential imaging sessions to obtain the TAC as compared to those of PET. Moreover, modern combined SPECT/CT scanners provide an improved attenuation map from CT for attenuation correction (AC) and scatter correction (SC) in SPECT reconstruction. The anatomical information from CT also improves volume-of-interest delineation and image registration in later TRT dosimetry.

The quantitative errors could be <10% for SPECT, depending on the compensation techniques used in the reconstructions. He et al. proposed a quantitative SPECT reconstruction method [17] using CT for AC, effective source scatter estimation (ESSE) for SC, perturbation-based geometric transfer matrix (pGTM) for partial volume compensation (PVC) [18], and Monte Carlo simulation (MCS)-based CDR compensation. The ESSE requires effective scatter source kernel and scatter attenuation coefficient kernel convolutions for each projection [19]. Errors less than 6.5% could be achieved for all organs except the small sphere in a radiology support device torso phantom study [18]. The long acquisition time of SPECT is its main obstacle for clinical TRT dosimetry purpose. The same research group later showed that the SPECT acquisition time could be shortened by a factor of 2 with a change in mean error of <1% [20]. When the scan time was further reduced to 1.5 min, the accuracy and precision in large and hot organs were still acceptable. However, even if the scanning time can be shortened, multiple bed positions are still required to cover the torso for whole-body quantification, increasing the difficulties in designing the scanning protocol and actual implementation. Nevertheless, one bed position could be sufficient if only critical organs are of interest in some applications, further reducing the acquisition time.

Dewaraja et al. developed a regularized reconstruction method to reduce the edge artifacts caused by CDR compensation after a large number of updates and improved the accuracy of activity distribution within the targets [21]. The penalized likelihood function employing CT side information (PL-CT) was incorporated to the reconstruction process after certain updates of ordered subset expectation maximization (OS-EM) reconstruction. In both simulation and phantom studies with uniform activity distribution, the PL-CT outperformed both the regularized reconstruction without CT and the conventional OS-EM reconstruction in visual assessment, image profile and target activity distribution.

Shcherbinin et al. proposed the interpolated analytical photon distribution (APDI) [22] method which used the Klein-Nishina cross section to analytically calculate the scatter distribution in the forward projection of the OS-EM reconstruction [23], shortening the computation time compared with the MCS-based SC method. Errors of activity estimation were within 10% for Tc-99m, In-111, I-123, and I-131.

Since gamma cameras are mostly optimized for imaging low and monoenergetic isotopes whose emitted photons are more likely to be detected correctly (Fig. 7.2, 1), problems may happen when imaging the therapeutic isotopes emitting high-energy gamma rays or particles, particularly collimator penetration (Fig. 7.2, 3), contamination from higher-energy peaks, and secondary X-rays. As the collimator septa are designed for low-energy peaks, a relatively large fraction of high-energy photons will penetrate the collimator. For example, I-131 emits 364 keV photons, and a large amount of penetration occurs when used in combination with medium energy collimators. Dedicated high-energy collimators can be used to reduce penetration, but this typically results in poor spatial resolution. Also, the photons that scatter in the patients or collimator/detector (Fig. 7.2, 2) can still end up in the energy window of the main photopeak. Even if these photons pass through both collimator and detector, they can still backscatter from the remaining parts of the gamma camera to the detector (Fig. 7.2, 4), affecting the quantitative accuracy.

Moreover, the attenuation and scatter corrections also need to be adapted for TRT isotopes. For example, some isotopes have two low-energy peaks for imaging, but each requires a different attenuation factor. For AC, one can simply discard photons from one of the energy windows, which would lead to a huge loss of information especially for isotopes whose two peaks have similar abundance, e.g., In-111 and Lu-177. Another approach would be to acquire photons from two peaks separately or enable list-mode acquisition, with two reconstructions followed by combination

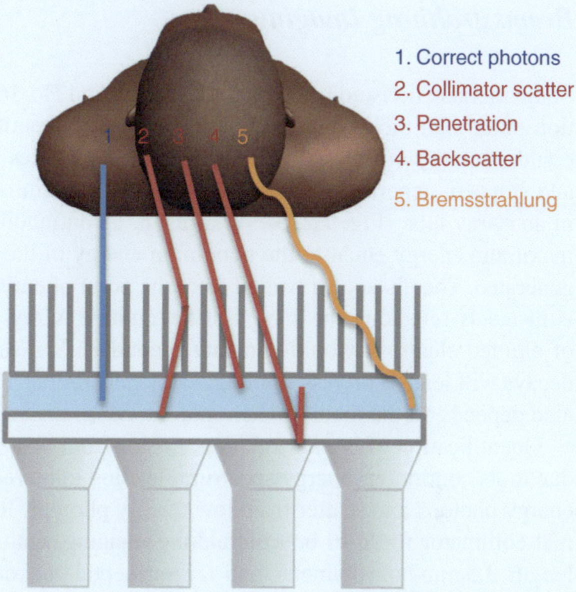

Fig. 7.2 High-energy photons and bremsstrahlung X-rays penetrate and scatter in the collimator and other parts of detector. (Image courtesy of Prof. Stefaan Vandenberghe)

of the two images. However, this approach suffers from increased computer storage, acquisition or computational time. One solution is to use an effective attenuation coefficient that regards the photopeaks as a single photon energy, which could make maximal use of the available information with no extra computational burden [24]. Model-based SC, such as ESSE, estimates scatter using an effective scatter source [19] by pre-calculating the blurring kernels from MCS. This method could be superior to energy window-based SC for clinical TRT, with reasonable reconstruction time.

A recent MIRD pamphlet presents a set of guidelines for data acquisition protocols and image reconstruction techniques recommended for quantitative Lu-177 SPECT for TRT dosimetry [25]. Medium energy collimators are recommended for their good signal-to-noise ratio (SNR) due to reduced septal penetration of high-energy photons. An energy window of 15–20% centered on the 208 keV photopeak is suggested for acquisition. Occasionally the 113 keV peak can be acquired as well if counts collected in the 208 keV window are insufficient. However, self-scattered 113 keV photons and down-scatter of 208 keV photons into this 113 keV energy window should be taken into consideration, and triple energy window (TEW) SC method is a potential solution. Uribe et al. evaluated the MIRD recommendations for Lu-177 SPECT and found the errors to be <5% for large objects [26]. He et al. applied their quantitative SPECT method for Lu-177 in a physical phantom study [27]. Independ image reconstructions were performed based on a 20% energy window for photopeaks of 208 keV, 113 keV, and the combination of both peaks. Errors were <3.2% for all organs using the 208 keV energy window, up to 40% using only the 113 keV energy window, and up to 14% for the combined photopeaks.

Bremsstrahlung Imaging

Some theranostic isotopes, e.g., Y-90, Sr-89, and Ho-166, present secondary radiation other than their own decay. For example, the emitted electrons or β particles could interact with the surrounding charged particles before being deaccelerated and stopped, generating bremsstrahlung photons similarly to the X-ray generation in an X-ray tube (Fig. 7.2, 5). As a result, a continuous spectrum of X-ray with a maximum energy equal to the maximum energy of the emitted electrons would be generated. The distance travelled from the point of emission before bremsstrahlung is inversely related to the energy of the emitted X-ray. Usually only a few percent of emitted electrons would generate secondary X-rays, e.g., about 2–4% of Y-90 decays will lead to bremsstrahlung X-ray generation. The amount of X-rays generated depends on the medium, i.e., more in dense materials like bone.

Quantification of bremsstrahlung images from beta emitters is very challenging due to its continuous energy spectrum, leading to increased penetration from high-energy photons and scatter from low-energy photons. Rong et al. designed an optimal collimator for Y-90 bremsstrahlung imaging, with parameters of 84 mm hole length, 3.5 mm hole diameter, and 1.4 mm septal thickness [28]. Compared with the commercial high-energy general purpose (HEGP) collimator, their design improved spatial resolution by 27%. Another challenge is that an effective attenuation coefficient is needed for AC due to the wide photon energy range [29]. Since there is no pronounced photopeak in the energy spectrum for bremsstrahlung radiation, choice of an optimal energy window is critical for quantification. Furthermore, traditional SC methods such as TEW are not suitable since the scattered photons cannot be distinguished from the primary photons in a continuous energy spectrum. The same group proposed an OS-EM reconstruction algorithm incorporating multi-range SC and CDR modeling methods which can provide accurate estimates of organ activities [30]. They separated modeling of the primary bremsstrahlung and scattered photons with multiple-energy ranges. The ESSE scatter kernels, attenuation and CDR were also modeled and compensated for each subrange in the forward and back projection. This reduced the Y-90 activity quantitation error for all organs of interest, especially the kidneys, down to −6.4±5.0%. Roshan et al. reviewed the energy window selection, collimator design, and reconstruction algorithm for Y-90-labeled microsphere bremsstrahlung imaging [31]. With a conventional medium energy general purpose collimator, a multiple-energy window with three energy peaks centered at 75 keV, 120 keV and 185 keV with CT-based AC and SC could achieve the highest system sensitivity and the lowest imaging acquisition time. Siman et al. proposed an energy window-based background compensation (BC) method to improve the Y-90 bremsstrahlung imaging quantitative accuracy [32] and found that the most appropriate energy window range for imaging was 90–125 keV. Dewaraja et al. implemented an MCS-based scatter correction for Y-90 bremsstrahlung imaging without increasing image noise or computational burden [33].

Although it is mostly for qualitative evaluation purpose, bremsstrahlung imaging is feasible to estimate organ activities in TRT with the development of advanced techniques to improve image quality and quantitation. Currently, bremsstrahlung imaging is still limited by inferior spatial resolution, low number of counts, broad energy distribution and severe scatter. Pinhole or multi-pinhole collimators could improve the tradeoff between sensitivity and resolution in comparison with the conventional parallel-hole collimator for bremsstrahlung SPECT [34]. The better attenuating material used for pinhole collimation, e.g., tungsten rather than lead, may improve the bremsstrahlung SPECT performances. High-energy X-rays would down-scatter into the acquisition energy window, which would lead to a higher count rate and substantial dead time effect. Scattering within the pinhole collimator is less of a problem for its empty cone geometry as compared to parallel-hole collimators. However, the small field of view (FOV) of pinhole collimators is still a major problem for whole-body TRT dosimetry, and further evaluation is warranted to confirm its clinical feasibility.

Quantitative PET/CT

PET is well-recognized to provide more accurate in vivo activity quantification due to its superior spatial resolution, sensitivity, and specificity for tumor detection, as compared to SPECT and bremsstrahlung imaging. Image degradation factors in PET include random coincidences, detector normalization, dead time, attenuation, and scatter [35]. Similar to SPECT/CT, the co-registered X-ray CT in PET/CT or segmented MR images in PET/MR can be used for AC and organ delineation. Time-of-flight (TOF) imaging method is now a common specification in new PET scanners to improve image SNR [36], lesion detectability, and uptake measurements. This advantage can also be traded for reduced acquisition time or injection dose [37]. Moreover, immuno-PET was a quantitative imaging procedure to investigate the biological effect and pharmacokinetics of radioimmunotherapy agents, e.g., radiolabeled antibody in targeted and nontargeted tissues with high resolution and sensitivity [38, 39]. This strategy can be used to improve patient selection and schedule adaption.

Similar to SPECT, the higher therapeutic doses required for TRT can also be challenging for PET scanners with limited count rate capability. The photons coming from secondary radiation or high-energy photons from non-pure annihilation effects lead to a higher random fraction, especially for Y-90 where the single rate is relatively high and the positron branching ratio is very low. With a proper energy and coincidence window, this effect can be alleviated but it still contributes to the background signal.

Most PET theranostic isotopes emit high-energy positrons with longer positron ranges as compared to F-18 with mean positron range of 0.64 mm, limiting the best possible spatial resolution and quantification accuracy. This should be less of a problem for the latest generation of clinical PET systems whose reconstructed spatial resolution is about 4–6 mm. In preclinical dosimetry using small animal imaging system with a typical 1–2 mm reconstructed spatial resolution, this factor has a crucial impact. Several groups have investigated the impact of nonconventional isotopes on both spatial resolution and image contrast using high-resolution preclinical and clinical PET and have proposed positron range correction [40–42]. Derenzo et al. removed the blurring in the FBP reconstructed images by Fourier deconvolution based on measured positron range functions [43]. Recently, methods incorporating isotope-specific positron range modeling into the MAP or OS-EM reconstruction algorithms were developed [44–47]. Jødal L et al. provided the positron range distribution for some conventional and nonconventional isotopes by MCS [116, 117]. These results could be applied to image reconstruction algorithms to improve spatial resolution and quantitative accuracy.

In order to fit the time activity curves (TAC) for TRT agents with half-lives of typically 2–4 days [48], positron emitters with longer half-lives such as I-124 (100.2 h), Y-86 (14.7 h), and Y-90 (64.1 h) are preferred in preclinical and clinical studies. Ideally, the positron emitters used for PET imaging are isotopes of the radionuclides in therapy, e.g., I-124 for I-131 and Y-86 for Y-90. However, I-124 and Y-86 are not pure positron emitters, and they are associated with spurious coincidences such as prompt gamma coincidences (PGC), gamma-gamma cascades, bremsstrahlung radiation, and high-energy gamma rays that result in pair production [49]. Although most prompt gamma emissions have energy peaks higher than the upper bound of the PET energy window, they may still be downscattered in the main PET energy window and degrade image contrast [50]. For example, about 50% of the positrons are emitted with a 603 keV gamma photon simultaneously for I-124. Three gamma photons with energies of 1077/1854 keV, 628 keV, and 443 keV are emitted simultaneously per Y-86 decay whose positron abundance is 32%. Background subtraction in the sinograms [51], empirical or analytical kernels for sinogram convolution [52], and recovery coefficient [53] have been proposed to resolve PGC. For Y-86 quantitation, Warland et al. proposed a patient-dependent method based on sinogram tail fitting with a Y-86 point spread function (PSF) library [52] to correct for PGC. The background and kidney activity errors were reduced from 117% to 9% and 84% to 5%, respectively, in a phantom study. In the patient studies, the activity difference between total body scanning and urine sample was reduced from 92% to 7%. Buchholz et al. developed a scanner-dependent background subtraction method for PGC [54]. They showed that quantification of Y-86-labeled radiotracers was feasible for simple cylindrical phantoms. Jentzen et al. estimated the RCs for I-124 in different PET/CT scanners [53]. Their results showed that after applying the RC, the activity estimation error was ±10% for sphere diameter ≥12.6 mm. However, RCs depend on different radionuclides, scanners, and post-processing parameters which need to be determined, respectively.

Lovqvist et al. compared the accuracy of biodistribution estimation between Y-86 PET and In-111 planar images in a nude mouse model [55] when they acted as Y-90 imaging surrogates. The results showed that the uptakes of In-111 and Y-86 were generally similar within the first 2 days postinjection but the activity of Y-86 was significantly higher than In-111 in most tissues at 4 days postinjection.

Instead of using Y-86 as surrogate, Y-90 also emits a few positrons via internal pair production, and they are sufficient to be detected by PET. Gates et al. [56] and D'Arienzo M et al. [57] used conventional PET/CT scanners to detect the deposition of Y-90 microsphere directly. Comparing the performance of quantitative Y-90 bremsstrahlung and PET, Kao et al. concluded that Y-90 PET with advanced compensation techniques is superior in the aspects of image resolution, sensitivity, and quantitation [58, 59], accordant with the results from Elschot et al. [60]. Sample Y-90 PET and bremsstrahlung images are shown in Fig. 7.3. Padia et al. showed that TOF Y-90 PET provided less scatter for comparable spatial resolution [61]. However, L(Y)SO, which is the most common scintillator in PET nowadays, contains Lu-176, which is intrinsically radioactive and leads to a small background signal in the coincidence measurement. This effect is a potential limitation associated with Y-90 quantification due to the low abundance of internal pair production for Y-90.

Motion blurring artifacts from patients' voluntary and involuntary motion, e.g., respiratory and cardiac motion, also affect image quantification. The motion influence on PET is more significant as compared to SPECT and bremsstrahlung imaging due to its superior resolution. The use of respiratory gating with PET imaging has proven to be an efficient way to reduce motion blurring with minimal count loss or increase in scan time. Osborne et al. have shown that amplitude-based gating on Y-90 PET/CT images can be used to realize respiratory motion correction, which may further improve post-therapy dosimetry accuracy [62].

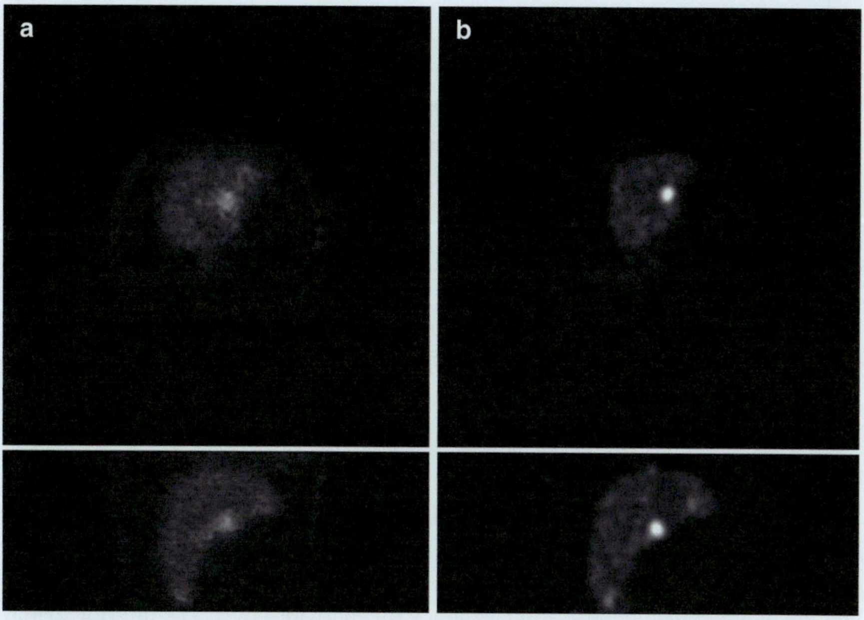

Fig. 7.3 (The grayscale of the fig is bad) Sample Y-90 (**a**) bremsstrahlung and (**b**) PET images for an anthropomorphic torso phantom. (Image courtesy of Prof. Stefaan Vandenberghe)

The quantitative accuracy for different imaging modalities would depend on the implemented compensations and the isotopes, though it is generally accepted that the quantitative accuracy for PET would be better than SPECT and bremsstrahlung imaging. Whole-body PET [63] and SPECT scanners with high sensitivity are expected to be the new gateways for fast and quantitative imaging solutions for voxel-based TRT dosimetry.

3D Dosimetric Methods

In order to convert the voxel count to 3D absorbed dose (Gy) information, there are a couple of pre- and post-imaging processing steps that need to be considered and practiced carefully to ensure the accuracy of the dose estimates. Each step is explained in details as follows.

Dose Calibration

To obtain quantitative biokinetic information of the radiopharmaceutical, it is essential to determine a calibration factor (cps/MBq) to convert the reconstructed voxel values into activity. The uncertainty caused by the determination of this calibration factor is dominant for quantitative SPECT imaging-based dosimetry [64].

Generally, there are two ways to measure the calibration factor. The first is to acquire an image of a uniform phantom with known activity concentration [65]. The calibration factor is equal to the known concentration in the phantom divided by the count in the ECT images. It can be used for other studies acquired using the same protocol and post-processing method. The second is to measure the calibration factor using a planar image of an in-air calibration source [66, 67]. In this method, the calibration factor is defined as the ratio between the background-corrected count rate in the whole image and the known source activity. The first approach using phantom calibration measurements is a more common approach. For SPECT imaging, if a parallel-hole collimator is used, then the measured calibration factor could be applied to all voxels within the FOV regardless of the source-to-collimator distance.

Volume-of-Interest (VOI) Delineation

Determination of the VOI is one of the most important steps in treatment planning and might affect the quantification accuracy by up to 30% [23]. The inferior spatial resolution and statistical noise on nuclear medicine images impede the accuracy of image segmentation for VOI definition. Therefore, it is suggested that this step be performed on high-resolution anatomical images such as CT and MRI and then applied the VOIs to the registered ECT images after interpolations. Zhou et al. proposed an accurate and robust interactive contour delineation method using a curve fitting approach to manually refine the automatic segmentation result [68]. Various groups showed that the combination of functional and anatomical information can improve segmentation accuracy [69–71]. Han et al. demonstrated that the use of a graph cut segmentation method based on both PET and CT data can yield 10% higher accuracy than using sole PET or CT data for tumors [71]. Besides, it should be noted that the CT and the emission images should be registered before delineating the VOIs; otherwise, the mismatch would be affecting not only the organ delineation but the corresponding attenuation correction and scatter correction [72]. Our study showed that organ activities' estimation errors are about proportional to the shift of the images in x- and y-directions. The errors are larger for small and cold organs, and they are more sensitive to the shift in the lateral (x-) and anterior-posterior (y-) directions than rotation in z-axis (Fig. 7.4).

A well-designed segmentation method satisfies three conditions: accuracy, repeatability, and efficiency. According to different operational methods, segmentation for VOIs can be categorized as manual, semiautomatic, and automatic methods. The accuracy of manual VOI may easily be affected by blurred boundary due to the image resolution, partial volume effect, and operator's experience. Thus, automated or semiautomated techniques are often suggested for reducing inter- and intraoperator variation and time. Many state-of-the-art interactive segmentation algorithms for medical imaging applications have been proposed and are covered in several comprehensive reviews [73–75].

Image Registration

In TRT, patients usually need to be imaged at different time points to obtain the TAC and calculate organs' cumulative activity. However, patient movement and organ deformation happen between scans which may lead to reduced accuracy, especially for 3D dosimetry where cumulative activity needs to be generated on a voxel-by-voxel basis. Papavasileiou et al. showed that the differences in absorbed dose may be up to 90% even for small rigid misregistrations with translations <9.5 mm and rotations <6° [76]. These errors became more serious when the VOIs were distant from the center of the images. Therefore, registrations between serial nuclear medicine scans are essential for improved TRT dosimetry. The same research group developed a 4D rigid image registration scheme in which each scan of the series is registered to its immediate predecessor for registration of SPECT scans at different time points [77]. This method used the spatial information and the voxel-based similarity criteria. Sequential 3D registration resulted in residual registration errors of 3.5 ± 2.5, 3.2 ± 2.0, and 7.0 ± 3.5 mm, whereas the corresponding 4D method gave errors of 2.4 ± 1.6, 1.9 ± 1.1, and 5.3 ± 2.9 mm for the correlation coefficient, mutual information, and sum-of-absolute difference criteria, respectively. The

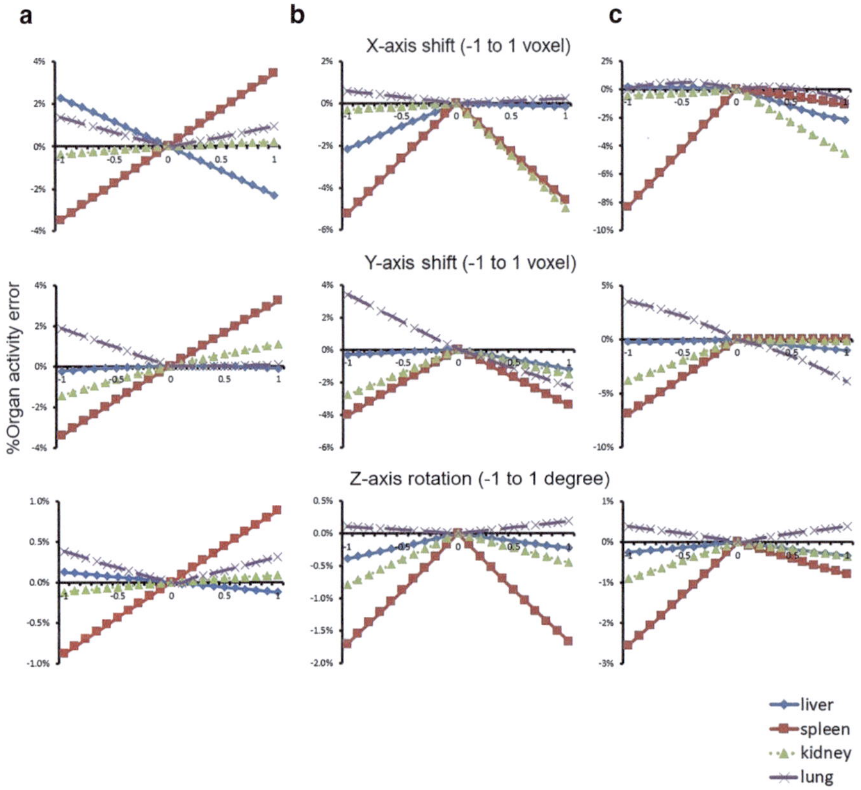

Fig. 7.4 ECT and CT mismatch effect of (**a**) attenuation correction, (**b**) VOI definition, and (**c**) combined attenuation correction and VOI definition on organ activity estimation, when the mismatch was along the *x*- (top), *y*- (middle), and *z*- (bottom) directions for different organs

algorithm incorporated the time information which was proven to be more robust and accurate comparing to the sequential voxel-based 3D registration.

Registration on quantitative functional images is feasible yet challenging due to the lack of anatomic information, statistical noise after a large number of updates, and isotope decay especially for later time points [78]. Modern multimodality scanners acquiring both ECT and high-resolution anatomical images provide a feasible solution for this problem [79]. Our previous studies showed that using sequential CT images for registration is superior to sequential SPECT images in terms of better activity and absorbed dose estimate. The use of CT improves quantitative image reconstruction, organ delineation, and image registration. Moreover, organ-based registration where organs are segmented out individually before registrations outperformed whole-body registrations, with the cost of more times of segmentations for each organ and each time point (Fig. 7.5) [80]. Fully automatic segmentation

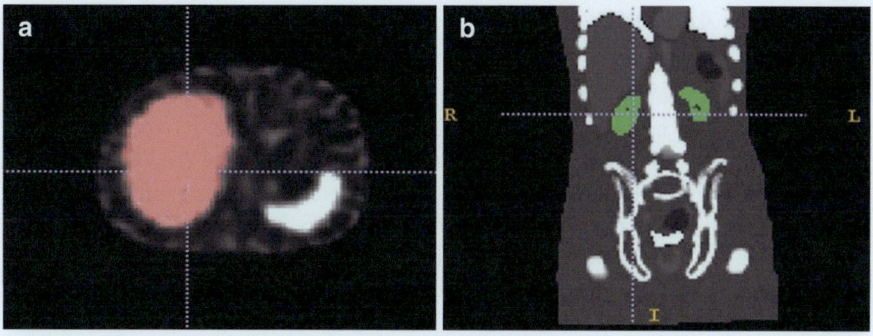

Fig. 7.5 Sample segmentation of (**a**) the liver on simulated SPECT and (**b**) kidneys on simulated CT images

method would be preferred for organ-based registration in TRT dosimetry to improve the clinical feasibility.

On the other hand, nonrigid deformation in organ or tumor is more likely to happen in the clinical circumstances, and rigid registration may not be adequate especially for small organs or lesions. Sjogreen et al. studied the impact of rigid or nonrigid registration of serial SPECT/CT images for TRT accuracy [81]. They performed rigid or nonrigid registration on the CT images, and the deformation field obtained from the CT-CT registration was then used to transform the corresponding SPECT images. They found that the activity estimation was more consistent after both rigid and nonrigid registrations. The differences between rigid and nonrigid registrations for residence time and absorbed dose in organs were small, but nonrigid registration had better precision especially in the anatomical regions where nonrigid movement was more likely to present, e.g., neck and shoulder region. Employing CT-derived spatial transformation avoids time-varying activity distribution in SPECT, but the CT deformation field may change the SPECT intensity distribution. Ao et al. investigated the effect of using nonrigid organ-based registration on 3D dosimetric estimation [78]. They used the normalized absolute error (NAE%) of differential dose volume histogram (DDVH) for 3D dosimetry evaluation. The results showed that the NAE% of DDVH was 8.18, 32.31, 16.28, and 7.02% for nonrigid registration whereas the corresponding rigid registration gave errors of 41.68, 77.41, 36.25, and 17.80% for the liver, spleen, kidneys, and lungs respectively, indicating the superior performance for the nonrigid registration.

As multimodality imaging techniques have shown merits for both segmentation and registration, sequential anatomical scans, e.g., low-dose CT, might be considered to be included in the standard clinical TRT protocol. To further reduce the CT radiation dose with similar dosimetric accuracy of sequential CT scans, our group proposed to generate virtual CTs at different time points based on a single CT acquisition and nonrigid registrations [82].

Cumulative Activity

Time-integrated activity coefficients can be generated either by fitting an exponential function to each voxel or integrating the values of each voxel analytically over time. One-phase, two-phase, and multiphase exponential decay models are used to describe the kinetic function of the targeted organs or tumors [20, 83, 84], depending on the number of data input and tracer kinetics. The sums of the exponentials are used as the model function of the TAC. Compartmental modeling is also proposed for the curve fitting [85], while Akaike and F-test can be used to evaluate the performance of the curve fitting [86]. Trapezoidal integration followed by extrapolation after the last time point following the physical decay is feasible if no curve fitting is available but errors are expected especially when fewer imaging sessions are acquired. More studies are yet to be performed to evaluate the substantial errors caused by the curve fitting process.

Dose Conversion

To achieve dosimetry at the voxel level, one can use either dose-point kernel (DPK) convolution [87], voxel S value (VSV) [96],or MCS [88, 89] for activity-absorbed dose conversion. The DPK convolution with the 3D activity distribution was widely recommended for its efficiency compared with the MCS in the late 1990s. The DPK for beta particles, electrons, and photons, i.e., the mean absorbed dose per transition at a given radial distance for an isotropic point source located within an infinite homogeneous medium, can be pre-calculated for different isotopes [90, 91]. This approach considers the absorbed dose from nearby voxels. The VSV approach was proposed to provide the corresponding S values to the geometry of the voxel imaging data and was adopted by the MIRD Committee [92, 93] (Fig. 7.6). Similar to DPK, VSV is defined as the mean absorbed dose to a target voxel per radioactive decay in a source voxel, again, by assuming source voxel and target voxel are both contained in an infinite homogeneous tissue medium. A series of strategies have been created for calculating the VSV including direct MCS [94–97], convolution [98], or numerical integration [99] of DPK. Moreover, Lanconelli et al. provided a free VSV database for seven common TRT radionuclides in several common voxel sizes for both soft tissues and bone [96]. The local energy deposition (LED) method was proposed by Bolch et al. to simplify the application of VSV for pure beta emitters. It assumed that all kinetic energy released from beta emissions is locally absorbed within the source voxel. Thus, the 3D dose distribution can be calculated by simply multiplying the cumulated activity in a voxel with a unique dosimetric factor. Pasciak et al. showed that conventional VSV method slightly underestimated the dose in the areas with the highest activity by about 15% and 10% for the voxel size

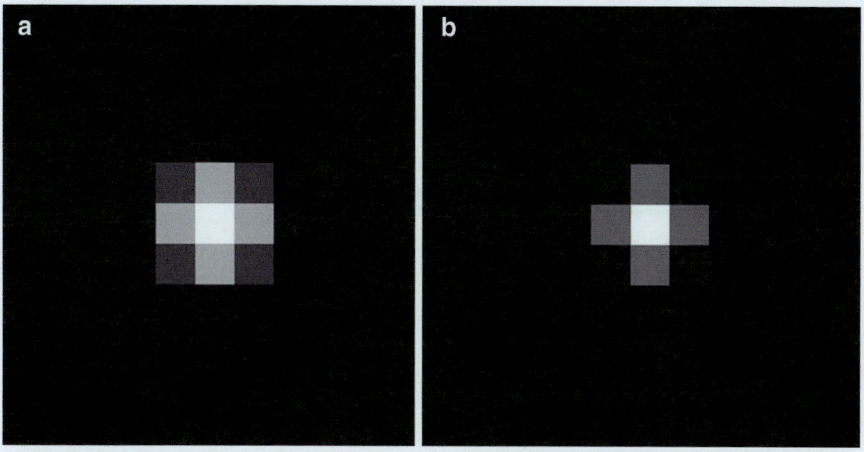

Fig. 7.6 Sample Y-90 VSV for (**a**) soft tissue and (**b**) bone for a voxel size of $4.22 \times 4.22 \times 4.22$ mm^3

of 6 mm^3 and 3 mm^3, respectively, while the LED method can reduce the blurring effects on the activity concentration and is more accurate compared to VSV using MCS method as the gold standard in a Y-90 microsphere SPECT study. This technique can further be applied to PET [100]. However, both DPK and VSV approaches cannot address the problem of tissue inhomogeneity. The MCS-based dosimetry [101] is more accurate since it considers all the tissue variations within the patients, simulating particle transportation and energy deposition from all possible source organs. Software including EGS4 and GATE can be used for the MCS dosimetric calculations, where the CT-derived density maps, activity, or cumulative activity images are input to calculate the absorbed dose. However, the intensive computation time impedes its clinical utility. Grimes et al. showed that the 3D dose distributions produced by the MCS and VSV approaches are nearly identical in a patient study [102].

Data Analysis

Conventional 2D dosimetric results include different average organ absorbed dose. They do not contain potential dose nonuniformity information within the tumors or the critical organs. The voxel-based dosimetry provides 3D absorbed dose information, including dose volume histogram, dose map, and isodose contour (Fig. 7.7). This information allows depicting the dose distribution, including minimum and maximum dose, for the treatment planning or dose verification. It can also be used to assess the potential toxicity to the critical organs, particularly for organs with tissues of potential different radiosensitivity.

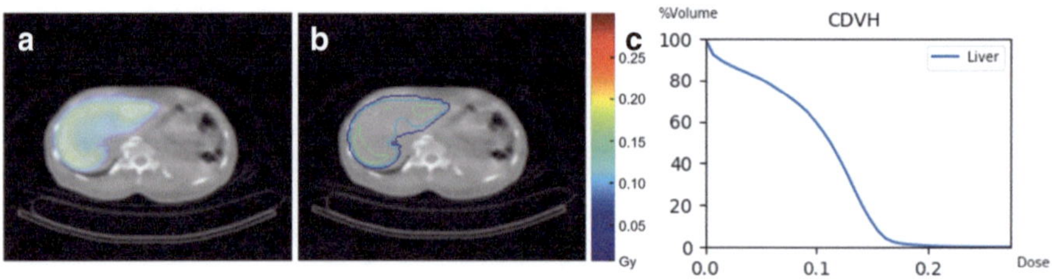

Fig. 7.7 Sample (**a**) dose map, (**b**) isodose contour, and (**c**) its corresponding cumulative dose volume histogram of the liver for a patient injected with In-111 octreotide

Dosimetric Software

Generally, a 3D internal dosimetric software involves steps of optional image registration, VOI segmentation, curve fitting for generating the time activity curve, dose conversion, and data analysis given the input of serial patient imaging data and a dose calibration factor. While early voxelized dosimetry software does not contain all five modules mentioned above and would need to be used together with other image processing or dosimetric software, more one-stop research and commercial dosimetric software packages are developed recently. Some software also provides options of quantitative reconstructions. A review of the recent codes for internal dosimetry can be found from the work of Ramos et al. [103]. Sample commercial and research voxelized TRT software is listed in Table 7.2.

Uncertainty Propagation for Image-Based Dosimetry

Uncertainties in image-based 3D dosimetry are attributed to many aspects including physical degradations during the imaging process, dose calibration for system sensitivity measurement, volume-of-interest delineation, image registration, curve fitting, and dose conversion. It is important to acknowledge the potential sources and amplitude of errors for the final dose assessment on the critical organs and tumors. Except for the uncertainties attributed to image acquisition and post-processing, differences between the dose calibration and dosage administration time, residual activity remaining in the delivery system post administration, radionuclide impurities, and operator's errors also contribute to the overall errors in absorbed dose assessment, which can introduce errors in the prescribed dose after treatment planning or efficacy assessment after dose verification.

Gustafsson J et al. investigated uncertainty propagation for image-based dosimetry by observing the decrease in standard deviation when removing a particular error source [114]. They used three anthropomorphic computer phantoms combined with a pharmacokinetic model of Lu-177-DOTATATE, modeling variations

Table 7.2 Overview of voxelized patient-specific dosimetry software

References	Software	Image registration	Image segmentation	Curve fitting model	Dose calculation
[104]	OEDIPE	N/A	Manual/semiautomatic/automatic segmentation by a user-defined threshold	N/A	MCNPX (MCS)
[105]	MrVoxel	Manual registration		Mono-exponential fitting	VSV or VOXnova (MCS)
[106]	RMDP	Semiautomatic or automatic registration using external landmarks		N-1 phases curve fitting (N is the number of SPECT scans)	MIRD voxel S value and DPK
[90]	3DID	N/A	Manual/automatic edge detection on CT/MRI images	Mono-exponential fitting	DPK and EGS4 (MCS)
[107]	RAYDOSE	Nonrigid registration	Manual segmentation on CT images	Mono-exponential/ linear+mono-exponential/ parallelogram method	Geant4 (MCS)
[108]	VRAK	Automatic rigid and nonrigid registration on CT images	N/A	Tri-exponential fitting	VSV
[109]	NUKDOS	N/A	Manual segmentation	Sums of exponential fitting	VSV
[110]	VIDA	Automatic rigid registration on CT images	Manual/semiautomatic segmentation on CT images	Mono- or bi-exponential fitting	Geant4 (MCS)
[111]	VoxelMed	Manual registration	Manual segmentation on CT images	Trapezoidal method followed by half-time mono-exponential tail integration	VSV
	Stratos	Rigid registration			VSV
[112]	PLANET Dose	Automatic/semiautomatic rigid/ nonrigid registration	Semiautomatic/ automatic segmentation	Mono-exponential fitting	VSV
[113]	HIRD	Manual or automated rigid body registration	Manual or semiautomatic segmentation	Numerical integration followed by trapezoid rule	Semi-MCS
[118]	BIGDOSE	Automated non-rigid body registration	Semi-automatic segmentation	Mono-/bi-/tri-exponential fitting or trapezoidal integration	VSV

in calibration factor, noise on the CT-derived density map, dynamic activity distribution during SPECT data acquisition, VOI delineation, and imaging starting time points. The absorbed dose of the left kidney was investigated by excluding variations in factors mentioned above. They showed that the highest uncertainty in kidney absorbed dose appears to be the PVC using a fixed recovery coefficient and gamma camera calibration. The uncertainty propagation in quantitative PET-based dosimetry, e.g., PGC, positron range correction, and PVC, has not been systematically studied yet.

Conclusion

Quantitative imaging for TRT is challenging since most of the therapeutic agents are not optimal for imaging [119]. The image reconstruction process for quantitative SPECT, bremsstrahlung imaging, and PET has to compensate many image degradation factors, including down-scatter, bremsstrahlung photons, and PGC, while researchers have obtained promising results for different isotopes. For gamma emitter imaging such as I-131 and In-111, quantification errors within 10% can been obtained with different combination of compensations. For imaging positron emitters like Y-86 and I-124, quantitative errors are within 7% [52]. However, it is hard to compare these methods as the studies were conducted using different phantoms, activity levels, and imaging protocols. For isotopes with more complicated energy spectrum (Ho-166) or pure beta emitters (Y-90), researchers could reach certain accuracy level with specific imaging hardware and reconstruction algorithms.

Nowadays, with the development of antibodies with high affinity and specificity, and the growing number of preclinical and clinical studies of a wide range of positron emitting radionuclides, PET is expected to play an important role in both diagnosis and therapeutic stage for individualized treatment planning and therapeutic monitoring in TRT applications, especially after the proposed concept of immuno-PET and its rapid development [48]. The studies in SPECT have built a firm foundation for the development of PET [115] whose nice features may make it become a good image protocol in TRT. Advanced correction algorithms need to be further developed for different PET isotopes with complicated decay scheme.

Still, more advanced post-processing techniques are required to pursue high dosimetric accuracy. For example, effective image registration, segmentation, and improved reconstruction algorithm are important for voxel-level dosimetry for nonuniform activity and tissue distribution. The optimization of imaging protocols with reduced imaging sessions and short acquisition times to cover the organs of interest or whole-body imaging is important for routine clinical implementation. Associated hardware improvements, e.g., choices of collimator and detector, are also essential to pursue high dosimetric accuracy. Finally, the optimal way for quantitative imaging in TRT may probably be task-dependent. With the advance in computing power and technology development, 3D absorbed dose calculation for tumor and organs at risk via quantitative emission tomography and one-stop dosimetric software is promising for the routine clinical practice in the near future.

Acknowledgments This work was supported by research grants from the University of Macau (MYRG2017-00060-FST). The author would like to thank Prof. Stefaan Vandenberghe from Ghent University for his contributions in related figures.

Competing Interests The author declares that she has no conflict of interest.

References

1. Yeong CH, Cheng MH, Ng KH. Therapeutic radionuclides in nuclear medicine: current and future prospects. J Zhejiang Univ Sci B. Oct 2014;15(10):845–63.
2. Jadvar H. Targeted radionuclide therapy: an evolution toward precision cancer treatment. AJR Am J Roentgenol. Aug 2017;209(2):277–88.
3. Eary JF, et al. Samarium-153-EDTMP biodistribution and dosimetry estimation. J Nucl Med. 1993;34(7):1031–6.
4. Waldherr C, et al. Tumor response and clinical benefit in neuroendocrine tumors after 7.4 GBq 90Y-DOTATOC. J Nucl Med. 2002;43(5):610–6.
5. Vallabhajosula S, et al. Pharmacokinetics and biodistribution of 111In-and 177Lu-labeled J591 antibody specific for prostate-specific membrane antigen: prediction of 90Y-J591 radiation dosimetry based on 111In or 177Lu? J Nucl Med. 2005;46(4):634–41.
6. Silberstein EB, et al. The SNMMI practice guideline for therapy of thyroid disease with 131I 3.0. J Nucl Med. 2012;53(10):1633–51.
7. Sinha V, Goyel V, Trehan A. Radioactive microspheres in therapeutics. Die Pharmazie- Int J Pharm Sci. 2004;59(6):419–26.
8. Committee on State of the Science of Nuclear Medicine, National Research Council. Advancing nuclear medicine through innovation. Washington (DC): National Academies Press (US); 2007; 59–74.
9. Prise KM. Bystander effects and radionuclide therapy. In: Targeted radionuclide tumor therapy: Springer; Berlin, Heidelberg. 2008. p. 311–9.
10. Ersahin D, Doddamane I, Cheng D. Targeted radionuclide therapy. Cancers. 2011;3(4):3838–55.
11. Ahmadzadehfar H, Biersack HJ, Ezziddin S. Radioembolization of liver tumors with yttrium-90 microspheres. Semin Nucl Med. 2010;40(2):105–21.
12. Kwekkeboom DJ, et al. Treatment of patients with gastro-entero-pancreatic (GEP) tumours with the novel radiolabelled somatostatin analogue [177Lu-DOTA0,Tyr3]octreotate. Eur J Nucl Med Mol Imaging. 2003;30(3):417–22.
13. Kabasakal L, et al. Pre-therapeutic dosimetry of normal organs and tissues of 177Lu-PSMA-617 prostate-specific membrane antigen (PSMA) inhibitor in patients with castration-resistant prostate cancer. Eur J Nucl Med Mol Imaging. 2015;42(13):1976–83.
14. Strigari L, et al. The evidence base for the use of internal dosimetry in the clinical practice of molecular radiotherapy. Eur J Nucl Med Mol Imaging. 2014;41(10):1976–88.
15. Ljungberg M, Gleisner KS. 3-D image-based dosimetry in radionuclide therapy. IEEE Transac Radiat Plasma Med Sci. 2018;2(6):527–40.
16. Loke KSH, Padhy AK, Ng DCE, Goh ASW, Divgi C. Dosimetric considerations in radioimmunotherapy and systemic radionuclide therapies: a review. World J Nucl Med. 2011;10(2):122–38.

17. Bin H, Yong D, Xiyun S, Segars WP, Eric CF. A Monte Carlo and physical phantom evaluation of quantitative in-111 SPECT. Phys Med Biol. 2005;50(17):4169.
18. Du Y, Tsui BM, Frey EC. Partial volume effect compensation for quantitative brain SPECT imaging. IEEE Transac Med Imaging. 2005;24(8):969–76.
19. Frey EC, Tsui B. A new method for modeling the spatially-variant, object-dependent scatter response function in SPECT. In: Nuclear science symposium, 1996. conference record, vol. 2: p. 1082–6.
20. He B, Frey EC. Effects of shortened acquisition time on accuracy and precision of quantitative estimates of organ activity. Med Phys. 2010;37(4):1807.
21. Dewaraja YK, Koral KF, Fessler JA. Regularized reconstruction in quantitative SPECT using CT side information from hybrid imaging. Phys Med Biol. 2010;55(9):2523–39.
22. Vandervoort E, Celler A, Wells G, Blinder S, Dixon K, Pang Y. Implementation of an analytically based scatter correction in SPECT reconstructions. IEEE Transac Nucl Sci. 2005;52(3):645–53.
23. Shcherbinin S, Celler A, Belhocine T, Vanderwerf R, Driedger A. Accuracy of quantitative reconstructions in SPECT/CT imaging. Phys Med Biol. 2008;53(17):4595–604.
24. Seo Y, Wong KH, Hasegawa BH. Calculation and validation of the use of effective attenuation coefficient for attenuation correction in in-111 SPECT. Med Phys. 2005;32(12):3628–35.
25. Ljungberg M, Celler A, Konijnenberg MW, Eckerman KF, Dewaraja YK, Sjögreen-Gleisner K. MIRD pamphlet No. 26: joint EANM/MIRD guidelines for quantitative 177Lu SPECT applied for dosimetry of radiopharmaceutical therapy. J Nucl Med. 2016;57(1):151–62.
26. Uribe CF, et al. Accuracy of 177Lu activity quantification in SPECT imaging: a phantom study. EJNMMI Phys. 2017;4(1):2.
27. He B, Nikolopoulou A, Osborne J, Vallabhajosula S, Goldsmith S. Quantitative SPECT imaging with Lu-177: a physical phantom evaluation. J Nucl Med. 2012;53(supplement 1):2407.
28. Rong X, Frey EC. A collimator optimization method for quantitative imaging: application to Y-90 bremsstrahlung SPECT. Med Phys. 2013;40(8):082504.
29. Clarke LP, et al. Bremsstrahlung imaging using the gamma camera: factors affecting attenuation. J Nucl Med. 1992;33(1):161–6.
30. Rong X, Du Y, Ljungberg M, Rault E, Vandenberghe S, Frey EC. Development and evaluation of an improved quantitative 90Y bremsstrahlung SPECT method. Med Phys. 2012;39(5):2346–58.
31. Roshan H, Azarm A, Mahmoudian B, Islamian J. Advances in SPECT for optimizing the liver tumors radioembolization using Yttrium-90 microspheres. World J Nucl Med. 2015;14(2):75.
32. Siman W, Mikell J, Kappadath S. Practical reconstruction protocol for quantitative 90Y bremsstrahlung SPECT/CT. Med Phys. 2016;43(9):5093–103.
33. Dewaraja YK, et al. Improved quantitative 90Y bremsstrahlung SPECT/CT reconstruction with Monte Carlo scatter modeling. Med Phys. 2017;44(12):6364–76.
34. Walrand S, Hesse M, Demonceau G, Pauwels S, Jamar F. Yttrium-90-labeled microsphere tracking during liver selective internal radiotherapy by bremsstrahlung pinhole SPECT: feasibility study and evaluation in an abdominal phantom. EJNMMI Res. 2011;1(1):1.
35. Zanzonico P. Positron emission tomography: a review of basic principles, scanner design and performance, and current systems. Semin Nucl Med. 2004;34(2):87–111.
36. Karp JS, Fletcher JW. Time-of-flight PET. In: PET Center of Excellence Newsletter; 2006.
37. Surti S. Update on time-of-flight PET imaging. J Nucl Med. 2015;56(1):98–105.
38. Boerman OC, Oyen WJ. Immuno-PET of cancer: a revival of antibody imaging. J Nucl Med. 2011;52(8):1171–2.
39. Van Dongen GA, Visser GW, Lub-de Hooge MN, De Vries EG, Perk LR. Immuno-PET: a navigator in monoclonal antibody development and applications. Oncologist. 2007;12(12):1379–89.
40. Laforest R, Rowland DJ, Welch MJ. MicroPET imaging with nonconventional isotopes. IEEE Trans Nucl Sci. 2002;49(5):2119–26.

41. Liu X, Laforest R. Quantitative small animal PET imaging with nonconventional nuclides. Nucl Med Biol. 2009;36(5):551–9.
42. Disselhorst JA, et al. Image-quality assessment for several positron emitters using the NEMA NU 4-2008 standards in the Siemens Inveon small-animal PET scanner. J Nucl Med. 2010;51(4):610–7.
43. Derenzo SE. Mathematical removal of positron range blurring in high resolution tomography. IEEE Trans Nucl Sci. 1986;33(1):565–9.
44. Bai B, Ruangma A, Laforest R, Tai Y-C, Leahy RM. Positron range modeling for statistical PET image reconstruction. In: Nuclear science symposium conference record, 2003 IEEE, vol. 4: p. 2501–5.
45. Bai B, Laforest R, Smith AM, Leahy RM. Evaluation of MAP image reconstruction with positron range modeling for 3D PET. In: Nuclear science symposium conference record, 2005 IEEE, vol. 5: p. 2686–9.
46. Fu L, Qi J. A novel iterative image reconstruction method for high-resolution PET imaging with a Monte Carlo based positron range model. In: Nuclear science symposium conference record, 2008 IEEE: p. 3609–12.
47. Cal-González J, Herraiz J, España S, Desco M, Vaquero JJ, Udías JM. Positron range effects in high resolution 3D PET imaging. In: Nuclear science symposium conference record (NSS/MIC), 2009 IEEE: p. 2788–91.
48. Verel I, Visser GW, van Dongen GA. The promise of immuno-PET in radioimmunotherapy. J Nucl Med. 2005;46(1 suppl):164S–71S.
49. Conti M, Eriksson L. Physics of pure and non-pure positron emitters for PET: a review and a discussion. EJNMMI Phys. 2016;3(1):1–17.
50. Lubberink M, Herzog H. Quantitative imaging of 124I and 86Y with PET. Eur J Nucl Med Mol Imaging. 2011;38(S1):10–8.
51. Lubberink M, Schneider H, Bergström M, Lundqvist H. Quantitative imaging and correction for cascade gamma radiation of 76Br with 2D and 3D PET. Phys Med Biol. 2002;47(19):3519.
52. Walrand S, et al. Quantitation in PET using isotopes emitting prompt single gammas: application to yttrium-86. Eur J Nucl Med Mol Imaging. 2003;30(3):354–61.
53. Jentzen W, et al. Iodine-124 PET dosimetry in differentiated thyroid cancer: recovery coefficient in 2D and 3D modes for PET (/CT) systems. Eur J Nucl Med Mol Imaging. 2008;35(3):611–23.
54. Buchholz HG, et al. PET imaging with yttrium-86: comparison of phantom measurements acquired with different PET scanners before and after applying background subtraction. Eur J Nucl Med Mol Imaging. 2003;30(5):716–20.
55. Lövqvist A, et al. PET imaging of 86Y-labeled anti-Lewis Y monoclonal antibodies in a nude mouse model: comparison between 86Y and 111In radiolabels. J Nucl Med. 2001;42(8):1281–7.
56. Gates VL, Esmail AA, Marshall K, Spies S, Salem R. Internal pair production of 90Y permits hepatic localization of microspheres using routine PET: proof of concept. J Nucl Med. 2011;52(1):72–6.
57. D'Arienzo M, et al. 90Y PET-based dosimetry after selective internal radiotherapy treatments. Nucl Med Commun. 2012;33(6):633–40.
58. Kao Y-H, et al. Post-radioembolization yttrium-90 PET/CT-part 1: diagnostic reporting. EJNMMI Res. 2013;3(1):56.
59. Kao Y-H, et al. Post-radioembolization yttrium-90 PET/CT-part 2: dose-response and tumor predictive dosimetry for resin microspheres. EJNMMI Res. 2013;3:57.
60. Elschot M, Vermolen BJ, Lam MG, de Keizer B, van den Bosch MA, de Jong HW. Quantitative comparison of PET and Bremsstrahlung SPECT for imaging the in vivo yttrium-90 microsphere distribution after liver radioembolization. PLoS One. 2013;8(2):e55742.
61. Padia SA, Alessio A, Kwan SW, Lewis DH, Vaidya S, Minoshima S. Comparison of positron emission tomography and bremsstrahlung imaging to detect particle distribution in patients

undergoing yttrium-90 radioembolization for large hepatocellular carcinomas or associated portal vein thrombosis. J Vasc Interv Radiol. 2013;24(8):1147–53.
62. Osborne DR, Acuff S, Neveu M, Kaman A, Syed M, Fu Y. 90Y liver radioembolization imaging using amplitude-based gated PET/CT. Clin Nucl Med. 2017;42(5):373–4.
63. Cherry SR, Jones T, Karp JS, Qi J, Moses WW, Badawi RD.Total-Body PET: Maximizing Sensitivity to Create New Opportunities for Clinical Research and Patient Care. J Nucl Med. 2018;59(1):3–12.
64. Zeintl J, Vija AH, Yahil A, Hornegger J, Kuwert T. Quantitative accuracy of clinical 99mTc SPECT/CT using ordered-subset expectation maximization with 3-dimensional resolution recovery, attenuation, and scatter correction. J Nucl Med. 2010;51(6):921–8.
65. Koral KF, et al. CT-SPECT fusion plus conjugate views for determining dosimetry in iodine-131-monoclonal antibody therapy of lymphoma patients. J Nucl Med. 1994;35(10):1714–20.
66. Ljungberg M, Frey E, Sjögreen K, Liu X, Dewaraja Y, Strand S-E. 3D absorbed dose calculations based on SPECT: evaluation for 111-In/90-Y therapy using Monte Carlo simulations. Cancer Biother Radiopharm. 2003;18(1):99–107.
67. Anizan N, Wang H, Zhou XC, Hobbs RF, Wahl RL, Frey EC. Factors affecting the stability and repeatability of gamma camera calibration for quantitative imaging applications based on a retrospective review of clinical data. EJNMMI Res. 2014;4(1):67.
68. Zhou W, Xie Y. Interactive contour delineation and refinement in treatment planning of image-guided radiation therapy. J Appl Clin Med Phys. 2014;15(1):141.
69. Li H, Bai J, Wu X, Bhatia S, Abu-Hejleh T, Sun W. Semi-automated co-segmentation of tumor volume using multimodality PET-CT in Non-Small Cell Lung Cancer (NSCLC). Austin J Cancer Clin Res. 2014;1(3):1013.
70. Ju W, Xiang D, Zhang B, Wang L, Kopriva I, Chen X. Random walk and graph cut for co-segmentation of lung tumor on PET-CT images. IEEE Transac Image Process. 2015;24(12):5854–67.
71. Han D, et al. Globally optimal tumor segmentation in PET-CT images: a graph-based co-segmentation method. In: Information processing in medical imaging: Springer; 2011. p. 245–56.
72. He B, Frey EC. The impact of 3D volume of interest definition on accuracy and precision of activity estimation in quantitative SPECT and planar processing methods. Phys Med Biol. 2010;55(12):3535–44. Published online 2010 May 28. https://doi.org/10.1088/0031-9155/55/12/017.
73. Schenk A, Prause G, Peitgen H-O. Efficient semiautomatic segmentation of 3D objects in medical images. In: Medical image computing and computer-assisted intervention–MICCAI 2000: Springer; 2000. p. 186–95.
74. Zhang H, Fritts JE, Goldman SA. Image segmentation evaluation: a survey of unsupervised methods. Comput Vis Image Underst. 2008;110(2):260–80. https://doi.org/10.1016/j.cviu.2007.08.003.
75. McGuinness K, O'connor NE. A comparative evaluation of interactive segmentation algorithms. Pattern Recogn. 2010;43(2):434–44.
76. Papavasileiou P, Divoli A, Hatziioannou K, Flux GD. The importance of the accuracy of image registration of SPECT images for 3D targeted radionuclide therapy dosimetry. Phys Med Biol. 2007;52(24):N539–48.
77. Papavasileiou P, Divoli A, Hatziioannou K, Flux GD. A generalized 4D image registration scheme for targeted radionuclide therapy dosimetry. Cancer Biother Radiopharm. 2007;22(1):160–5.
78. Ao EC, Wu NY, Wang SJ, Song N, Mok GS. Improved dosimetry for targeted radionuclide therapy using nonrigid registration on sequential SPECT images. Med Phys. 2015;42(2):1060–70.
79. Townsend DW, Carney JP, Yap JT, Hall NC. PET/CT today and tomorrow. J Nucl Med. 2004;45(1 suppl):4S–14S.

80. Li T, Wu N-Y, Song N, Mok GS. Evaluation of sequential SPECT and CT for targeted radionuclide therapy dosimetry. Ann Nucl Med. 2018;32(1):34–43.
81. Sjögreen-Gleisner K, Rueckert D, Ljungberg M. Registration of serial SPECT/CT images for three-dimensional dosimetry in radionuclide therapy. Phys Med Biol. 2009;54(20):6181–200.
82. Li T, Mok GSP. Technical note: virtual CT for reducing CT dose in targeted radionuclide therapy dosimetry. Med Phys. 2018;45:5138.
83. He B, et al. Evaluation of quantitative imaging methods for organ activity and residence time estimation using a population of phantoms having realistic variations in anatomy and uptake. Med Phys. 2009;36(2):612–9.
84. He B, et al. Comparison of residence time estimation methods for radioimmunotherapy dosimetry and treatment planning—Monte Carlo simulation studies. IEEE Transac Med Imaging. 2008;27(4):521–30.
85. Nickel M, Strand SE, Linden O, Wingardh K, Tenvall J, Gleisner KS. Development and evaluation of a pharmacokinetic model for prediction of radioimmunotherapy based on pretherapy data. Cancer Biother Radiopharm. 2009;24(1):111–22.
86. Glatting G, Kletting P, Reske SN, Hohl K, Ring C. Choosing the optimal fit function: comparison of the Akaike information criterion and the F-test. Med Phys. Nov 2007;34(11):4285–92.
87. Loevinger R, Japha E, Brownell G. Discrete radioisotope sources. In: Radiation dosimetry. New York: Academic Press; 1956. p. 693–799.
88. Furhang EE, Chui CS, Sgouros G. A Monte Carlo approach to patient-specific dosimetry. Med Phys. 1996;23(9):1523–9.
89. Furhang EE. A Monte Carlo-based dosimetry method for patient-specific internal emitter therapy. New York: Columbia University; 1996.
90. Tagesson M, Ljungberg M, Strand S-E. A Monte Carlo program converting activity distributions to absorbed dose distributions in a radionuclide treatment planning system. Acta Oncol. 1996;35(3):367–72.
91. Ferrer L, Chouin N, Bitar A, Lisbona A, Bardiès M. Implementing dosimetry in GATE: dose-point kernel validation with GEANT4 4.8. 1. Cancer Biother Radiopharm. 2007;22(1):125–9.
92. Liu A, Williams LE, Wong JY, Raubitschek AA. Monte Carlo-assisted voxel source kernel method (MAVSK) for internal beta dosimetry. Nucl Med Biol. 1998;25(4):423–33.
93. Bolch WE, Bouchet LG, Robertson JS, Wessels BW. MIRD pamphlet No, 17: the dosimetry of nonuniform activity distributions--radionuclide S values at the voxel level. J Nucl Med. 1999;40(1):S11.
94. Strigari L, Menghi E, D'Andrea M, Benassi M. Monte Carlo dose voxel kernel calculations of beta-emitting and Auger-emitting radionuclides for internal dosimetry: a comparison between EGSnrcMP and EGS4. Med Phys. 2006;33(9):3383–9.
95. Pacilio M, et al. Differences among Monte Carlo codes in the calculations of voxel S values for radionuclide targeted therapy and analysis of their impact on absorbed dose evaluations. Planning. 2009;5:8.
96. Lanconelli N, et al. A free database of radionuclide voxel S values for the dosimetry of non-uniform activity distributions. Phys Med Biol. 2012;57(2):517.
97. Amato E, Italiano A, Minutoli F, Baldari S. Use of the GEANT4 Monte Carlo to determine three-dimensional dose factors for radionuclide dosimetry. Nucl Instrum Methods Phys Res, Sect A. 2013;708:15–8.
98. Erdi AK, Yorke ED, Loew MH, Erdi YE, Sarfaraz M, Wessels BW. Use of the fast Hartley transform for three-dimensional dose calculation in radionuclide therapy. Med Phys. 1998;25(11):2226–33.
99. Franquiz J, Chigurupati S, Kandagatla K. Beta voxel S values for internal emitter dosimetry. Med Phys. 2003;30(6):1030–2.
100. Pasciak AS, Erwin WD. Effect of voxel size and computation method on Tc-99m MAA SPECT/CT-based dose estimation for Y-90 microsphere therapy. IEEE Transac Med Imaging. 2009;28(11):1754–8.

101. Furhang EE, Chui CS, Kolbert KS, Larson SM, Sgouros G. Implementation of a Monte Carlo dosimetry method for patient-specific internal emitter therapy. Med Phys. 1997;24(7):1163.
102. Grimes J, Celler A. Comparison of internal dose estimates obtained using organ-level, voxel S value, and Monte Carlo techniques. Med Phys. 2014;41(9):092501.
103. Ramos S, Thomas S, Pinheiro M, Coelho A, Albernaz M. Internal radiation dose and modeling codes in nuclear medicine: a fresh look at old problems. Int J Radiol Radiat Ther. 2017;4(5):00111.
104. Petitguillaume A, Bernardini M, Broggio D, de Labriolle Vaylet C, Franck D, Desbrée A. OEDIPE, a software for personalized Monte Carlo dosimetry and treatment planning optimization in nuclear medicine: absorbed dose and biologically effective dose considerations. Radioprotection. 2014;49(4):275–81.
105. McKay E. A software tool for specifying voxel models for dosimetry estimation. Cancer Biother Radiopharm. 2003;18(3):379–92.
106. Guy MJ, Flux GD, Papavasileiou P, Flower MA, Ott RJ. RMDP: a dedicated package for 131I SPECT quantification, registration and patient-specific dosimetry. Cancer Biother Radiopharm. 2003;18(1):61–9.
107. Marcatili S, et al. Development and validation of RAYDOSE: a Geant4-based application for molecular radiotherapy. Phys Med Biol. 2013;58(8):2491.
108. Jackson PA, Beauregard JM, Hofman MS, Kron T, Hogg A, Hicks RJ. An automated voxelized dosimetry tool for radionuclide therapy based on serial quantitative SPECT/CT imaging. Med Phys. 2013;40(11):112503.
109. Kletting P, et al. The NUKDOS software for treatment planning in molecular radiotherapy. Z Med Phys. 2015;25(3):264–74.
110. Kost SD, Dewaraja YK, Abramson RG, Stabin MG. VIDA: a voxel-based dosimetry method for targeted radionuclide therapy using Geant4. Cancer Biother Radiopharm. 2015;30(1):16–26.
111. Grassi E, et al. Quantitative comparison between the commercial software STRATOS® by Philips and a homemade software for voxel-dosimetry in radiopeptide therapy. Phys Med. 2015;31(1):72–9.
112. Dieudonné A, et al. Correlation between average absorbed dose and metabolic response in the radio-embolization of liver colorectal metastases with resin microspheres. J Nucl Med. 2015;56(supplement 3):1237.
113. Hippeläinen ET, Tenhunen MJ, Mäenpää HO, Heikkonen JJ, Sohlberg AO. Dosimetry software Hermes internal radiation dosimetry: from quantitative image reconstruction to voxel-level absorbed dose distribution. Nucl Med Commun. 2017;38(5):357–65.
114. Gustafsson J, Brolin G, Cox M, Ljungberg M, Johansson L, Gleisner KS. Uncertainty propagation for SPECT/CT-based renal dosimetry in 177Lu peptide receptor radionuclide therapy. Phys Med Biol. 2015;60(21):8329.
115. Pecking AP, Bellet D, Alberini JL. Immuno-SPET/CT and immuno-PET/CT: a step ahead to translational imaging. Clin Exp Metastasis. 2012;29(7):847–52.
116. Jødal L, Le Loirec C, Champion C. Positron range in PET imaging: an alternative approach for assessing and correcting the blurring. Phys Med Biol. 2012;57(12):3931.
117. Jødal L, Le Loirec C, Champion C. Positron range in PET imaging: non-conventional isotopes. Phys Med Biol. 2014;59(23):7419.
118. Li T, Zhu L, Lu Z, Song N, Lin KH, Mok GS. BIGDOSE: software for 3D personalized targeted radionuclide therapy dosimetry. Quant Imaging Med Surg 2020;10(1):160–70.
119. Li T , Ao ECI, Lambert B, Brans B, Vandenberghe S, Mok GS. Quantitative Imaging for Targeted Radionuclide Therapy Dosimetry - Technical Review. Theranostics. 2017 Oct 13;7(18):4551–65.

Chapter 8
Locoregional Unsealed Radionuclide Cancer Therapy: Experimental Findings

Franklin C. L. Wong

Introduction

As described further in Chap. 5, the use of radionuclides for human cancer therapy is exemplified by systemic administration of I-131 sodium iodide for the treatment of thyroid cancer and hyperthyroidism (Graves' disease). Other examples are lymphoma therapy using anti-CD20 monoclonal antibodies labeled with Y-90 (Zevalin) or I-131 (Bexxar), lutetium 177 somatostatin analogue for therapy of neuroendocrine tumor, Sr-89 chloride and samarium-153 EDTMP for cancer metastasis pain palliation and radium 223 chloride, as well as lutetium 177 PSMA for the treatment of prostate cancer. The systemic use of radionuclides for cancer therapy, while established as the standard of care, suffers from the disadvantage of limited delivery (typically less than 1%) of radionuclide to the target tumor while the rest of the body is subject to potential adverse effects of the rest of the dose (typically greater than 99% of administered dose). This disadvantage effectively restrains the therapeutic window to narrow ranges. The therapeutic windows can be nevertheless vastly expanded by pharmacokinetic advantages from locoregional delivery because the majority of the radiopharmaceuticals are delivered to the target before diffusion, perfusion, or lymphatic drainage and the radiopharmaceuticals would be diluted into the systemic circulation to cause less harm than from systemic administration.

The main concern for locoregional therapy would be locoregional toxicity which would potentially be caused by chemical toxicity from the formulated drug in the vicinity and from radiotoxicity of the radionuclide. As for chemical toxicity of the drug itself, the typical physical amount of radiopharmaceutical may be a concern of low specific activity formulation, but the actual amount is typically much less than micrograms and not likely to cause substantial harm. Radiotoxicity arises from the

F. C. L. Wong (✉)
Department of Nuclear Medicine, University of Texas, M. D. Anderson Cancer Center, Houston, TX, USA
e-mail: fwong@mdanderson.org

F. C. L. Wong (ed.), *Locoregional Radionuclide Cancer Therapy*,
https://doi.org/10.1007/978-3-030-56267-0_8

radionuclide of the radiopharmaceutical and is the intended consequence to treat the tumor and should be considered effective. Nevertheless, these potential locoregional toxicities need to be monitored in animal experiment and in clinical trials before a specific locoregional radionuclide cancer therapy becomes an acceptable form of treatment.

The choice of radiopharmaceuticals for therapeutic use largely depends on the radionuclide because of the need for larger radiation-absorbed doses than for diagnostic use. Examination of the target dosimetry and depth dosimetry of commercially available radionuclides with beta and gamma emissions as in Chap. 6 would allow rational choices of the radionuclide. The choice of radiopharmaceuticals also depends on the available radiochemistry and logistics to produce/attach the radionuclide to result in a relatively stable final product for human use.

The requirement of a therapeutic agent or device to be useful in the clinics is the assurance of efficacy and low acceptable toxicity profiles, as exemplified by federal requirements from agencies including the FDA and NRC. Before any drug or device is approved for routine human use, the safety and efficacy need to be demonstrated. Radiopharmaceuticals certainly need to fulfill those requirements. In vivo animal experiments are therefore needed.

This chapter reviews the LRCT animal experiments performed under the support of several federal grants from the NIH (R21CA89891 and R21CA97729) and US DOD Army Breast Cancer Research Grant (BC020808) and an MDACC University Cancer Fund Grant (#94712). Parts of the data were used to apply for a US Patent "Locoregional Internal Radionuclide Ablation of Abnormal Tissues," United States, 8329141, issued on 12/11/2012.

The choices of radiopharmaceuticals were made from commercially available radionuclides that are readily accessible in an ordinary radiopharmacy. The hypothesis is that commercially available radiopharmaceuticals in relatively low-dose range (less than 5 mCi) are able to suppress tumor growth when injected locoregionally inside solid tumors in animals.

Methodology

Upon approval from institutional animal use committee on each of the animal tumor model protocol, intratumoral injections of radionuclides were performed in three tumor models in the rats (13762 rat mammary tumor in F344 rats) [1, 2], mice (B16-OVA tumor in C57BL/6 mice), [3] and dogs (canine venereal transmissible tumor (cTVT)) [4, 5]. Excerpts from approved protocols are enclosed for reference as in Appendices I and II for small animal models, rat and mice, respectively, and in Appendix III for large animal model. Available animal tumor models are further discussed in Chap. 9.

For rat and mice experiments, tumors are typically implanted subcutaneously over the right hind limb, and the tumors were measured daily, and the general health was observed by veterinary staff. Serial tumor size measurements (length, width, and height) were made for at least 4 weeks or until clinical deterioration requiring euthanasia. Dogs were implanted with cTVT in the lungs and/or prostates and monitored using CT and T1- and T2-weighted MRI. Selected animals were chosen for additional imaging studies including CT and/or F-18 FDG PET scan and other imaging studies before and after intratumoral injection. Most of the radiopharmaceuticals used were purchased from radiopharmacies, but combinations with nonradioactive components were prepared by proprietary methods. Interstitial injections were also performed in subcutaneous tissues and/or muscle as controls for therapy and imaging.

Sample size estimation for measuring tumor size was obtained from earlier experiments and found to be triplicate (Appendix IV) based on a control experiment on rats with 13762 tumors. Groups of triplicate rats were studied. Therapy outcomes are tumor sizes at 20 days (S20) after injection. The survival rate estimation is unreliable because of the limited sample size of 3 and intervening events including reuse of the animal for additional experiments. Retention of radionuclides is detected by gamma camera (Siemens M-CAM) and PET (Siemens Inveon and Gamma Medica) scanner. Optical imaging was acquired using Luminal II XR instruments (IVIS, now PerkinElmer, Waltham, MA, USA) [6].

Results

Small Animal LRCT: 13762 Breast Cancer in F344 Rats

Suppression of tumor growth was observed following the intratumoral injection of radiopharmaceuticals as low as 0.5 mCi using yttrium-90 chloride, F-18 FDG, In-111- chloride, and I-131 sodium iodide and radioactivity between 0.5 mCi and 3 mCi (Fig. 8.1a, b). Serial images of triplicate rats receiving intratumoral injection of 0.5 or 2 mCi of I-131 sodium iodide showed a progressive transit of I-131 from the injection site to the systemic circulation (early visualization of the stomach and urinary bladder) and the rest of the body followed by clearance from the rest of the body (Fig. 8.2). Radiation dosimetry in the injection site (0 cm) and depth dosimetry (distance from the edge of injection) are estimated in Table 8.1 based on image-derived residence time of 0.7 hour and dosimetry models as in Chap. 6.

Retention rates of intratumoral injection of sodium iodide can also be estimated using CT to detect intratumoral injection of I-125 and sodium iodide as in Fig. 8.3. While there is a faster effective half-life for intramuscular retention of sodium iodide at 0.25 hour, the effective half-life for intratumoral sodium iodide is 0.5 hour. Therefore, the residence time should be ($0.5 \times 1.4 = 0.7$ hour).

Differential intramuscular retention of F-18 FDG is also noted with a residence time of 0.7 hour compared with F-18 NaI at 0.5 hour (Fig. 8.4). Tumor growth suppression by intratumoral injection of radionuclide can also be accomplished with positron emitters including Ga-68 and Cu-64 (as well as F-18) at injection doses of

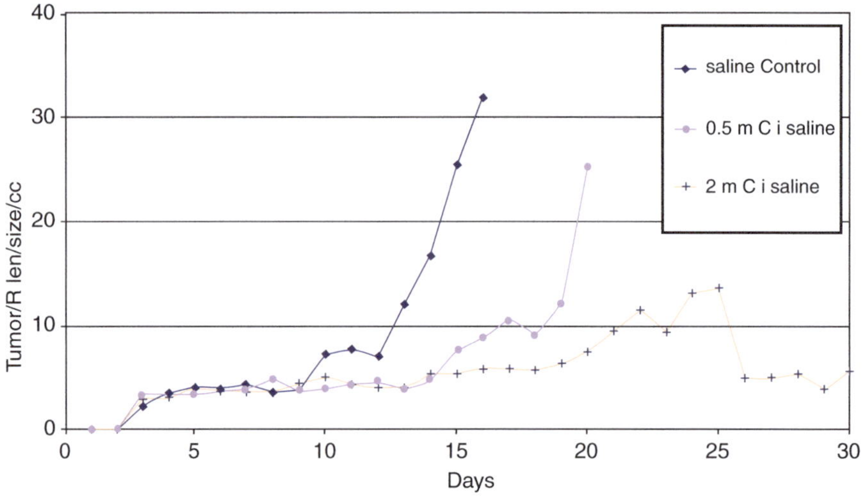

Fig. 8.1 (**a**) Suppression of tumor growth in rat 13762 tumor using I-131 NaI. (**b**) Suppression of tumor growth using F-18 FDG, In-111 Cl, and Y-90 Cl

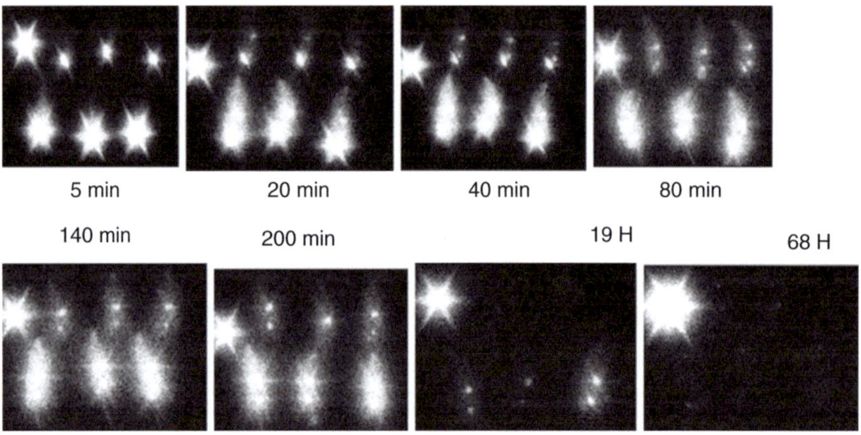

Fig. 8.2 Serial scintigrams of rats injected with 0.5 and 2 mCi of I-131 NaI

0.5–2 mCi in 0.2–0.5 ml (Fig. 8.5) [7] because of the ionizing beta energy before the subsequent annihilation adding to the annihilation ionizing gamma radiation.

The intratumoral residence times and tumor sizes at day 20 after inoculation (S20) are listed for commercially available radiopharmaceuticals of Tl-201 chloride, Sm-153 EDTMP, Tc99m-pertechnetate, and Re-188 perrhenate in Table 8.2. Various intervention schemes including change of pH and addition of ferric chloride, nonradioactive sodium iodide, and epinephrine were tested to derive the image-based residence time and outcome-based S20. The addition of ferric chloride or epinephrine increased the residence. However, at the dose range of 2.5 mCi, there was not sufficient effect to increase tumor suppression. This type of preliminary data may be helpful to design intervention schemes.

Table 8.1 Radiation dosimetry estimate of intratumoral injection of I-131 NaI

Radiation absorbed dose cGy	I-131 NaI	0.5 mCi	2 mCi
Physical half-life (h)	193.1		
Residence time (h)	0.7		
	Distance (cm)		
Distance from edge of 0.4 cc volume	Inside injectate		
	0	335.8	1343.2
	0.026	58.9	235.6
	0.075	8.9	35.6
	0.125	3.05	12.2
	0.175	2.2	8.8
	0.225	1.85	7.4
	0.3	1.45	5.8

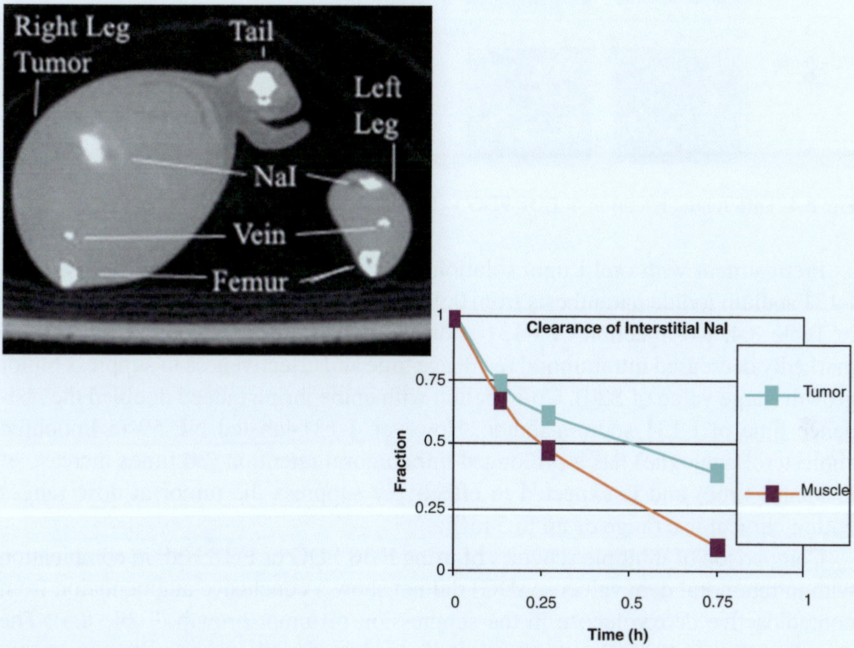

Fig. 8.3 Serial CT of rat following injection of 1 mg of NaI in Tumor/Muscle

A similar scheme can be used to test the interaction with other intervention schemes such as Photofrin II, addition of human serum albumin (HSA) or cytokines (IL-12 or GM-CSF), or intraperitoneal injection of DTPA to evaluate the potential interaction with LRCT on Table 8.3. Whether via intratumoral injection or intraperitoneal injection, Photofrin II did not have additive effects, while the addition of HSA, IL-12, or GM-CSF proved effective in tumor suppression by yttrium-90 or Ga-67 chloride. Pretreatment with injection of DTPA indeed reversed the effectiveness of yttrium-90 chloride but did not change the effectiveness of Y-90 chloride in the presence of HSA.

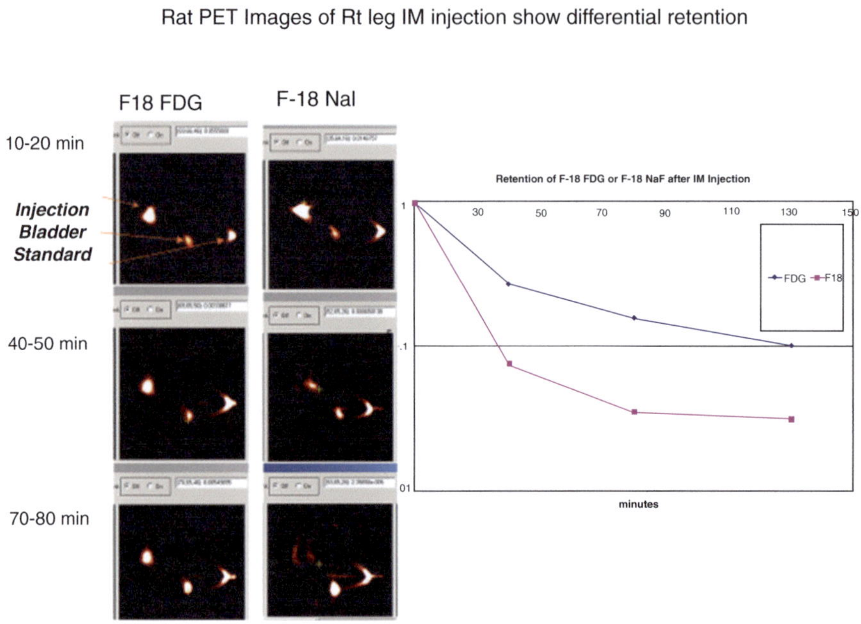

Fig. 8.4 Differential retention of F-18 FDG vs F-18 NaF after IM Injection

Pretreatment with oral Lugol solution decreased intratumoral residence time of I-131 sodium iodide parenthesis from 0.96 to 0.35 hour in a dose-dependent manner in Table 8.4. Co-injection of I-131 sodium iodide and I-127 sodium iodide also markedly decreased intratumoral residence time and effectiveness to suppress tumor growth (large value of S20). Co-injection with epinephrine indeed doubled the residence time of I-131 sodium iodide. However, I-131-labeled NP 59 (a lipophilic cholesterol analogue) has a prolonged intratumoral retention (20 times increase of residence time) and is expected to effectively suppress the tumor at dose ranges within clinical use range of up to 5 mCi.

Comparison of multiple schemes of using F-18 FDG or F-18 NaF in combination with intratumoral deoxyglucose (DG) did not show a conclusive augmentation from nonradioactive deoxyglucose in the suppression of tumor growth (Table 8.5). The combination of F-18 FDG and epinephrine indeed was found to suppress tumor growth.

Ga-67 gallium iron macroaggregate (GIMA) has been found to remain in the injection site for multiple days and be detectable by MRI up to 17 days and has a dose-dependent relationship in terms of its ability to suppress tumor growth (Table 8.6) [8, 9]. Ga-67 citrate had a shorter intratumoral residence time (17.8 hours) than gallium 67 chloride (27.3 hours). Ga-67 citrate's intratumoral residence time was not prolonged with the addition of ferric chloride, while the addition of ferric chloride tool Ga-67 chloride markedly increased the residence time to 37.6 hours.

Indium-111 DTPA has a rapid clearance from the tumor with a residence time of 0.4 hour, while indium chloride has larger residence time of 20 hours, when the pH of the injectate is between 5 and 9. With the addition of ferric chloride, intratumoral residence time is prolonged to 36–40 hours and effective in suppressing tumor

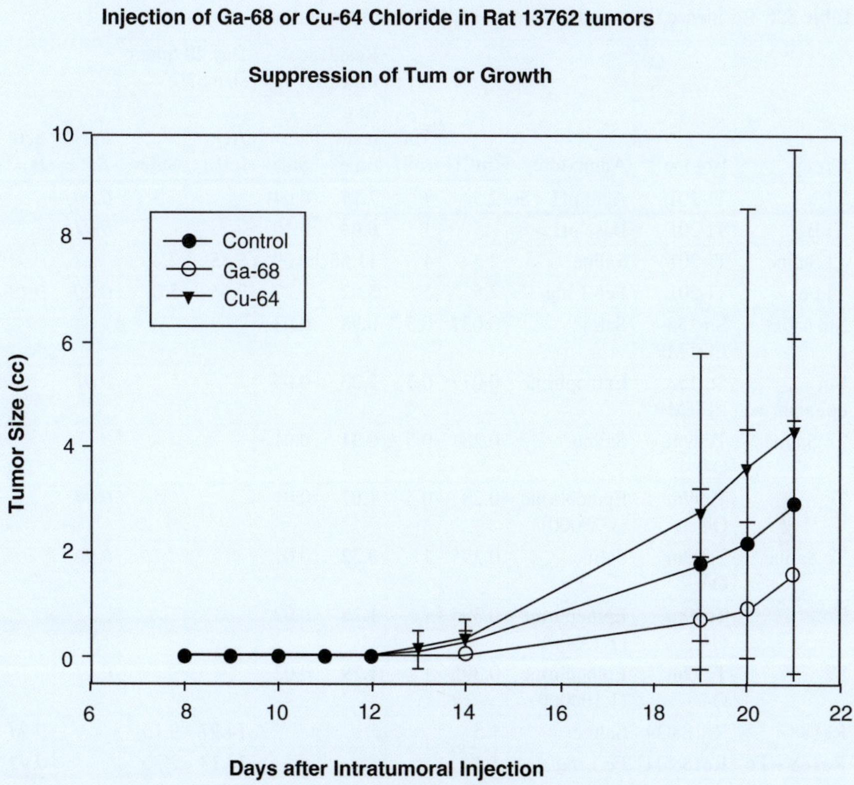

Fig. 8.5 Suppression of tumor growth by Ga-68 and Cu-64 chloride

between 1.5 and 2.2 mCi (Table 8.7). Co-injection with Gd-DTPA provides a rapid clearance of In-111 residence time of 1.3 hour but managed to provide significant tumor suppression. Pre-injection of intraperitoneal DTPA followed by indium-111-labeled biotin results in a moderate decrease of residence time to 11.9 hours. The addition of ferric chloride, gadolinium chloride, or HSA markedly increased residence times of In-111-chloride to provide tumor suppression better than the control. In-111-chloride injection test dose of In-111-Zevalin (monoclonal antibodies against CD20 in lymphoma) also demonstrates good retention in the breast tumor with a residence time of 19.9 hours. These findings suggest that prolonged interstitial or intratumoral retention of radionuclides may be accomplished by choosing biochemical properties of the radiopharmaceutical including molecular sizes (e.g., Zevalin and human serum albumin (HSA)) or coprecipitation (In-111 chloride, or with iron chloride) or lipophilicity (in the case of I-131 NP59 as in Table 8.4). Such an increase in retention may increase the efficacy of tumor suppression. In these days of molecular targeting, ligand binding or antibody binding (e.g., Zevalin for lymphoma) is certainly another alternative to increase retention time of the radionuclide for better efficacy. Whether these latter types of molecular targeting by ligand binding provide better efficacy than by other mechanisms such as lipophilicity (NP59) or coprecipitation (In-111 chloride with ferric chloride) or large molecular

Table 8.2 Residence times and outcome of LRCT and intervention

					Residence time (h)		Day 20 tumor size S20			
Group	Isotope	Admixture	(mCi)	Vol (ml)	Avg resid time	Stdev	Avg (mL)	Stdev.	*Resid T P =*	*S20 P =*
TI A	TI-201	Acid pH < 5	2.5	1	**7.77**	0.04			*0.00*	
TI B	TI-201	Base pH > 8	2.5	1	**6.04**	0.10			*0.01*	
TI Saline	TI-201	Saline	2.5	1	**11.65**	0.69	**5.35**	2.46		*0.01*
TI Fe	TI-201	Fe# 1 mg	2.5	1	**5.02**	1.39	**9.66**	5.07	*0.00*	*0.13*
Sm saline	Sm153 EDTMP	Saline	0.037	0.5	**0.98**	0.03				
Sm epinephrine	Sm153 EDTMP	Epinephrine	0.037	0.5	**2.23**	0.05			*0.01*	
Tc Saline	Tc99m O4	Saline	0.28	0.5	**0.31**	0.01				
Tc	Tc99m O4	Epinephrine (1:25000)	0.28	0.5	**1.07**	0.01			*0.04*	
Tc Saline	Tc99m O4	Saline	0.395	1	**0.32**	0.01			*0.96*	
Tc	Tc99m O4	Epinephrine (1:12500)	0.395	1	**1.28**	0.02				
Tc	Tc99m O4	Epinephrine (1:100000)	0.395	1	**1.79**	0.03			*0.01*	
Re188	Re188O4	Saline	1.5				**14.97**	9.15		*0.93*
Re188 + Fe	Re188O4	Fe 1 mg	1.5				**14.13**	2.90		*0.92*
Re188	Re188O4	Saline	0.1	0.2	**0.35**	0.02				
Re188 Fe	Re188O4	Fe# 1 mg	0.1	0.2	**0.81**	0.02			*0.18*	
Re188 Saline	Re188O4	Saline	0.144	0.5	**0.39**	0.01			*0.31*	
Re188 Epinep	Re188O4	Epinephrine	0.144	0.5	**1.60**	0.02			*0.00*	
Re188 Saline	Re188O4	Saline	0.18	1	**0.45**	0.02			*0.05*	
Re188 Epinep	Re188O4	Epinephrine 1:50000	0.18	1	**1.51**	0.02			*0.00*	
Re188 NaI	Re188O4	NaI-100 mg/ml	0.18	1	**0.44**	0.01			*0.13*	
Re188 NaI	Re188O4	NaI + Epinephrine	0.18	1	**1.32**	0.02			*0.02*	
Control							**14.39**	3.22		

size retention needs to be empirically verified in animal models. Perhaps, a more convenient predictor would be the interstitial retention time measurement that could be accomplished in hours instead of days as in tumor growth curves.

Yttrium-90 is a powerful radionuclide that has been used for therapy. It is a beta emitter that does not directly emits photons for imaging. Nevertheless, analysis of the Bremsstrahlung radiation by scintigraphy (as described in Chap. 7) was able to derive residence times. Intratumoral injection of yttrium-90 chloride at doses of

Table 8.3 Residence times and outcome of LRCT using Y-90 and Ga-67

					Day 20 tumor S20		*P (T-test)*
Group	Isotope	Subgroups	Amount (mCi)	Remarks	Avg vol	Stdev.	*vs Control*
		Photofrin II vol		Photofrin II route			
Control		0	0		**55.50**	0.86	
Ga67	Ga67	0.8	1	IP	**27.87**	8.27	*0.03*
Y90	Y90	0.8	1	IP	**17.58**	2.27	*0.00*
Ga67	Ga67	0.8	1	IT	**16.61**	6.15	*0.01*
Y90	Y90	0.8	1	IT	**24.95**	13.88	*0.06*
Ga67	Ga67	0.4	1	IT	**25.43**	8.17	*0.02*
Y90	Y90	0.4	1	IT	**28.45**	10.33	*0.04*
Y90	Y90	0	1	Control	**10.55**	9.82	*0.01*
Ga67	Ga67	0	1	Control	**26.31**	11.71	*0.05*
Photofrin II control		0.8	0	IT	**78.07**	29.99	*0.48*
Photofrin II control		0.8	0	IP	**33.27**	11.45	*0.22*
Control					**10.11**	2.10	
Bilat tumor control					**12.06**	6.74	*0.67*
Y90HSA	Y90		0.2	HSA	**244**	0.22	*0.02*
Y90HSA-IL	Y90		0.2	IL12 + HSA	**253**	0.06	*0.02*
Y90HSA	Y90		0.2	HSA	**S38**	5.35	*0.26*
Y90HSA-IL	Y90		0.2	IL12	**4.27**	2.09	*0.03*
GmCSFY90ILHSA	Y90		0.2	GmCSF + IL12	**3.75**	2.74	*0.04*
GmCSFY90HSA	Y90		0.2	GmCSF + HAS	**13.89**	10.17	*0.59*
		DTPA days					
Y90 Cl	Y90	0	0.1		**34.53**	8.26	*0.10*
Y90 Cl	Y90	0	0.6		**27.00**	33.81	*0.35*
Y90 Cl	Y90	7	0.1		**17.63**	8.62	*0.01*
Y90 Cl	Y90	7	0.6		**19.87**	17.74	*0.07*
Y90 HSA	Y90	1	0.1	HSA	**3.88**	0.79	*0.01*
Y90 HSA	Y90	1	0.6	HSA	**9.32**	10.22	*0.01*
Y90 HSA	Y90	7	0.1	HSA	**52.20**	17.94	*0.92*
Y90 HSA	Y90	7	0.6	HSA	**9.22**	8.14	*0.01*
Control		7	0		**50.87**	9.90	
Y90 Cl	Y90	7	0.3		**2.04**	0.79	*0.01*
Y90 Cl	Y90	1	0.3		**25.3**	0.10	*0.01*

0.1–0.5 mCi in 1 mL was able to suppress tumor growth (Table 8.8). However, animals failed to thrive with 100% lethality between days 25 and 30, and necropsy results demonstrating a loss of bone marrow and liver function. Injection of yttrium-90 chloride after intraperitoneal injection of gadolinium-DTPA also suppressed tumor growth with a residence time of 10.8 hours. Additional ferric chloride

Table 8.4 Residence times and outcome of LRCT using I-131 and intervention

Group	Isotope	Admixture	(mCl)	Vol (ml)	Residence time (h) Avg resid time	Stdev	Day 20 tumor size S20 Avg (mL)	Stdev.	*Resid T P =*	*S20 P =*
I131 po Lugol	I-131	Lugol po (1:10 0.3 ml)	0.1	1	**0.74**	0.03			*0.17*	
I131 po Lugol	I-131	Lugol po (1:10 0.3 ml)	0.5	1	**0.35**	0.00	**3.78**	0.04	*0.01*	*0.00*
I131 po Lugol	I-131	Lugol po (1:10 0.3 ml)	2	1	**0.39**	0.01	**5.04**	1.42	*0.03*	*0.00*
I131 NaI	I-131	Saline	0.0612	1	**0.96**	0.02				
I131 NP59	I-131	Saline	0.0612	1	**20.34**	0.32			*0.02*	
IDA	I-131	Diatrizoic acid	0.09	0.4	**0.61**	0.03			*0.12*	
I131AAI	I-131	Saline	0.05	0.5	**0.34**	0.01			*0.02*	
I131 + 1127	I-131	NaI 40 mg	0.041	0.5	**0.28**	0.01			*0.01*	
I131 + 1127 SSKIpo	I-131	NaI 40 mg SSKI 1:10,0.3 ml po	0.041	0.5	**0.35**	0.02			*0.01*	
I131 + Conray	I-131	Conray	0.11	0.4	**0.16**	0.01			*0.01*	
I131 + Ethoidol	I-131	Ethiodol	0.11	0.4	**0.56**	0.04			*0.18*	
I131 + DG	I-131	DG	2	0.5			**10.90**	4.73		*0.01*
I131 repeat	I-131	Saline	0.1	0.5	**0.37**	0.01			*0.02*	
I131 + I127 repeat	I-131	NaI 40 mg	0.1	0.5	**0.28**	0.00			*0.02*	
I131 HSA	I-131	Saline	0.0387	1			**3.36**	0.42		*0.00*
I131 + 1127	I-131	NaI 100 mg/ml 1 ml (in 10 min)	3	1	**0.42**	0.01	**20.35**	3.03	*0.02*	*0.01*
I131 Epinephrine	I-131	Epinephrine 1:25000 SSKI po	0.5	1	**3.39**	0.02			*0.00*	
I131 Saline	I-131	Saline SSKI po (1:10 0.3ml)	0.21	1	**0.76**	0.02			*0.19*	
I131 NaI	I-131	NaI 100 mgl-/ml SSKI po	0.21	1	**0.67**	0.01			*0.10*	
I131 Epinephrine	I-131	Epinephrine 1:25000 SSKI po	0.21	1	**2.07**	0.07			*0.00*	
I131 NaI Epinephrine	I-131	18 + 19	0.21	1	**2.02**	0.05			*0.05*	

Table 8.4 (continued)

Group	Isotope	Admixture	(mCl)	Vol (ml)	Residence time (h) Avg resid time	Stdev	Day 20 tumor size S20 Avg (mL)	Stdev.	*Resid T P =*	*S20 P =*
I131 Epinephrine	I-131	Epinephrine	3mCi	1			**29.79**	6.23		*0.60*
I131 NaI	I-131	NaI	3mCi	1			**32.16**	2.34		*0.97*
I131 NaI Epinephrine	I-131	NaI Epinephrine	3mCi	1			**36.93**	6.78		*0.34*
Control							**32.07**	2.74		*1.00*

or gadolinium chloride did not further enhance the ability to suppress tumor and substantially increased the residence time. Small activities of yttrium-90-labeled Zevalin were able to suppress tumor growth and retained in the tumor for a longer residence time of 15 hours suggesting a potential efficacy in treatment.

Small Animal LRCT: B16-OVA Tumor in C57BL/6 Mice

Intratumoral injection of radionuclide for suppression of tumor was also accomplished in a mice melanoma model according to established methods. A group of six mice were studied. Tumor size was measured up to 15 days after tumor inoculation. Following intratumoral injection of up to 1.5 mCi of F-18 FDG, Cu-64 chloride, or Ga-68 chloride, suppression of tumor growth was noted, more pronounced with Cu-64 and F-18 and less with the Ga-68 group as seen in Fig. 8.6 [7]. These experiments further confirm the findings of tumor suppression by positron emitters in the rat model. It also allows the evaluation of possible splenic T cell activation and recruitment if there were successful immune recognition and amplification in the mice model with human melanoma graft. However, further analysis including splenic T cell immunostaining could not confirm the increase in activated T cell as immune response to tumor treatment. Further experiment will be required to characterize this model that involves immunocompromised mice and human tumors.

Large Animal LRCT Model: cTVT in Dogs

Animals larger than rats provide better approximation to human dimensions in terms of pharmacokinetics and in terms of radiation dosimetry. The canine transmissible venereal tumor model has been established for radiologic investigations to allow intervention experiments and was chosen for expiration of LRCT. This model requires an initial suppression of the immune system, specifically the T cells, using

Table 8.5 Residence times and outcome of LRCT using F-18 and intervention

Group	Isotope	Admixture	(mCi)	Day 20 tumor size S20 Avg (mL)	Stdev.	*S20 P* =
FDG	F18	Saline (0.2 mL)	0.2	**46.82**	15.46	*0.74*
FDG + DG	F18	DG (0.2 mM, 0.2 ml)	0.2	**41.84**	21.29	*0.95*
FDG + DG	F18	DG (2 mM, 0.2 ml)	0.2	**33.07**	10.38	*0.32*
FDG	F18	Saline (0.2 mL)	1	**19.13**	0.83	*0.01*
FDG + DG	F18	DG (0.2 mM, 0.2 ml)	1	**37.91**	8.75	*0.58*
FDG + DG	F18	DG (2 mM, 0.2 ml)	1	**29.54**	1.10	*0.10*
F18	F18	Saline (0.2 mL)	0.2	**33.99**	12.81	*0.42*
F18 + DG	F18	DG (0.2 mM, 0.2 ml)	0.2	**29.27**	2.84	*0.09*
F18 + DG	F18	DG (2 mM, 0.2 ml)	0.2	**27.57**	2.52	*0.06*
F18	F18	Saline (0.2 mL)	1	**25.76**	7.46	*0.07*
F18 + DG	F18	DG (0.2 mM, 0.2 ml)	1	**32.73**	4.42	*0.21*
F18 + DG	F18	DG (2 mM, 0.2 ml)	1	**20.83**	4.32	*0.02*
F18	F18		3	**33.71**	9.80	*0.34*
F18 + DG	F18	DG (5 mM)	3	**46.48**	17.30	*0.78*
FDG	F18		2.7	**37.38**	10.91	*0.58*
FDG + DG	F18	DG (5 mM)	2.7	**40.00**	2.69	*0.70*
FDG	F18		1.35	**44.59**	8.02	*0.84*
FDG	F18		1	**40.08**	2.57	*0.71*
FDG	F18		2	**24.45**	2.26	*0.03*
FDG	F18		3	**17.00**	15.38	*0.07*
FDG + DG	F18		2	**19.97**	3.34	*0.01*
FDG	F18		2	**19.14**	12.24	*0.05*
FDG	F18		2	**29.13**	0.31	*0.09*
FDG + NaI	F18	NaI	0.1	**20.47**	5.28	*0.02*
FDG + NaI + Epinep	F18	FDG + NaI + Epinephrine	2	**14.56**	0.11	*0.00*
DG 2 mM (0.2 mL)				**28.96**	12.87	*0.22*
Saline (0.2 mL)				**44.97**	22.58	*0.89*
Control				**27.51**	2.63	*0.07*
Control				**50.95**	22.01	*0.61*

cyclosporine A for 2 weeks, followed by implantation of stored tumor trunks from the previous animal host. It also required a continuous and indefinite maintenance of cyclosporine A treatment to allow continuous tumor growth. If cyclosporine A was interrupted, the animal would acquire tumor immunity so the implanted tumor and future tumor inoculation would not grow. By itself this tumor model is interesting in that exposure of the tumor to an animal confers tumor immunity. The cancer biology of such mechanism may be further explored for application to human defense against tumors.

Table 8.6 Residence time and outcome of LRCT using Ga-67 and intervention

					Residence time (h)		Day 20 tumor size			
Group	Isotope	Admixture	(mCl)	Vol (ml)	Avg resid time	Stdev	Avg (mL)	Stdev.	*Resid T P =*	*S20 P =*
Ga67	Ga67cit		0.50				**18.45**	7.19		*0.03*
Ga67	Ga67cit		2.00				**17.94**	12.75		*0.13*
Ga67A	Ga67cit	Acid pH < 5	0.60		**3.04**	0.05			*0.19*	
Ga67B	Ga67cit	Base pH > 8	0.60		**4.28**	0.36			*0.01*	
Ga67cit Fe	Ga67cit	Fe	0.05	0.10	**2.80**	0.08			*0.07*	
Ga67cit	Ga67cit		0.05	0.10	**1.97**	0.04			*1.00*	
Ga67cit IT	Ga67cit		0.07	0.10	**17.82**	1.26			*0.04*	
Ga67cl Fe	Ga67 cl	Fe# 1 mg	1.70	0.50	**37.63**	1.07	**29.18**	7.72	*0.00*	*0.34*
Ga67 Fe	Ga67	Fe# 1 mg	2.50	1.00	**31.00**	1.77	**18.92**	13.76	*0.00*	*0.17*
Ga67	Ga67	Saline	2.50	1.00	**17.55**	0.73	**16.47**	11.32	*0.00*	*0.08*
Ga67	Ga67	Saline	0.10	1.00	**5.94**	0.23			*0.04*	
Ga67Gd	Ga67	Gd# 1 mg	0.10	1.00	**3.93**	0.16			*0.18*	
Ga67cl IM	Ga67 cl	Saline	3.00	1.00	**5.49**	0.96			*0.04*	
Ga67cl IT	Ga67 cl	Saline	3.00	1.00	**27.29**	0.50			*0.09*	
Ga67cl IM	Ga67 cl	Saline	0.25	0.50	**2.28**	0.01			*0.24*	
GIMA	Ga67		0.10				**20.69**	8.42		*0.07*
GIMA	Ga67		0.20				**20.78**	5.56		*0.02*
GIMA	Ga67		0.50				**17.74**	2.59		*0.00*
GIMA	Ga67		1.00				**15.22**	10.63		*0.06*
GIMA	Ga67		2.00				**2.50**	0.75		*0.00*
GIMA	Ga67						**4.00**	0.74		*0.00*
PBS							**36.28**	11.71		*0.88*
PBS							**33.88**	2.48		*0.74*
Control							**50.95**	22.01		*0.34*
Control							**32.07**	2.74		*0.42*

Under institutional animal use committee approval with the protocol with which an excerpt is on Appendix II, six animals were studied and inoculated with cTVT after 2 weeks of immunosuppression using cyclosporine A. Tumors were inoculated under image guidance to the left lung, right lung, left prostate, and right prostate (Fig. 8.7a, b). In one animal, supply of cyclosporine A was interrupted for several days and ongoing tumor regressed. Subsequent implantation of tumor did not grow in spite of reinstitution of immunosuppression with cyclosporine A.

Table 8.7 Residence time and outcome of LRCT using In-111 and intervention

					Residence time (h)		Day 20 tumor size			
Group	Isotope	Admixture	(mCi)	Vol (ml)	Avg resid time	Stdev	Avg (mL)	Stdev.	*Resid TP =*	*S20 P =*
In	In-111		0.1	0.5	**20.06**	0.37			*0.16*	
In DTPA	In-111	DTPA	0.1	0.5	**0.43**	0.00			*0.00*	
In A	In-111	Acid	0.6	0.5	**19.81**	0.87			*0.01*	
In B	In-111	Base	0.6	0.5	**21.47**	0.63			*0.00*	
In Cl	In-111	Saline	1	0.5	**27.01**	0.41	**41.69**	7.92	*0.29*	*0.98*
In Cl	In-111	Saline	4	0.5			**23.56**	10.02		*0.09*
Incl PBS	In-111	PBS	1	0.5	**33.66**	0.32				
In Fe	In-111	Fe# 1 mg	2.2	1	**39.97**	0.82	**3.30**	0.69	*0.03*	*0.00*
In Fe	In-111	Fe# 1 mg	2.2	1	**37.52**		**2.95**	0.59	*0.04*	*0.00*
In	In-111	Saline	2.2	1	**29.38**	1.03	**7.42**	7.32	*0.30*	*0.00*
In Fe	In-111	Fe# 1 mg	1.5	1	**36.82**	8.82	**4.33**	1.32	*0.30*	*0.00*
In Gd	In-111	Gd# 1 mg	1.5	1	**27.44**	0.49	**3.95**	0.74	*0.00*	*0.00*
In GdDTPA	In-111	Gd DTPA 1:2000	1.5	1	**1.26**	0.11	**3.86**	0.31	*0.00*	*0.00*
In Bio ipDTPA	In-111	DTPA ip	0.05	1	**11.89**	0.85			*0.00*	
In I127 IM	In-111	I127 (50 mg - I/ml)	0.167	0.5	**3.62**	0.50				
In I127 IT	In-111	I127 (50 mg - I/ml)	0.167	0.5	**18.92**	0.43			*0.01*	
I127 then In	In-111	I127 (50 mg - I/ml)	0.167	0.5	**9.43**	0.80			*0.09*	
In Saline	In-111	Saline	0.167	0.5	**11.64**	0.38			*0.01*	
EC In	In-111	EC	0.176	0.5	**0.67**	0.01			*0.00*	
Ec-Biotin In	In-111	EC-Biotin	0.176	0.5	**0.86**	0.01			*0.00*	
DOTA In	In-111	DOTA	0.176	0.5	**0.62**	0.01			*0.00*	
DOTA-Biotin In	In-111	DOTA-Biotin	0.176	0.5	**0.61**	0.01			*0.00*	
In Saline	In-111	Saline	1.75	1	**26.90**	0.26	**14.59**	4.28	*0.02*	*0.01*
In Fe	In-111	Fe# 1 mg	1.75	1	**38.05**	0.45	**6.50**	5.23	*0.03*	*0.00*
In Gd	In-111	Gd# 1 mg	1.75	1	**24.24**	1.21	**5.19**	1.96	*0.04*	*0.00*
In Serum	In-111	Serum	0.2	0.5	**29.45**	0.74			*0.17*	
In Zavelin	In-111	Saline	0.2	0.5	**19.90**	1.01			*0.00*	
Control							**32.07**	2.74		*0.25*
Control							**50.95**	22.01		*0.56*

Table 8.8 Residence time and outcome of LRCT using Y-90 and intervention

					Residence time (h)		Day 20 tumor size S20			
Group	Isotope	Admixture	(mCi)	Vol (ml)	Avg res time	Stdev	Avg (mL)	Stdev.	*Resid T P =*	*S20 P =*
Y90 Saline	Y90	Saline	0.1	1			**3.83**	0.17		*0.00*
Y90 Saline	Y90	Saline	0.2	1			**3.26**	0.26		*0.00*
Y90 Saline	Y90	Saline	0.5	1			**3.61**	0.68		*0.00*
Y90 Fe	Y90	Fe (1 mg)	0.5	1			**3.69**	0.16		*0.00*
Y90 Gd	Y90	Gd (1 mg)	0.5	1			**3.94**	0.71		*0.00*
Y90 DTPA	Y90	Gd DTPA 1:2000	0.5	1	**10.76**	1.14	**3.68**	0.75	*0.01*	*0.00*
Y90 DTPA	Y90	Gd DTPA 1:1000	0.2	1			**3.87**	0.88		*0.00*
Y90 Zevaline	Y90	Saline	0.45	1	**14.48**	0.86			*0.00*	
Y90 Zevaline	Y90	Saline	0.225	1	**15.72**	2.25			*0.00*	
Y90 Zevaline	Y90	DG	0.05	1			**23.00**	7.56		*0.18*
Y90 Zevaline	Y90		0.02	1			**14.29**	10.93		*0.11*
Y90 Zevaline	Y90		0.1	1			**10.44**	5.09		*0.01*
Y90 Zevaline	Y90		0.05	1			**24.47**	9.96		*0.34*
Y90 Zevaline	Y90		0.1	1			**11.02**	6.16		*0.02*
Y90 IM	Y90	Saline	0.4	0.5					*0.49*	
Y90 IT	Y90	Saline	0.4	0.5					*0.51*	
Y90 Saline	Y90	Saline	0.475	1			**5.20**	1.48	*0.24*	*0.00*
Y90 Fe	Y90	Fe# 1 mg	0.475	1	**46.45**	0.71	**2.99**	0.10	*0.00*	*0.00*
Y90 Gd	Y90	Gd# 1 mg	0.475	1	**47.41**	0.90	**3.10**	0.26	*0.00*	*0.00*
Y90 Ca#	Y90	Ca# 1 mg	0.3	1	**26.67**	0.67			*0.00*	
Y90 Ca#	Y90	Saline	0.3	1	**1.19**	0.04			*0.02*	
Y90	Y90	Ca# 1 mg	0.3	1	**43.14**	0.28			*0.00*	
Y90Fe#DTPA	Y90	Fe# 1 mg	0.3	1	**44.60**	0.14			*0.00*	
Y90 Saline	Y90	Saline	0.3	1	**1.14**	0.04			*0.02*	
Y90	Y90	Epinephrine	1	1			**3.66**	0.31		*0.00*
Y90 NaI	Y90	NaI	1	1			**3.88**	0.49		*0.00*
Y90 NaI	Y90	NaI Epinephrine	1	1			**3.71**	0.42		*0.00*
YIMA	Y90		0.1	1			**1.64**	0.24		*0.00*
YIMA	Y90		0.2	1			**3.21**	2.08		*0.00*
YIMA	Y90		0.5	1			**1.47**	0.37		*0.00*
YIMA	Y90		1	1			**1.58**	0.22		*0.00*
YIMA	Y90		0.2	1			**6.97**	0.18		*0.00*
Cold YIMA				1			**26.06**	3.24		*0.07*
Control				1			**30.10**	4.15		

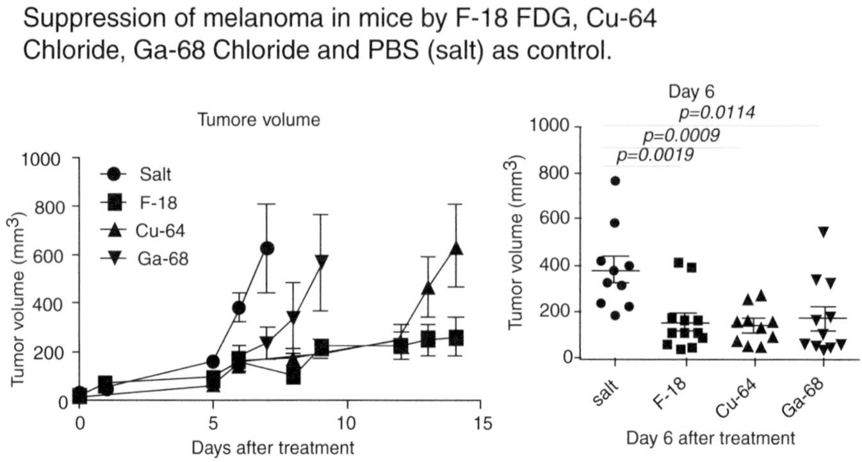

Fig. 8.6 Suppression of melanoma by F-18 FDG, Cu-64, and Ga-68 chloride

In one animal, 0.5 mCi of Ga-68 GIMA was injected under MRI guidance into the cTVT implanted into the right prostate. PET-CT of the pelvis revealed an intense initial tracer retention with SUV of 3144 (Fig. 8.8a). In another experiment, following the interstitial injection of 0.1 mCi of F-18 FDG, serial PET-CT images of the thorax show a persistent tracer retention at the injection site throughout the serial scanning with a residence time of 2 hours (Fig. 8.8b).

For another animal, cTVT were implanted into the left and right lungs after immunosuppression using cyclosporine A and confirmed by F-18 FDG PET-CT (Fig. 8.9a). Both tumors were localized, and their SUV were 6.2 and 6.5 in the left and right tumors, respectively (Fig. 8.9a) [10]. Intratumoral injection of Ga-68 GIMA was under MRI guidance to the right lung tumor, using the paramagnetic property of iron in GIMA. A dose of 0.27 mCi of Ga-68 GIMA was injected into the right lung cTVT, and the immediate Ga-68 PET-CT showed an SUV or greater than 1600 throughout the study of 2 hours (Fig. 8.9b). Retention of iron in the right lung tumor allowed measurement of the volume to be 0.5 ml. Together with radiation dosimetry models in Chap. 6, radiation dosimetry to the tumor and the surrounding tissues could be estimated. The 7-day follow-up F-18 FDG PET-CT (Fig. 8.9c) revealed a stable tumor SUV (6.6) in the right, while the untreated left tumor had continual increasing SUV (8.8), consistent with radiation dosimetry calculation of a moderate radiation-absorbed dose of 235 cGy to the right lung tumor as illustrated in Chap. 6. In this animal, partial necrosis of the right lung tumor was noted on necropsy.

Monitoring of Radionuclides in Animal LRCT Model Using Optical Imaging (Cherenkov Light Imaging, or CLI)

High-energy beta radionuclide emissions in water may produce visible light (Cherenkov light) of relatively low but measurable intensities that could be quantified by prolonged exposure and photon counting. Imaging is possible for

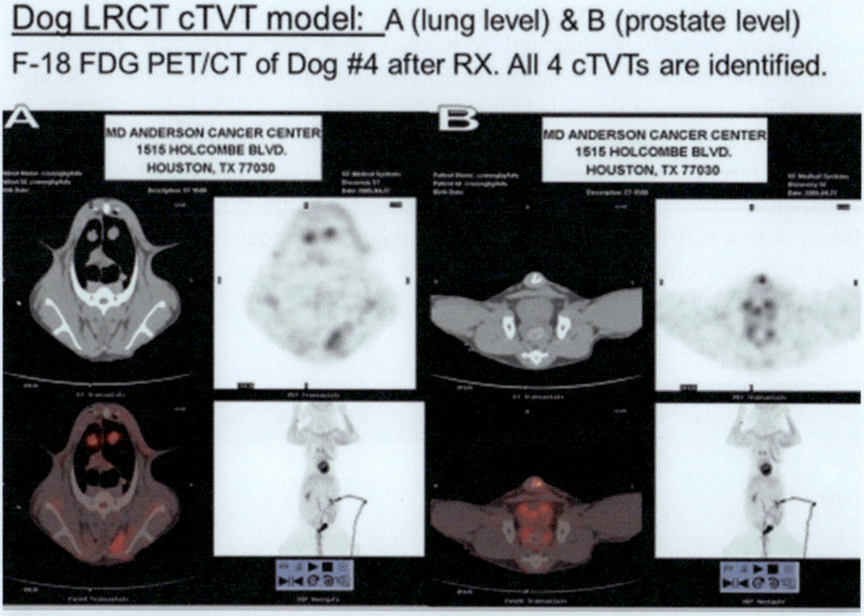

Fig. 8.7 PET-CT of cTVT tumors implanted in lungs (**a**) and prostate (**b**)

radionuclides such as I-131, Ga-68, F-18, Zr-89, and Cu-64 for sub-millicurie levels [6].

For instance, using a Luminal instrument, an anesthetized rat was injected with 1 mCi of Ga-68 compound A over the right shoulder and 0.2 mCi of Ga-68 compound B in the shaved skin over the left upper back as shown in Fig. 8.10. Quantification was accomplished with the use of a reference syringe with 0.4 mCi of Ga-68 standard. Serial scans from 5 to 180 minutes were acquired as in Fig. 8.10, and the photo counts of region of interests were tabulated. The effective half-lives from the plotted curves were calculated to be 69, 35, and 63 minutes for the Ga-68 standard, compound A in the right shoulder, and compound B in the left upper back, respectively. The respective residence times are 98, 50, and 91 minutes. The measured effective half-life findings (69 hours) in the Ga-68 standard inside the syringe have validated the use of Cherenkov light imaging in LCRT by approximating the physical half-life of 68 hours for Ga-68. Pharmacokinetics and radiation dosimetry profiles of different radiopharmaceuticals of the same radionuclides can thus be estimated and contrasted by comparing their half-lives and residence times.

This experiment indicated that compound A is subject to substantially faster clearance with a biologic half-life of 72 minutes (residence time of 50 minutes) compared to compound B with a longer biologic half-life of 854 minutes (residence time of 91 minutes). In that case, compound B would remain longer in the injection site to deliver higher radiation-absorbed dose. This method can be used to screen for potentially efficacious radiopharmaceuticals for LRCT based on residence times/effective half-lives. Potential limitations of CLI include tissue attenuation of light that renders less sensitive detection of photons from injection site deep to the surface as well as recirculating radionuclides that render less specific counting of photons.

Pharmacokinetic data from CLI in the above example can also help in designing radiopharmaceuticals. Compound A labeled with Ga-68 (physical half-life of 68 minutes) has a biological halftime of 72 minutes and residence time of 50 minutes, while compound B labeled with Ga-68 has a biological halftime of 854 minutes and residence time of 91 minutes. Since the radiation dosimetry depends on the residence time and the S value (a constant for the two compounds), the difference in radiation dosimetry from compound A versus compound B is 72/91, or 1:1.26. If Ga-67 with a half-life of 78 hours is used to label compound A and compound B, their respective effective half-lives would be 1.2 hour and 11.29 hours. Their residence time would be 1.7 hour and 16.26 hours, respectively. The difference in

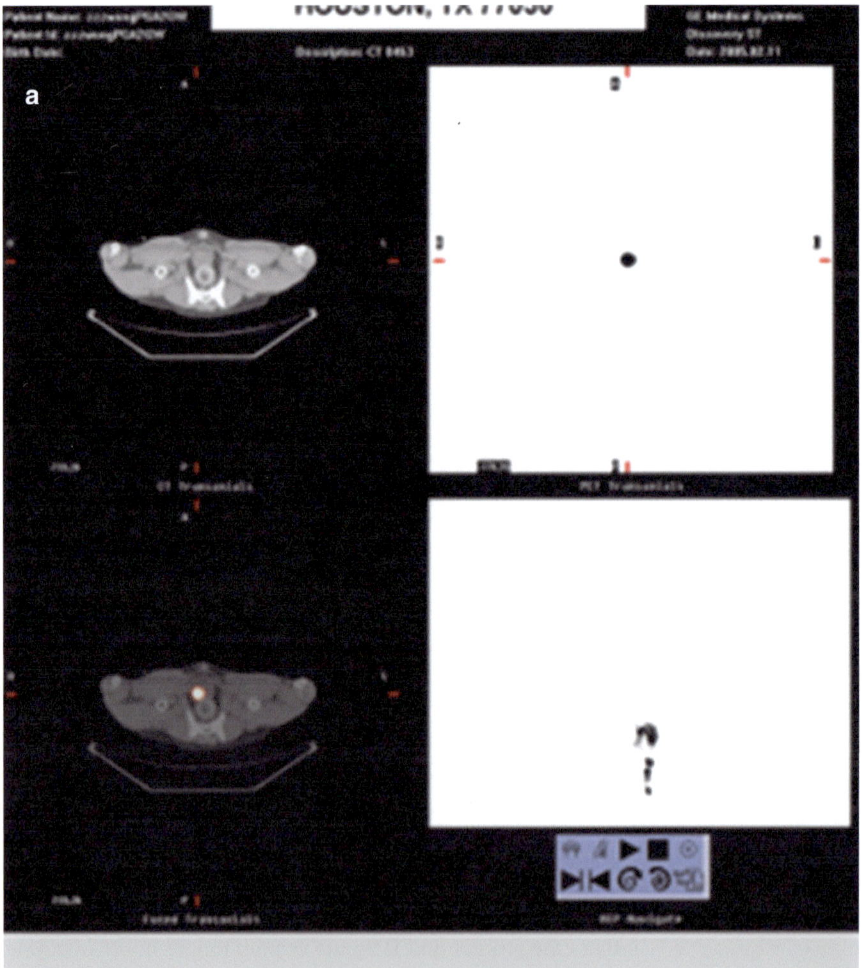

Fig. 8.8 (**a**) PET-CT of Ga-68 GIMA injected in the right prostate cTVT. (**b**) Serial PET after interstitial injection of F-18 FDG in lungs

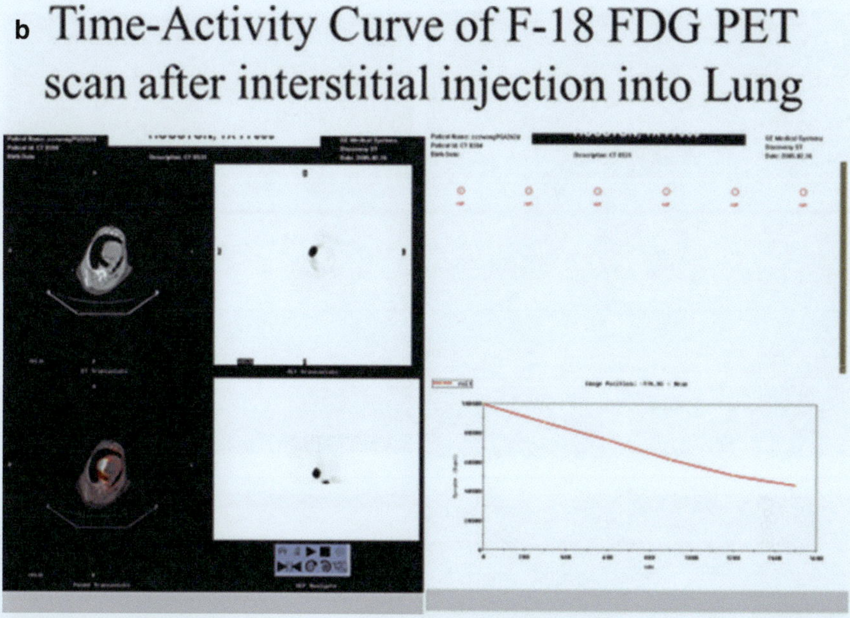

Fig. 8.8 (continued)

radiation dosimetry from compound A versus compound B would be 1.7/16.26, or 1:9.6, indicating that compound B labeled with Ga-67 would be a much more potent therapeutic agent than compound A, if they are labeled with Ga-67 instead of Ga-68. If the S values were also included for comparison, compound B labeled with Ga-67 will certainly be the choice for LRCT. When other radionuclides are contemplated to substitute Ga-68 to label compound A or compound B, radiation dosimetry can be also estimated. As long as there is good justification of similar biologic behavior or biologic half-life, effective half-life (hence residence time) of the new radiopharmaceutical can be calculated as a first approximation (the harmonic mean of biologic half-life of the radiopharmaceuticals and physical half-life of the radionuclide). More exact estimates of residence time require image-based time-activity curves of the region of interest on serial scans using CLI, scintigrams, PET, or SPECT.

Induction of Tumor Immunity in Animals After LRCT: Quest for Radionuclide Tumor Vaccine In Situ

Activation of immune system could be an effective mechanism to eradicate tumors and prevent cancer recurrence, as demonstrated by the example of the cTVT model. Solid tumors establish themselves by escaping immune surveillance via multiple mechanisms through creation of barriers, excretion of tumor growth factors,

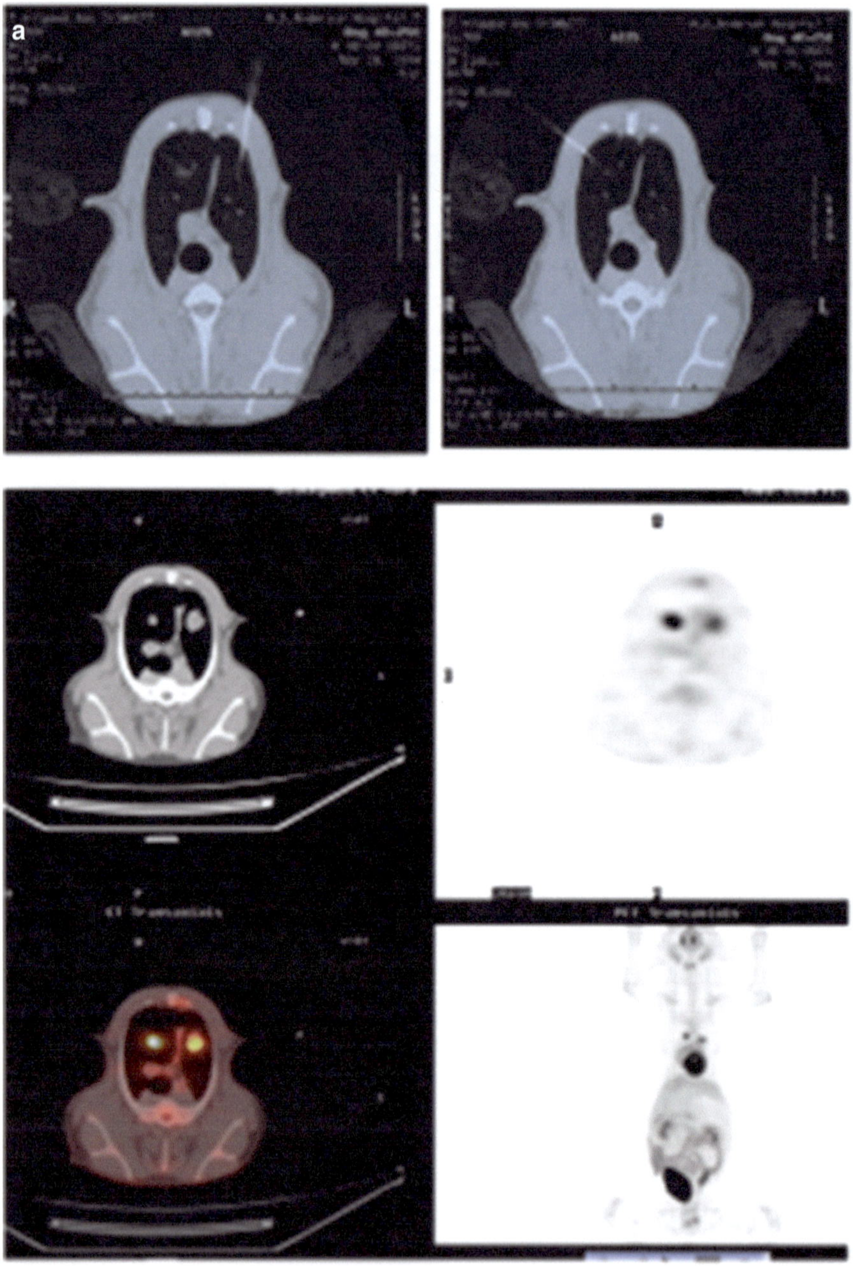

Figs. 8.9 (**a**) CT-guided implantation of cTVT in left and right lungs. (**b**) MRI-guided injection of Ga-68 GIMA and Ga-68 PET-CT. (**c**) MRI monitoring of GIMA, F-18 FDG PET monitoring of tumors

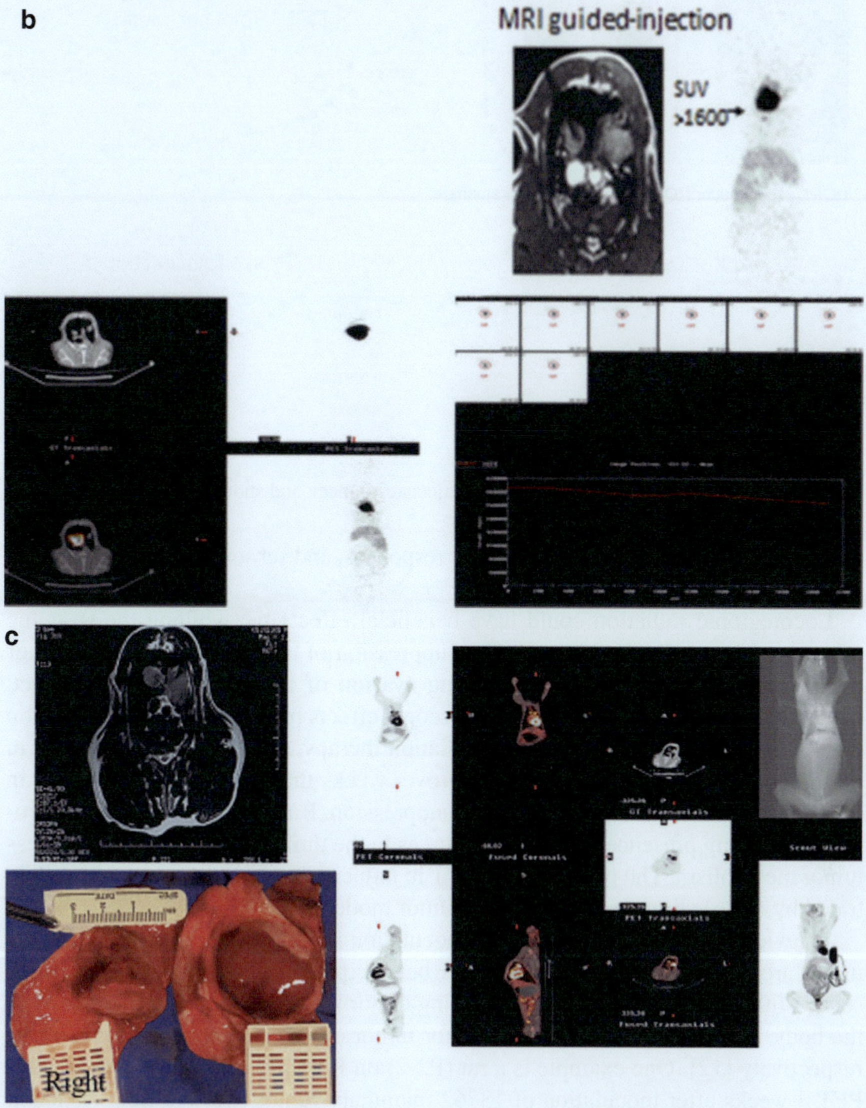

Fig. 8.9 (continued)

inhibition of APC immune recognition, and amplification of circulating immune cells. Reestablishment of immune surveillance including immune recognition to treat a cancer patient could be complicated by multiple factors including adverse effects from chemotherapy on immune cells and the stimulatory effects of inflammation and infection. Therapeutic modalities including alkylating chemotherapeutics, radiofrequency ablation, cryoablation, and absolute alcohol injection could interrupt the orderly mechanism of immune recognition by macrophages and APC,

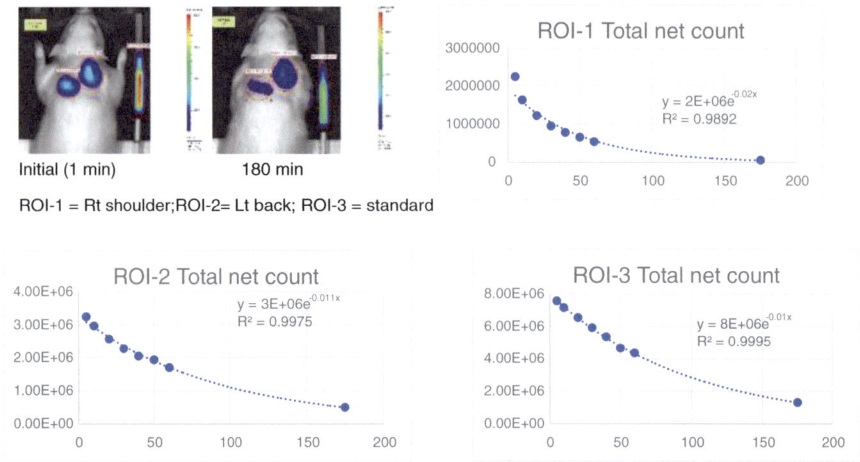

Fig. 8.10 Cherenkov light imaging of Ga-68 injectates in neck and shoulder

amplification and recruitment of cellular responses, and serous response to establish effective tumor eradication.

Locoregional radiation could have beneficial effects by avoiding the systemic effects on immune cells and rendering suppression of tumor replication and tumor metabolism that contribute to continuing evasion of immune responses. In fact, there are ongoing trials to explore the abscopal effects from external beam radiation therapy [11]. Current external beam radiation therapy, in practice, is performed in multiple short sessions of minutes daily over weeks that may allow tumor cells in different phases of cell cycles to escape suppression. Radionuclide therapy can provide continuing presence of radiation sources in the tumor to continuously suppress tumor metabolism. The potential of LRCT in inducing tumor immunity can be illustrated by observations in the rat 13762 tumor model.

A review of tumor incidence after inoculation of 13762 tumor showed that the tumor arose in 93% rats that have never been exposed to the tumor cells. After a successful LRCT, success rates of inducing tumor by inoculation into other parts of the body were 6/25, 0/15, 0/8, and 0/3 for tumor exposure of 1, 2, 3, and 4 times, respectively [12]. One example is a rat (P2-2) on Fig. 8.11 showing the F-18 FDG PET 3 weeks after inoculation of 13762 mammary tumor over the right shoulder. The control (P1-1) and two other rats treated with intratumoral absolute ethanol (P3-3) and Ga-67 GIMA (P4-1) also underwent F-18 FDG PET. Having been treated successfully twice with LRCT with two prior tumor inoculations, P2-2 did not show neither tumor presence nor growth in the right shoulder. Serial PET images over 4 weeks did not show a significant rise in the ratio of right to left forelimb in P2-2, compared with rising ratios over 4 weeks for other rats. These PET images also demonstrate no abnormal uptakes in other body parts in P2-2 in 3 weeks, further supporting the idea of exposure to tumor and successful intratumoral radionuclide therapy (or LRCT) as a potential means to produce a lasting immunity against tumors. Therefore, nuclear tumor vaccine in situ (NuTuVIS) should be further explored for human applications.

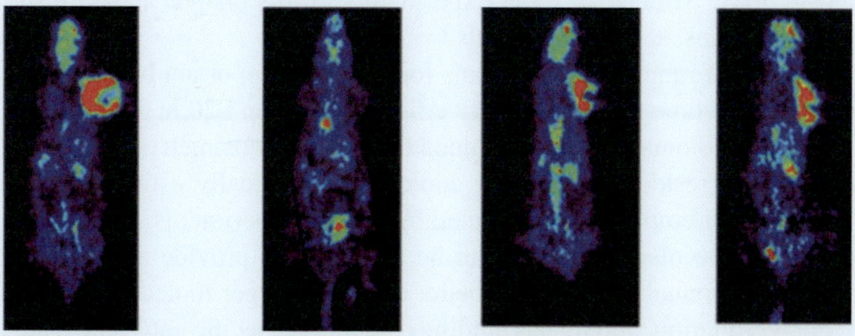

Ratio of Tumor to Lt forelimb	Week 1	Week 2	Week 3	Week 4
P1-1	0.86	15.36	21.35	euthanized
P2-2	*0.70*	*0.85*	*0.52*	*0.75*
P3-3	1.10	4.25	6.39	8.31
P4-1	1.80	8.85	6.78	13.23

Fig. 8.11 F-18 FDG PET images of rats 3 weeks after tumor innoculation

Conclusion

Animal models are necessary and convenient means to test radiopharmaceuticals for LRCT before human use to establish the efficacy and safety profiles. Three different animal models of LRCT in mice, rats, and dogs were reviewed. Tumor suppression was accomplished with LRCT in rat and mice models with relatively small level of radioactivity (0.1–5 mCi). Tumor suppression was also observed in large animal experiment using dogs showing sufficient suppression of lung tumor metabolism and confirming prolonged retention of tracer in the selected radiopharmaceuticals. The locoregional distribution of radionuclide can also be studied using Cherenkov light imaging (CLI) for convenient screening and comparison of potential LRCT candidly radiopharmaceuticals. Incidental findings of tumor growth suppression from prior exposure to tumor and successful LRCT have opened opportunities for intratumoral injection of radionuclide for successful treatment and induction of immunity and, hence, nuclear tumor vaccine in situ (NuTuVIS).

Discussion

Animal models have demonstrated that LRCT is possible in mouse, rat, and dog tumor models. Whether it is feasible to apply to human cancer treatment depends on whether the radiopharmaceuticals are available, accessible, efficacious, or with acceptable toxicity profiles. An effective delivery of the radiopharmaceutical to the tumor target is crucial but can be made possible by image guidance using ultrasonography, CT, MRI, PET, or SPECT. Monitoring of the radiopharmaceutical is also important to assure sufficient target coverage over space and time can be accomplished by PET, SPECT, or CLI. Experiments in this chapter have illustrated the above possibilities, at least in animals.

The choice of radiopharmaceuticals for LRCT is important but could be guided by the residence time and preliminary efficacy based on S20 in the enclosed tables. The choice of radionuclide can be guided by radiation dosimetry models in Chap. 6, assuming good residence time that could be theoretically estimated by biologic characteristics or empirically confirmed by animal experiments.

Multiple molecular properties can be exploited to provide a longer interstitial retention of radionuclides to effect better efficacy. Larger molecular sizes, lipophilicity, coprecipitation, and ligand binding (including specific antibodies) are all possible means to increase retention time and hence increase efficacy. Radionuclide retention times can be measured by scintigraphic imaging including planar images, PET, SPECT, and CLI.

The use of commercially available radiopharmaceuticals has the advantage that systemic toxicity profiles are published and available. Systemic toxicity will be less an important concern as long as the total LRCT dose is below the published upper limits of dose approved for systemic administration. Typically, the physical material of the radiopharmaceutical is minute, less than micrograms. Therefore, locoregional chemical toxicity should not be significant. Locoregional radiotoxicity is indeed the concern but would be the intended result to the target tumor. Monitoring will be important to quantify retention of the radiopharmaceutical to estimate the geographic coverage and radiation-absorbed dose to the target tumor.

Multiple interventional schemes could be tested and applied including adding other compounds and pretreatment as well as posttreatment medication such as DTPA, Lugol solution, epinephrine, or human serum albumin. This type of interventional schemes to alter or augment pharmacokinetics of radiopharmaceuticals in LRCT will allow further applications to increase efficacy and to decrease toxicity of radiopharmaceuticals for LRCT.

Acknowledgments and Disclosure The author is indebted for skillful assistance and thoughtful discussions to each team member: Kamran Arhar MD, Gary Whitman MD, Jason Staford PhD, Shuang Wang MD, Leonard Chow MD, Yuetang Wang MD, Vicenzo Wong MD, Osama Mawlawi PhD, Adres Fonnegra DDS, Mei Song MD, Farrah Chickerneo DDS, Meiling Zhuang MD, Charles Kinsley PhD, Peggy Tingley DVM, Suzzane Craig DVM, LaToya Ingram MS, Patrick Hwu MD, and Sharon Davis.

The funding of experiments of this study was partly provided by US NIH grants R21CA89891 and R21CA97729, a US DOD Army Breast Cancer Research Grant BC020808, and a Univ. of Texas MDACC University Cancer Foundation Grant (#94712), as well as royalty from licensing of an issued US Patent (8329141) to the author as the sole inventor and UTMDACC as the assignee.

Competing Interests The author declares that he has no conflict of interest.

Appendix I: Excerpts/Flowchart from Rat 13762 Tumor Model Protocol

Specific Aim: To evaluate the tumor response to internal radiation targeted therapy in tumor-bearing animal models by radiation detection and dosimetry.

F-344 rats (10 rats/compound[1]/cell-line[2])

Rats will be inoculated subcutaneously with 0.1 ml of a tumor cell-line suspension (10^5 cells/0.1 ml/rat) into the right hind leg, intrascapular space, or in the right or left shoulder or axillary space using a 25-guage needle. Rats will be chemically restrained with isoflurane less than 5 minutes for this procedure.

Studies will be performed once tumor volume is between 0.8 and 1 cm in diameter. Tumor volume is usually reached between days 14–17.

Rats will be anesthetized and imaged[3] (baseline)

Treatment[4]

Group I	Group II
5 rats	5 rats
(2 mCi/compound/rat; i.t.)	(10 mCi/compound/rat; i.t.)
Radiation monitoring[5**]	Radiation monitoring[5**]
Tumor size measurment[3]	Tumor size measurment[3]
CO_2 euthanization[6]	CO_2 euthanization[6]

1. Compound (14 compounds, 10 rats per compound, 2 cell-lines; total *280* rats):
   ^{177}Lu-chloride, ^{177}Lu-HSA (human serum albumin), ^{177}Lu-DTPA (diethylenetriamine penataacetic acid), ^{188}Re (perrheneate, control), ^{67}Ga-chlroide, ^{67}Ga-HSA, ^{68}Ga-chloride, ^{68}Ga-HSA, ^{90}Y-chloride, ^{90}Y-DTPA, ^{90}Y-HSA, ^{111}In-chloride, ^{111}In-HSA, and ^{18}F-FDG (14 compounds).
2. Cell-lines: 13726 (rat mammary cell-line) and IL-45 (rat mesothelioma cell-line)
3. Two rats from all groups will get FDG for either microPET imaging in rooms SB.8005 and SB.8015, PET/CT imaging in room G3.3579, or PET imaging in room G3.3673. Tumor volume will be measured ([l × h × w]/2) daily by calipers. Tumor tissue specimen will be used for immunohistochemical analysis. Rat will be anesthetized by ketamine cocktail (ketamine/xylazine/acepromazine; 75–100 mg/kg, 2–6 mg/kg, 1–2 mg/kg, respectively, inject (ip) 20–30 minutes during imaging.
4. Treatment: Agents listed above will be administered intratumorally (i.t.).
5. Radiation monitoring will be performed using external radiation detectors immediately after intratumoral injection until complete decay of isotope.

   A pilot study of up to ten rats will be performed to determine feasibility of continuous data collection via externally applied dosimeters. InLight nanoDot dosimeters (Landauer Inc) will be taped with Steri-strips over the injection site. These dosimeters are approved for use in humans for single point radiation measurement. The device measures 10 mm × 10 mm × 3 mm. Rat jackets will be placed on rats to minimize movement of the devices and protect them from removal by the animal. In the pilot we will use a short half-life radioisotope; dosimeters will be removed within 8 hours. No additional animals are required for this pilot.

   After 3 months of observation, all rats resistant to 13762 tumor implantation will be re-inoculated (subcutaneously, intramuscularly, or intravenously) with either 13762 or IL45 cells. This step will be repeated every 3 months until resistance is overcome and rats develop tumors, or until rats are 2 years of age.
6. Rats will be euthanized by CO_2 if tumor exceeds 2 cm or beyond 2 years. For rats weighting more than 200 grams, euthanasia will be performed by injection with Nembutal at 100 mg/kg following by cutting open the chest.

Appendix II: Excerpts/Flowchart from Mice Melanoma Tumor Model Protocol

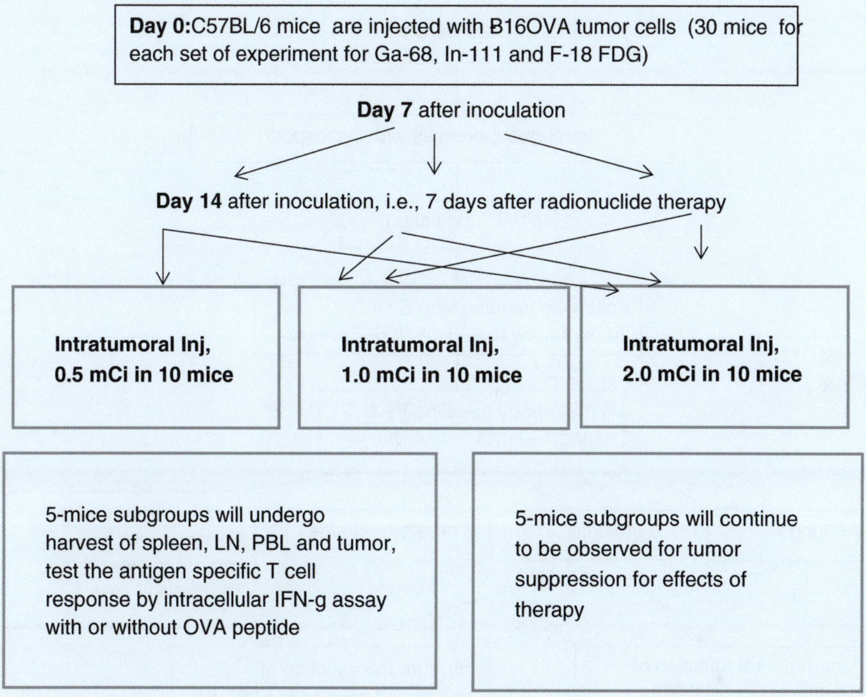

B16-OVA subcutaneous inoculation 4×10^5 B16-OVA cells in 0.1 ml PBS s.c. injection on the flank of mice using 27G1/2 needle.

Tissue collecting 50 μl blood/mouse will be collected from tail vein bleeding before euthanization and all other organs will be collected immediately after mice euthanize.

Euthanize CO_2 on day 10 when isolate BM cells from donor mice; CO_2 when sacrifice receipt mice; a second method of cervical dislocation will be added. For the group in which suppression is successful, observation will be extended up to 8 months or until euthanasia criteria is met. For those mice with successful tumor suppression, reinoculation of tumor may be performed after tumor free for 3 months from initial inoculation.

Objective, readouts, and comparisons The objective is the antigen-specific CD8 T cell response induced; the readout will be the percentage of IFN-g secreting CD8 T cell upon in vitro OVA stimulation in total lymphocytes gate in each tissue.

Appendix III: Flowchart from Dog cTVT Tumor Model Protocol

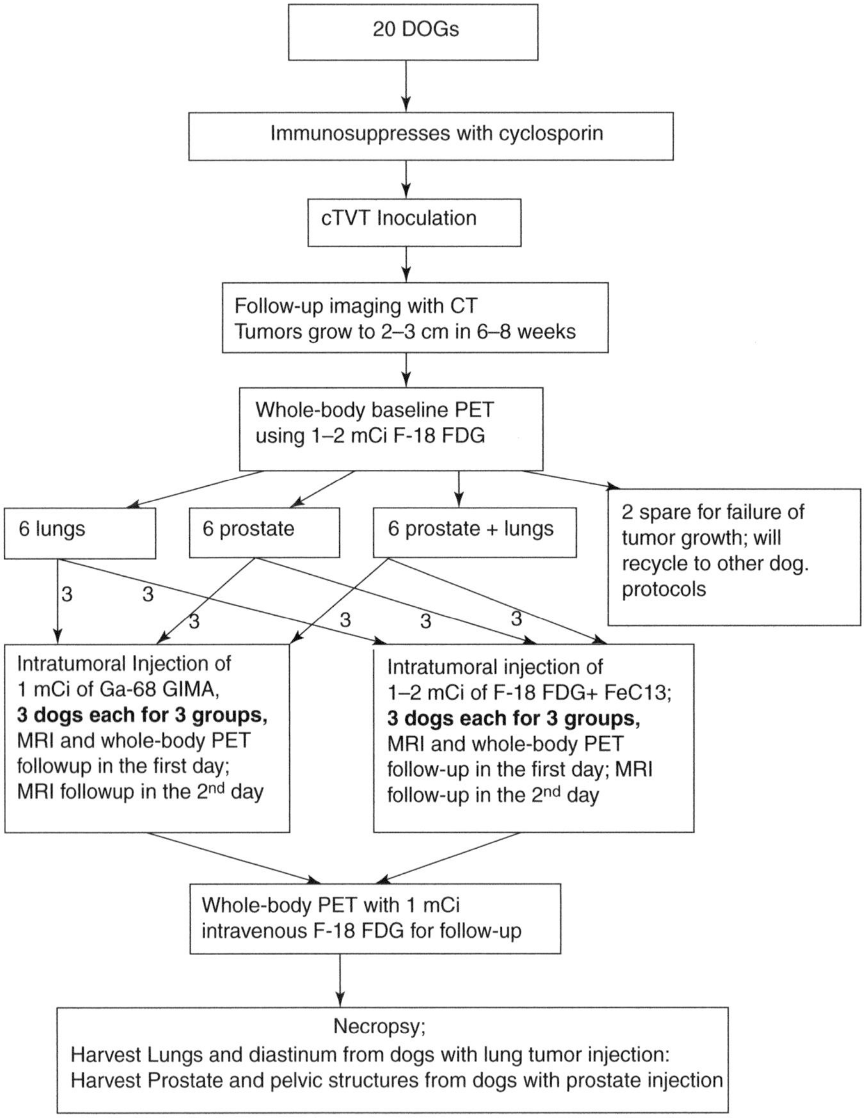

Appendix IV: Sample Size Estimation for Rat Tumor Suppression Experiments

Statistical Justification for the sample size of three rats per group in Protocol #03-03-03641

The sample size was calculated using a Statistical Software: *PS Power and Sample Size Calculation version 2.1.31* provided by the Vanderbilt University Medical Center http://biostat.mc.vanderbilt.edu/twiki/bin/view/Main/PowerSampleSize

The assumptions are as follows:

1. Tests group and control group have independent means
2. Alpha of 0.05
3. Power of 0.95
4. Mean of 8.4 cc on day 14 or 22.2 cc on day 17
5. Standard deviation of 2.4 cc on day 14 or 6.3 cc on day 17
6. Identical number of test group and control group, or, $M = 1$
7. (4) and (5) are based on a set of 6/2003 experimental results from the control group of rats injected intratumorally with phosphate buffered saline only. This calculation set derives the number of rats required to show statistically (Student's T-test) different tumor growth pattern than those of the control rats at the end of the 2nd week between day 14 and day 17.

The calculation proceed as following:

PS logging enabled 4/7/2005 8:14:02 PM

Type of study: T-test
Requested output: Sample size
Design: Independent
alpha = 0.05 power = 0.95 DIFF = 8.4 SIGMA = 2.4 M = 1
Sample size = 3

Type of study: T-test
Requested output: Sample size
Design: Independent
alpha = 0.05 power = 0.95 DIFF = 22.2 SIGMA = 6.3 M = 1
Sample size = 3

Reference

Dupont WD, Plummer WD. Power and sample size calculations: a review and computer program. Control Clin Trials. 1990;11:116–28. or

Dupont WD, Plummer WD. Power and sample size calculations for studies involving linear regression. Control Clin Trials. 1998;19:589–601.

This calculation is based on a Control Experiment in June 2003.

References

1. Schecter RL, Woo A, Duong M Batist G. In vivo and in vitro mechanisms of drug resistance in a rat mammary carcinoma model. Cancer Res. 1991;51(5):1434–2.
2. Biouin S, Basue MF Chappard D. Rat models of bone metastases. Clin Exp Metastasis. 2005;22(8):605–14.
3. Rodriguez AB, Peske JD, Englehard VH. Identification and characterization of tertiary lymphoid structures in murine melanoma. Methods Mol Biol. 2018;1845:241–57.
4. Ahrar K, Madoff DC, Gupta S, et al. Development of a large animal model for lung tumors. J Vasc Interv Radiol. 2002;13(9 Part 1):923–8.
5. Zayas YR, Molina MAF, Guerra RT, Padilla CR. Evaluation of a canine transmissible venereal tumour cell line with tumour immunity capacity but without tumorigenic property. J Vet Res. 2019;63(2):225–33.
6. Komarov S, Zhow D, Liu Y, Tai YC. Cherenkov luminescence imaging in transparent media and the imaging of thin or shallow sources. J Biomed Opt. 2015;20(3):06011.
7. Wong FC, Naff K, Liu C, Ferguson A, Hwu P. Intratumoral positron emission cancer therapy (IPECT) using F-18 FDG, Cu-64 Cl and Ga-68 Cl. J Nucl Med. 2013;54(Supp 2):313P.
8. Wong FC, Wang S. Locoregional ablation of rat breast cancer using Ga-67 iron macroaggregates (GIMA) and Y-90 iron macroaggregates (YIMA). Eur J Nucl Med Imaging. 2004;31(2Suppl):S297.
9. Wong FC, Wang S. Paramagnetic radiopharmaceuticals of Iron and gadolinium macroaggregates. Eur J Nucl Med Imaging. 2004;31(2 suppl):S387.
10. Wong FC, Kim EE. Molecular imaging: translation from rats to dogs and humans. Curr Med Imaging Rev. 8/2009;5(3):137–43.
11. Liu Y, Dong Y, Kong L, et al. Abscopal effect of radiotherapy combined with immune checkpoint inhibitors. J Hematol Oncol. 2018;11:104.
12. Wong FC. Successful intratumoral radionuclide cancer therapy (IRCT) prevents growth of subsequently re-innoculated 13762 mammary tumors in rats. J Nucl Med. 2012;53(Supp 1):54P.

Chapter 9
Animal Cancer Therapy Models: Ready Translation to Humans

V. Behrana Jensen and Suzanne L. Craig

Introduction

Radionuclides have been used in the early 1900s for the treatment of skin lesions associated with tuberculosis. A few years later, radium was suggested for the treatment of cancer. In the mid-1900s, ^{131}I was used for the treatment of thyroid cancer. Later, in the 1980s, malignant melanoma was treated with radionuclides labeled with monoclonal antibodies. In the 1990s, strontium-89 was used to treat bone pain. Radioimmunotherapy (RIT) is the use of radiotherapy in combination with immunotherapy. A well-known example is the treatment of non-Hodgkin's lymphoma with the RIT combination of ^{90}Y ibritumomab tiuxetan. More recently, in 2013, the RIT combination therapy radium-223 dichloride was approved by the FDA for use in certain patients with prostate cancer. The ultimate goal of radiopharmaceutical therapy is to deliver cytotoxic levels of radiation and drug to the tumor while sparing the surrounding normal tissue [1].

Radionuclides have been used for diagnosis, staging, and treatment of cancer. Clinically, to use radionuclides, one must consider the half-life, additional products formed, tissue retention, safety, and toxicity. Animal models with and without cancer are required to study the effect of various radionuclides alone and in combination with other moieties prior to their use in clinical studies in humans. Animal models also assist in predicting efficacy. Through the process of testing, some of

V. B. Jensen (✉)
UT MD Anderson Cancer Center, Department of Veterinary Medicine and Surgery, Houston, TX, USA
e-mail: VBJensen@mdanderson.org

S. L. Craig
Medical University of South Carolina, Division of Laboratory Animal Resources, Charleston, SC, USA
e-mail: CraigS@MUSC.edu

F. C. L. Wong (ed.), *Locoregional Radionuclide Cancer Therapy*,
https://doi.org/10.1007/978-3-030-56267-0_9

these agents are used in animals to cure, diagnose, and modulate spontaneous or xenographic growths. Although pigs, dogs, hamsters, and rabbits have been used as animal models, rodents are by far the most common animal model for preclinical testing particularly for efficacy testing [1, 2]. Studies using animal models have demonstrated that there is a relationship between exposure to radon and lung cancer. Review of radium used in the luminizing industry proved that radium led to the formation of bone sarcoma and sinus carcinoma in many of the workers [3, 4].

There are several methods used to treat tumors. The most common strategies are shown in Table 9.1.

Animal models often serve as surrogates to study the effect of agents or procedures prior to their use in humans. Early studies using animals and radioisotopes looked at various doses, routes of administration, promotion of neoplasia by other substances, and the potential of radioisotopes for causing cancer [5–16]. Other studies were performed to decrease the biological effects of radiation [17]. In August 1945 during World War II, atomic bombs were dropped on Hiroshima and Nagasaki. These bombs instantly killed over 120,000 people. Others later died of radiation exposure. The effects of radiation in humans is often studied by reviewing incidents such as the atom bomb and miner exposure to radon and comparing direct administration of various radioisotopes to animals.

There are several types of studies that animal models have been utilized such as in drug development. Biodistribution studies are basic studies that determine via varying routes of administration where drugs are deposited in tissues and clearance rates through direct measurement [2]. Brachytherapy utilizes a form of radiotherapy where a sealed radiation source is placed inside or next to the area requiring treatment. It can provide a long-term antitumor effect with less damage to surrounding normal tissue [18, 19]. There also is the use of radionuclide probes for monitoring drug efficacy. Nuclear probes can be used for early detection and monitoring posttreatment of cancer. Examples of this sort of molecular imaging would be the use of single-photon emission computed tomography (SPECT) and positron-emission tomography (PET). These imaging modalities have high specificity and high sensitivity and can be quantified. SPECT and PET have the ability to measure tumor metabolism. PET does have the advantage over SPECT in that PET has greater capacity for spatial resolution and sensitivity, shorter scans, and improved image quality [20]. Radionuclides can be used as drugs due to their cytotoxic effect of radiation itself. Therapeutic beta- or alpha-emitter radiopharmaceuticals protect the surrounding tissue due to their short emission range. Positron-emitting radionuclides can be used for labeling diagnostic pharmaceuticals. The ability of gamma-emitters to penetrate tissue allows them to be used as tags for therapeutic cells. RIT which is the combination of monoclonal antibodies with a radionuclide is used to target and damage tumors. Common examples of RIT use

Table 9.1 Tumor treatment strategy

Tumor treatment strategy
Target blood vessel support (angiogenesis)
Target necrosis using necrosis-avid compound
Target the tumor proliferating cells

Table 9.2 Radioisotope half-lives and type of emitter

Radioisotope	Type of emitter	Half-life
Uranium-238 (^{238}U)	Alpha	4.46 billion years
Radon-222 (^{222}Rn)	Alpha	3.8 days
Polonium-218 (^{218}Po)	Alpha	3 minutes
Polonium-214 (^{214}Po)	Alpha	1.6×10^{-4} seconds
Radium-226 (^{226}Ra)	Alpha	1600 years
Radium-224 (^{224}Ra)	Alpha	3.66 days
Bismuth-213 (^{213}Bi)	Alpha	45 minutes
Holmium-166 (^{166}Ho)	Beta	26.8 hours
Yttrium-90 (^{90}Y)	Beta/gamma	64.1 hours
Phosphate-32 (^{32}P)	Beta	14.5 days
Strontium-89 (^{89}Sr)	Beta	50.5 days
Iodine-131 (^{131}I)	Beta/gamma	8.04 days
Iodine-125 (^{125}I)	Gamma	60.14 days
Iodine-123 (123I)	Gamma	13.22 hours
Samarium-153 (^{153}Sm)	Beta	46.3 hours
Lutetium-177 (^{177}Lu)	Beta/gamma	6.73 days
Technetium-99m (^{99m}Tc)	Gamma	6.02 hours
Fluorine-18 (^{18}F)	Positron	109.7 minutes
Copper-64 (^{64}Cu)	Positron/gamma	12.7 hours
Copper-67 (^{67}Cu)	Beta	61.83 hours
Gallium-68 (^{68}Ga)	Positron	68 minutes
Indium-111 (^{111}In)	Electron capture	67.32 hours
Rhenium-186 (^{186}Re)	Beta/gamma	90 hours
Rhenium-188 (^{188}Re)	Beta	16.98 hours

are for treatment of thyroid cancer and treatment of metastasis of prostate cancer to bone [21]. Table 9.2 lists several radioisotopes used in the treatment, diagnosis, and staging of cancer.

This chapter discusses the use of radioisotopes in animal models as various diagnostics and radionuclide therapies to further be translated into clinical use for the human patient population.

Rodent Animal Models

Brain Cancer

Despite gliomas and glioblastomas being two different types of brain tumors, both tumor types have high levels of morbidity and mortality. This is due to their recurrence rates and resistance to cancer therapy because of the blood-brain barrier. Newer and more curative therapies are needed.

Many different methods have been employed in mouse models utilizing radionuclides. One such example is the use of chlorotoxin as a new approach for targeted imaging and therapy for gliomas. Buthus martensii Karsch chlorotoxin (BMK CT) is a chlorotoxin-like peptide which was labeled with ^{131}I (^{131}I-BmK CT). This radiolabeled chlorotoxin was shown to inhibit glioma cell growth in a dose- and time-dependent manner. Intratumoral and intravenous injections of ^{131}I-BmK CT exhibited significant tumor inhibition efficacy and prolonged the life of tumor-bearing mice [22].

^{131}I is considered one of the radionuclides for theranostic use due to its relatively long half-life, radiation energy, and γ-emission for SPECT imaging. To study the intratumoral retention of ^{131}I-BmK CT, BALB/c female nude mice were administered a subcutaneous injection of C6 glioma cells into the right flank. When tumors reached a volume of 0.5–1.0cm^3, SPECT scans were performed at various time points post-intratumoral injections of ^{131}I-BmK CT or Na^{131}I. The results indicated the ^{131}I-BmK CT group had the radiolabeled peptide accumulated within the tumor during the entire period with low levels of radioactivity concentrated in the urinary system or other tissues. In contrast, Na^{131}I had rapid exclusion at 5 minutes postinjection from the tumor followed by accumulation in various organs [22].

The antitumor effects of intratumoral injection of ^{131}I-BmK CT was also compared to Na^{131}I-injected mice. The mice treated with ^{131}I-BmK CT had a survival rate of 25% after day 69, whereas those treated with Na^{131}I was day 34. In addition, H&E staining showed necrotic regions of the tumors of the group treated with ^{131}I-BmK CT when compared to no necrosis of the Na^{131}I group as well as no apparent organ damage to major organs [22].

In the exploration for new therapeutic approaches for brain tumors, the direct injection of ^{131}I-BmK CT into the tumor itself provided maximum radiation damage to the target area with minimal toxicity to surrounding tissues. Furthermore, the single injection showed no major toxicities to other major organs. The benefit of ^{131}I-BmK CT is it offers not only diagnostic data but therapeutic results as well [22].

Intralesional ^{131}I-labeled hyaluronectin glycoprotein is another substance which may be utilized for cancer therapy. A number of studies suggest hyaluronan (HA), the principal glycosaminoglycan in the extracellular matrix of the brain, is a critical factor for glioma invasion [23]. The advantage of hyaluronectin (HN) is its high and specific affinity for the HA-target molecule. To study the effects of ^{131}I-HN, athymic (SWISS-nu/nu) mice were injected subcutaneously at the base of the skull with CB109 glioblastoma cells. Tumors were palpable on day 5; however, treatment was initiated on day 10 post tumor inoculation of a single intralesional injection of ^{131}I-HN solution. The growth rate of the CB109 tumor slowed down as early as 8 days after treatment. The difference in tumor size between treated and control groups was also apparent by day 30. Four out of 54 treated mice remained alive up to 3 months without reaching tumor volumes as other treated mice had. The assumption of HN inhibitory effect on tumor growth could be the result of HN binding to HA, thereby inhibiting proliferation. The high HN affinity for HA and the HA role in tumor invasion make ^{131}I-HN a worthwhile agent to be investigated deeper as a therapeutics for gliomas [24].

Nanomedicine is an area of science that may also impact radiation oncology. Nanotechnology has enhanced cancer radiotherapy in the area of treatment delivery. The large surface area of nanomaterials makes them modifiable for high stability, biocompatibility, and interaction with particular cells. They are able to reach the target tissue due to the prolonged period in the bloodstream and decreased penetration to normal tissues due to tumor vasculature. Once inside cancer cells, nano-sized therapeutics can accumulate and be retained in the tumor for an extended time frame [25].

In glioblastoma patients, T-cell suppression usually occurs, and therefore the use of LNC^{188}Re-SSS in T cell-deficient mice was utilized. This is a lipid nanocapsule loaded with a lipophilic complex of Rhenium-188. Female, nude NMRI mice received intracranial injections into the right striatum of Lab 1 glioblastoma (GB) cells. On day 12 and 19 after inoculation of cancer cells, the center of the tumor was injected with LNC^{188}Re-SSS via the use of a convection-enhanced delivery (CED) system and compared to a control of Blank-LNCs. Mice which received no treatment or Blank-LNCs died within 27 days; however, 50% of those treated with LNC188-Re-SSS survived up to 104 days. This was a median survival rate of 180% relative to the Blank-LNC or non-treated mice. In addition, the tumor growth was approximately half the size in treated mice 6 days after the first LNC^{188}Re-SSS compared to the Blank-LNC mice. In fact, there was no detectable brain tumor at day 100 in surviving mice as evidenced by MRI or histological analysis. These long-term mice were rechallenged with Lab 1 GB cells in the left striatum; however, there was no increase in longevity. These mice as well as control animals died within 27 days of tumor cell implantation [26].

Analysis of the periphery of the tumor of mice treated with LNC^{188}Re-SSS revealed similar structure of the contralateral hemisphere which was not injected along with well-organized vasculature. Retention analysis showed 70% of the LNC^{188}Re-SSS was retained in the tumor 24 hours after LNC injection. The tumor tissue displayed more apoptotic cells and greater infiltration of innate immune cells. The peri-tumoral tissue had normal histology after LNC^{188}Re-SSS treatment indicating minimal side effects on healthy brain tissue. LNC^{188}Re-SSS is a promising treatment for phase I patients with relapsed GB due to its function in an immunosuppressive environment exhibiting good distribution and retention through tumor tissue without toxicity to healthy brain tissue [26].

Rhenium-188-loaded nanocarriers with a functioning antibody 12G5 immunotargeting CXCR4 has also been evaluated. Cancer cell CXCR4 overexpression contributes to tumor growth, invasion, angiogenesis, metastasis, relapse, and therapeutic resistance. Antagonism to CXCR4 can disrupt tumor-stromal interactions, sensitize cancer cells to cytotoxic drugs, and decrease tumor growth and metastatic load. Targeting CXCR4 is a beneficial therapeutic approach [27].

Female Swiss Scid mice were intracerebrally injected into the right striatum with U87MG GB cells that were transfected by a lentivirus coding for CXCR4 expression. Animals received 12G5-LNC^{188}Re, a nanocarrier combined with not only rhenium but function-blocking antibody, 12G5, which is directed against the CXCR4 on the surface via CED on day 12 post tumor inoculation. Only this single injection into the mouse striatum directly into the tumor was performed. Control mice received CXCR4-negative tumor cells. In addition, when testing the survival of mice with treatments, control treatments consisted of saline or blank LNCs. The results indicated a median survival time of 36 days for blank LNCs and saline versus 39 days for 12G5-LNC; however, approximately 50 days of survival were seen in mice injected with LNC^{188}Re. Furthermore, in a comparison of LNC^{188}Re and 12G5-LNC^{188}Re, mice tumors had regressed or totally disappeared, but new masses were visible via MRI as early as 65 days and 100 days, respectively. This study exhibited overall no significant differences between any of the rhenium-treated group; however, the 12G5-LNC^{188}Re-treated mice had a significant survival benefit compared to non-radiated mice [28].

The preclinical feasibility and worth of 12G5-LNC^{188}Re single infusion treatment resulted in an increase in the median survival time suggesting CXCR4 targeting has value in glioblastoma treatment. In addition, it was noted the benefit of 12G5-LNC^{188}Re was the higher retention in a CXCR4-positive tumor compared to other nanocarriers which in turn irradiate tissue more efficiently. The use of intracerebral nanocarrier for active targeting of tumor tissue may have benefit in human clinical trials [28].

Overexpression of PARP1 exists in various cancers including glioblastoma; therefore, targeting PARP1 with radiotherapy makes for a potential therapeutic agent [29]. Malignant gliomas reportedly have alterations in the p53 tumor suppressor gene [30]. Female athymic nude CrTac:NCr-Fo mice were subcutaneously injected with U87-p53 cells (glioma cell line expressing the p53 gene) into the right shoulder and allowed to grow for 2 weeks. Treatment consisted of a PEG/PBS vehicle, nonradioactive ^{127}I-PARPi, or fractionated doses of ^{131}I-PARPi injected intratumorally on day 0, 3, and 6 after tumor growth. There was no statistical difference in tumor volume between the vehicle and ^{127}I-PARPi group; however, there was reduction in tumor volume in the ^{131}I-PARPi compared to the vehicle group. In addition, mice receiving the fractionated ^{131}I-PARPi had a median survival rate of 29 days compared to 22 days with the vehicle cohort and 20 days with ^{127}I-PARPi group [29]. The combination of Iodine-131 radioisotope with the poly(ADP-ribose) polymerase enzyme shows promise for increasing survival rate.

Breast Cancer

The mouse 4T1 mammary carcinoma is a highly tumorigenic and invasive cell line which can spontaneously metastasize from the primary tumor in the mammary gland to multiple distant sites. This spontaneous metastatic disease is similar to human breast cancer with many characteristics that allows it to be suitable for animal models of human mammary cancer [31].

Breast cancer is the most common cancer in women worldwide; therefore, new treatments are constantly evaluated [32]. Cyclopamine (CPA) has been found to boost tumor response to radiotherapy. CPA encapsulated in a liquid-lipid nanoparticle system (CPA-LLP) would enhance the response of tumor cells to lutetium-177 conjugated to core-cross-linked polymeric micelles (CCPM-^{177}Lu) [33].

Nu/Nu mice were subcutaneously injected with murine 4T1 breast cancer cells in the right flank. Mice were injected intratumorally at approximately 7 days when the tumor was 0.1cm^3. Control mice were injected with saline three times in 1 week, one group received a single injection of CCPM-^{177}Lu, and one group received a combination of three injections of CPA-LLP IV over 1 week along with a single injection of CCPM-^{177}Lu when the first dose of CPA-LLP was administered. At the end of the study (day 120), the group with the best survival rate of 5 out of 9 mice was the combination therapy group compared to the other groups. All mice in the saline control group died within the first 3 weeks. The combination therapy not only killed cancer cells but also delayed tumor growth. The monotherapy with CCPM-^{177}Lu also slowed tumor growth; however, the combination therapy slowed tumor growth rate by a twofold difference. This localized radiotherapy has the benefit of avoiding whole-body radiation while delivering an effective treatment. Further studies are warranted to study the efficacy of the combination in other breast cancers [33].

Combination therapies as indicated above have merit in overcoming the limitations of conventional cancer treatments. Dual modalities with the use of radiotherapy (RT) combined with photothermal (PTT) therapy facilitated with a nanosystem can be used to suppress breast cancer through the eradication of tumor initiating cells (TICs). Ionizing radiation can cause lethal DNA damage to tumor cells which is the basis for the use of RT [34]. Photothermal therapy often uses infrared wavelength to treat medical conditions such as cancer. Discriminatory delivery of optical energy into tumors to destroy cancer cells can be accomplished through nanoparticles which absorb light in the near-infrared (NIR) regions to provide an opportunity for photothermal conversion [35, 36].

Female Balb/c mice were injected with 4T1 tumor cells into the mammary fat pads. When tumors reached 50–150 mm^3, intratumoral injections of copper-64-labeled copper sulfide nanoparticle ([^{64}Cu]-CuS) were given to the RT and RT/PTT group. Mice in the PTT received intratumoral injection of nonradioactive CuS nanoparticle (NP), and the control group received no treatment. Mice in the PTT and RT/PTT treatment groups were also treated with NIR laser 24 hours post-NP injection. By day 10, none of the ten mice in the untreated group survived. The mice treated with RT, PTT, or the combination therapy had a longer mean survival time; however, not only did the RT/PTT treatment group have a mean survival time of 48.7 days in comparison with the non-treated group, but two of the ten mice were tumor-free at day 60. In addition, lung metastasis which is the primary cause of mortality in breast cancer patients was noted in the control groups, mice treated with RT alone, and those treated with PTT alone. However, no visible lung metastasis was noted in the surviving mice treated with the combination therapy of RT/PTT up to day 60 when mice were euthanized for analysis [37].

The enhanced antitumor effect of [64Cu]-CuS nanoparticles along with NIR laser treatment may be due to prolonged retention of the beta-emitting nanoparticle in the tumor and/or the synergistic interaction between radiotherapy and heat. The data supports the feasibility of a therapeutic approach of combination therapy to suppress tumor metastasis [37].

Gold nanoparticles have become popular due to their good biocompatibility, range of sizes, and the attachment of ligands required to target cancer cells [38]. Trastuzumab is a monoclonal antibody targeting HER-2 positive breast cancer [39]. The combination of trastuzumab-modified gold nanoparticles (AuNP) labeled with lutetium-177 (trastuzumab-AuNP-^{177}Lu) targeted to HER2 has been studied as a form of local radiation treatment for HER2-positive breast cancer.

Female NOD/SCID mice were injected subcutaneously with MDA-MB-361 human breast cancer (BC) cells 1 day after being implanted with a sustained release 17β-estradiol pellet subcutaneously. When tumors reached 5–8 mm in diameter, mice were injected intratumorally with trastuzumab-AuNP-^{177}Lu or AuNP-^{177}Lu, and the control group received normal saline. The trastuzumab-AuNP-^{177}Lu significantly inhibited tumor growth over a 16-day period compared to the saline control mice group. The tumor growth inhibition of the AuNP-^{177}Lu mice was not significantly different than the normal saline group. In addition, transmission electron microscopy and dark-field/wide-field fluorescence microscopy confirmed that targeting HER2 with trastuzumab enabled binding and internalization of trastuzumab-AuNP-^{177}Lu breast cancer cells. This internalization of trastuzumab-AuNP into the BC cells is possibly promoted by a multivalent cross-linking mechanism which enhances the HER2 internalization by the binding of trastuzumab-AuNP to the BC cells [40].

Gold nanoparticles administered intravenously has limitations due to sequestration by the liver and spleen causing quick removal from the blood and therefore lower tumor uptake [41]; however, there are benefits to nanomedicine in conjunction with cancer therapy via other routes, especially locally. AuNP modified with polyethylene glycol (PEG) chains linked to trastuzumab and diethylenetriamine-pentaacetic acid (DTPA) labeled with Indium-111 (trastuzumab-AuNP-^{111}In) is another therapeutic utilized in breast cancer experiments to inhibit tumor growth.

Female CD1 athymic mice were subcutaneously implanted with a sustained release 17β-estradiol pellet followed by MDA-MB-361 human BC xenografts subcutaneously 2 days post-pellet implantation. Tumors were then permitted to grow 5–8 diameters prior to intratumoral injection of trastuzumab-AuNP-^{111}In or normal saline. Treatment injections were administered at multiple sites of the tumor for a more homogenous distribution of the AuNP. Only these two groups were studied due to data (not provided) indicating that unlabeled trastuzumab-AuNP intratumor into CD1 athymic mice had no tumor growth inhibition. The treatment of the CD1 athymic mice injected intratumorally inhibited tumor growth over a 70-day period, whereas the untreated control mice tumors reached eight times the original size over the 70 days. Furthermore, biochemistry results indicated no toxicity to the liver, kidneys, or hematopoietic system as well [42]. These results are promising toward HER2-positive BC with a local treatment.

Gelatin microspheres, a type of derivative of collagen, are a suitable tool for drug delivery due to its biocompatibility [43]. The efficacy of Iodine-131-labeled gelatin microspheres (^{131}I-GMS) was studied against breast cancer cells MCF-7 in nude mice. Female nude mice were injected into the mammary fat pads with MCF-7 human breast cancer cells. When tumors reached 1.0–1.5 cm in diameter, either ^{131}I-GMS or nonradioactive microspheres suspended in a 25% glucose solution were injected into the center of the tumor. On day 21 post-treatment, the tumor volume of the ^{131}I-GMS group decreased, whereas in the control group, the tumor volume increased drastically causing animals to be sacrificed by day 21 [43].

Seven weeks postinjection of the ^{131}I-GMS, the tumor tissue showed a large area of necrosis with very small amounts of residual tumor cells evidenced by histological examination. In addition, radioactive evaluation showed higher intratumoral radioactivity than other tissues with the exception of the lung which decreased rapidly by day 8 postinjection. It is important to note, if gelatin microspheres are used as carriers of radionuclides, the degradation period should be regulated based on the half-life of the radionuclide to prevent radionuclide release as a result of early degradation of the microsphere. Despite the degradation of ^{131}I-GMS, the radioactivity concentration was quite low throughout the study making ^{131}I-GMS a viable candidate for breast cancer therapy [43].

As more local cancer radiotherapies are explored, biodegradable drug delivery systems need to be evaluated as feasible choices. However, macromolecules and nanoparticles do not distribute across tumors via diffusion adequately. This limits interstitial infiltration [44]. There is rapid clearance of soluble polymers and drugs from tumor interstitium [45] and normal tissue toxicity from drug diffusion outside the target tissue or by systemic reabsorption which generates obstacles [46–49]. To overcome some of the issues indicated above, thermally sensitive elastin-like polypeptide (ELP) manufactured to undergo a soluble-insoluble transition between room temperature and body temperature was conjugated to Iodine-131. This phase transition forms a viscous microparticle from the liquid state upon intratumoral injection.

Female nude mice (Balb/C/nu/nu) were inoculated with murine 4T1 tumor cells in the right lower leg subcutaneously. Tumors were permitted to grow approximately 150 mm^3 prior to treatment initiation. Treatment consisted of intratumoral injection of [^{131}I]ELP$_1$ which went through the soluble-insoluble state and, [^{131}I]ELP$_2$, the negative control which remained in a soluble state upon injection or administration of a NaCl solution into the tumor. The ELP$_1$ had a 57-fold greater tumor retention rate than the ELP$_2$ and exhibited tumor inhibition from days 3 to 11 after intratumoral injection when compared to the NaCl solution and [^{131}I]ELP$_2$. There was also prolonged survival time when compared to the two controls [50].

ELPs may be engineered to undergo a soluble to viscous transition slightly below body temperature. Upon intratumoral injection, a radionuclide-ELP conjugate can form a depot in the tumor. Thermally sensitive ELPs are promising substances for intratumoral drug delivery due to the prevention of deiodination of the conjugated radionuclide and longer retention when compared to a soluble polymer; however, experimentation remains to be performed to advance this system for providing complete tumor regression [50].

Melanoma

Malignant melanoma can be a lethal cancer that arises from melanocytes which is usually resistant to chemotherapy and radiotherapy [51, 52]. Due to the radioresistance of melanomas, external radiotherapy has its limitations as a primary therapeutics [53, 54]; however, the exploration of intratumoral locoregional therapy may pose a possible treatment.

Certain therapies use high-energy radiation, alpha particles, to kill cancer cells. Biologically, alpha irradiation is relatively insensitive to oxygen deficiency, a condition in solid tumors which curtails the effectiveness of radiation treatment [55]. A form of therapy using alpha particles named diffusing alpha-emitter radiotherapy (DaRT) has been developed as a form of brachytherapy for the treatment of melanoma in mice. The DaRT method is based on the use of implantable radioactive sources which carry small amounts of Radium-224 (^{224}Ra). As ^{224}Ra decays, it emits Radon-220, Polonium-216, and Lead-212 into the tumor. The concept of DaRT in cell death may be accomplished by the emitters at therapeutic distance keeping the parent ^{224}Ra in the primary tissue source [56].

Athymic nude mice were implanted with C32 human melanoma tumor cells subcutaneously into the low lateral side of the back. When tumors reached approximately 8 mm in diameter, mice were treated with ^{224}Ra-loaded or inert wires. These wires are 4–6 mm and placed into the tumor. The treatment did not affect tumor growth; however, it was noted that untreated mice died when tumors reached 1000 mm^3 but the ^{224}Ra-loaded wire treated mice did not die despite tumors reaching 1000 mm^3 [56]. This possibly indicates an involvement with the metastatic process, and it is worthwhile to further investigate this method of locoregional therapy.

Targeted alpha therapy (TAT) has the potential of selectively destroying pre-angiogenic clusters of melanoma cells, thus inhibiting the development of metastatic melanoma. Utilizing an α-emitting radioisotope bismuth-213 (^{213}Bi) to a melanoma monoclonal antibody (9.2.27) to form a α-immunoconjugate (AIC), experiments indicated the AIC is highly specific and cytotoxic to melanoma cells [57]. The monoclonal antibody 9.2.27 forms a potent and specific immunotoxins which can inhibit growth of established human melanoma in nude mice [58]. This antibody is expressed on $\geq$90% of melanoma cell lines [59–61].

BALB/c nude mice were inoculated subcutaneously with melanoma xenografts in the flank. Control mice received saline. At day 2 postinoculation of melanoma cells, mice received intratumoral injections of the AIC when tumor volume reached 20–300 mm^3. At doses between 150 and 200 µCi of the AIC, there was a 10–25% weight loss in the mice. However, intratumor injection at the high dose resulted in complete and permanent regression of established tumors between days 40 and 60 post AIC therapy. At day 14, only two of four mice showed tumor regression at a dose of 50 µCi. Intratumoral injection of 25 µCi caused some regression of small tumors but was not able to provide regression of large tumors. There is a dose-response effect with a shorter average regression time resulting from a larger injected volume. Also, multiple AICs were required over a 1–2 day period when treatment began. Tumors in the control mice continued to grow [57].

Overall, local TAT has a potential application as a complementary therapy to surgery. The local targeted alpha therapy in the range of 12.5–200 μCi exhibited a high level of tumorigenesis and regression of tumors.

Unsealed high-energy beta-emitter has arisen as a new technique for local therapy of tumor control as an alternative to external radiotherapy. Beta rays have a short soft tissue penetration range which enables precise large radioactivity to be delivered without effects to the underlying normal tissue [62]. Holmium-166 (^{166}Ho), a beta-emitter, has a short half-life with a soft tissue penetration range of 8.7 mm which makes it an ideal radiotherapy source [63].

B16 melanoma tumor cells were inoculated subcutaneously into the back of female C57BL/6 mice. When tumors measured approximately 1 cm along its long axis and volume reached 492–631 mm^3, intratumoral injections of ^{166}Ho were administered with normal saline as the control. None of the control mice lived for greater than 16 days following the saline injection with mean tumor volume reaching 30 times the original volume. However, the mean tumor volume of the treated group showed a slow decrease in tumor size. The median survival ranged from 29 to 33 days due to various combinations of saline volume and ^{166}Ho dose without statistical significance. H&E staining of melanomas injected bilaterally into the flank for a side-by-side comparison with saline control and ^{166}Ho showed necrosis with growth delay in ^{166}Ho injected tumors [63].

Gamma camera imaging indicated ^{166}Ho was retained in the tumor without much leakage up to 6 days postinjection; however, macro-autoradiography revealed the injected radiotracer did not distribute uniformly which can lead to tumor regrowth or marginal failure. In fact, most of the treated animals died of tumor regrowth or marginal failure creating a probable limitation. A larger volume of the vehicle with ^{166}Ho or multiple tumor injections at various sites of the tumor could reduce the technical limitation. It should be noted, though, that a larger volume can increase the potential of overlying skin damage [63].

Intratumoral injection of beta-emitting radionuclide ^{166}Ho has promise as an alternative for local control of malignant melanomas. It may be utilized as an additional therapy to the conventional external radiotherapy or chemotherapy. Further studies using continuous radiation via this method should be considered for investigation [63].

Since internal radiotherapy with Holmium-166 into B16 melanoma proceeded to decrease tumor size and growth rate but didn't produce complete remission, other treatments are researched such as dendritic cell (DC) therapy to determine if it could improve therapeutic results. Dendritic cells (DCs) are specialized antigen presenting cells in peripheral tissues such as the skin. Skin DCs migrate to draining lymph node where they interact with naïve T cells to generate an immune response to tumors [64]. The combined ^{166}Ho- and DC-based immunotherapy was investigated as a local radiotherapeutic. The hypothesis was intratumoral ^{166}Ho would release tumor antigen and decrease tumor size while the injected DCs would take up the tumor antigen and migrate to regional lymph nodes creating a T lymphocyte immune reaction [65].

Female C57Bl/6 mice were inoculated subcutaneously with malignant B16F10 melanoma cells. When tumors reach approximately 1 cm in diameter (10–14 days post melanoma cell injection), mice were treated with either 1) immature DC (D6) only or 2) ^{166}Ho only, 3) not treated, or 4) treated with D6 on day 7 after ^{166}Ho treatment (^{166}Ho + DC) directly into the tumor. Three cycles of DCs were injected in total at 2–3-day intervals after the ^{166}Ho injection. Decreased tumor growth was noted in the ^{166}Ho animals after 11 days compared to the non-treated controls, but after day 14, the inhibitory effect was not as pronounced. Contrarily, the tumor growth inhibitory effects of DC after ^{166}Ho administration continued after day 14 resulting in much smaller tumor size compared to the other treated mice. All mice in the non-treated and only mice in the DC treated group died before day 31 and 40, respectively. However, 3 of 16 mice in the ^{166}Ho treated and 10 of 19 in the ^{166}Ho + DC group survived until day 60. Additional B16F10 melanoma cells were injected into the contralateral side of the surviving mice on day 60 to assess if tumor-specific immunity was possible. Despite the longevity of mice after the original treatment, the ^{166}Ho-treated mice developed new tumors slowly 11 days after the challenge as well as the ^{166}Ho + DC group, but the ^{166}Ho + DC tumor challenge mice had approximately one-fourth the size [65].

^{166}Ho + DC treatment was found to bring about a greater potent immune reaction than DC treatment alone; therefore, demonstrating radiotherapy does compliment DC treatment. This study did exhibit that the combination of ^{166}Ho and immature DC could be used to treat unresectable melanoma or may be utilized as adjuvant therapy.

A different type of drug delivery system is a modular nanotransporter (MNT) which can penetrate into target cells and distribute therapeutics into their subcellular compartments, particularly into the nucleus. Auger electron emitters are known to be ineffective outside the cell nucleus but possess high cytotoxicity in the proximity of nuclear DNA [66]. Coupling MNT along with an Auger electron such as Indium-111 (^{111}In) was evaluated for targeted radiotherapy.

A modified MNT with p-SCN-Bn-NOTA and labeled with ^{111}In was designed to target melanocortin-1 receptor (MC1R)-targeted tDTox-HMP-NLS-MSH (MNT-MSH) which is overexpressed on cancer cell. Cytotoxicity of the ^{111}In-labeled MNT was assessed on the cancer cell line B16-F1 presenting the receptor target MC1R [67].

Female C57BL/6 J mice were inoculated with B16-F1 melanoma tumor cells into the flank via a subcutaneous injection. When tumor volume reached a mean of 88 mm^3, intratumoral injections of either ^{111}In-NOTA-MNT-MSH, ^{111}In-EDTA, unlabeled NOTA-MNT-MSH, or saline were administered. Using SPECT/CT imaging, ^{111}In-NOTA-MNT-MSH indicated good intratumoral retention of ^{111}In, while radioactivity of normal tissues was very low with almost an undetectable signal in kidneys and liver. Three different doses of ^{111}In-NOTA-MNT-MSH were used with the highest dose at 10.4 MBq resulting in 82% tumor growth inhibition compared to control groups receiving saline by day 15. The same dosages of control ^{111}In or non-labeled NOTA-MNT-MSH did not result in any tumor growth inhibition [67].

^{111}In-labeled MNT targeting MC1R provided specific activity for treatment. The ^{111}In-NOTA-MNT-MSH conjugate displayed cytotoxicity against cancer cells overexpressing the MC1R as evidenced by in vitro studies. This data suggests further that evaluation of MNTs is warranted for its use as a form of local radiotherapy.

Prostate Cancer

Prostate cancer is the second most common cause of death from cancer in men after lung cancer. It is a very slow-growing cancer in which early spread of cancer cells occurs before the disease is apparent clinically [68]. As previously discussed, targeted alpha therapy has valuable use in the brachytherapy arena, not just for melanoma but other cancers therapies as well. Prostate-specific membrane antigen (PSMA) is a cell surface glycoprotein expressed in prostate cancer cells. J591 is one of many monoclonal antibodies to the extracellular domain of PSMA. α-Particle emitting radioisotope ^{213}Bi conjugated to J591 monoclonal antibody (mab) creating an AIC was used in the treatment of prostate cancer in nude mice [69].

Metastatic human tumor cell line, LNCaP-LN3, is an androgen-sensitive human prostate cancer cell line established from LNCaP which has features of human prostate cells such as production of the prostate secretory protein, PSMA, and the androgen receptor [70–73].

Male athymic nude mice, BALB/c (nu/nu), were injected in the right flank with LN3 cells subcutaneously. Note that LN3 cells need additional stromal cells or factors to grow; therefore, it is necessary to co-inject the cells with a Matrigel [74, 75]. Multiple experiments were performed. At 2 days post-cellular inoculation, 50 μCi AIC (^{213}Bi conjugated to J591 mab), no treatment control, or nonspecific AIC was administered into the cellular injection site. At 10 weeks, the mice in the AIC group had complete inhibition of tumor growth, whereas at 3 weeks, six out of seven mice in the no treatment group and five out of seven in the nonspecific AIC group had measurable tumors. In a second experiment, 1 week after LN3 cellular injection when tumors reached 40–60 mm^3, treatment consisting of a single intratumoral injection of AIC at 50 μCi or 100 μCi or nonspecific AIC at 100 μCi was given. Results indicated non-palpable tumors at 2 weeks after treatment for the 100 μCi group and non-palpable tumors at 3 weeks posttreatment in the 50 μCi group; however, tumor growth was seen with the nonspecific AIC group. Lastly, in a third experiment when tumors reached 70–80 mm^3, treatment was initiated with an intralesional injection at the same dose and therapy as in the second experiment. The results indicated non-palpable tumors at 3 weeks after treatment in the 100 μCi group yet the 50 μCi and nonspecific AIC animal had increased tumor volumes. Overall, no weight loss was noted in the AIC treated groups [69].

In general, the results indicated that a single locoregional injection of AIC at 50 and 100 μCi can be used to regress early-stage prostate cancer with small tumors or a higher dose of 100 μCi may be used for slightly larger tumors. Enhancing the selectivity of tumor cell irradiation by labeling monoclonal antibodies with nuclides is one approach to cancer therapy. As demonstrated, ^{213}Bi-labeled α-particle emitting immunoconjugate had high levels of antigen-selective cytotoxicity when compared to the nonspecific AIC [69].

Thermoresponsive polymers which are soluble at room temperature and precipitated at body temperature and are slowly eliminated from a local depot have also been evaluated as therapy for prostate cancer. In one set of studies, a polymer [poly(N-isopropyl acrylamide) labeled with the radionuclide ^{131}I was utilized in mice with human prostate adenocarcinoma PC3 xenograft [76].

CD-1 male outbred nude mice were administered with PC3 cells subcutaneously into the right flank. When tumors reached 0.15 cm^3, mice were injected with 0.1 ml intratumorally with the ^{131}I-labeled polymer as a 2% wt solution in dimethyl sulfoxide (DMSO). The groups used a radiolabeled polymer at 2 MBq, radiolabeled polymer at 25 MBq, a non-labeled polymer, or a control of physiological saline. At day 46, all mice were humanely euthanized. Results indicated the tumor volume decreased for both radiolabeled polymer doses; however, at 2 MBq, the tumor growth was less when compared to the control and non-labeled group, but still kept growing. In comparison, the 25 MBq group tumor size continued to decrease until the end of the experiment [76].

There were no apparent signs of weight loss indicating radio- or chemotoxicity. Additionally, there was significant suppression of inflammation around the radioiodine-treated tumors compared to the untreated controls on histological assessment. Histologically, at the higher radionuclide dose, there was complete destruction of tumor cells with no signs of relapse. At the lower dose of the radionuclide group, the unlabeled polymer group, and the untreated control group, relapse and viable tumor cells were noted. This provides evidence that dose-dependent tumor growth inhibition may be attained with a single dose of an intratumoral injection of ^{131}I-labeled thermoresponsive polymer [76].

Different polymers may also be utilized or a combination of various polymers and/or radionuclides as therapeutics. A thermoresponsive polymer (polyoxazoline [POZ]) labeled with Yttrium-90 (^{90}Y) which self-aggregates above a specific transition temperature was used to study not only tumor growth suppression but also survival rate [77].

Human prostate cancer cells, PC-3, were inoculated subcutaneously into the right thigh of male BALB/c-nu/nu mice. When the tumor reached 0.7–1.0 cm in diameter, mice were treated intratumorally with either PBS, a nonradioactive yttrium-labeled Isp-PrPOZ, or three different doses (0.74 MBq, 1.85 MBq, or 3.70 MBq) of the ^{90}Y-Isp-PrPOZ. Animals in the ^{90}Y-Isp-PrPOZ had tumor suppression which was dose-dependent in comparison with the PBS group and the nonradioactive yttrium-labeled Isp-PrPOZ group. Cellular damage was most severe in the 3.70 MBq dose group. The survival period was also greatest in group injected with 3.70 MBq of ^{90}Y-Isp-PrPOZ. At day 90 posttreatment, 50% of the mice survived with no obvious loss of body weight or systemic side effects [77].

The retention of the radioactivity was noted to be dependent on the POZ molecular weight; however, a POZ formulation of 20 kDa may augment the POZ depots in the tumor tissue. Overall, injectable radiopharmaceutical ^{90}Y-Isp-PrPOZ has potential for brachytherapy [77].

Chitosan, a high-molecular-weight polymer of 2-deoxy-2-amino-D-glucose chelated with ^{166}Ho, is another complex utilized as a radiopharmaceutical drug. This ^{166}Ho-chitosan complex (DW-166HC) is an acidic solution which converts to a gel state when directly injected into tissue. Noble male rats were surgically inoculated with androgen-independent Noble rat prostate carcinoma cells (AIT) into the ventral prostate. Seven days later when the tumor reached 0.2–0.3 cm in diameter, another surgery was performed for local tumor treatment consisting of 1) normal saline, 2) ^{165}Ho-chitosan complex solution, 3) (18.5 MBq) ^{166}Ho-chitosan complex solution, and 4) (37 MBq) ^{166}Ho-chitosan complex solution. Rats were euthanized at 2 and 4 weeks. Results indicated prostate weights were significantly lower in groups 3 and 4 compared to groups 1 and 2 with no significant difference between groups 3 and 4 at both time points. Histopathology demonstrated tumor cell necrosis in the latter groups treated with the ^{166}Ho-chitosan complex solution. Furthermore, examination of various other organs showed no pathological lesions. It may be extrapolated that the injection volume of ^{166}Ho is a greater factor than the radiation dose and maximal tumor inhibition was reached at 18.5 MBq. Local treatment of prostate cancer without adverse effects on bordering tissues is an important consideration. Therefore, ^{166}Ho-chitosan complex warrants further exploration as a therapeutic option [78].

Additional peptide polymers have also been utilized for treatments in prostate cancer. Thermally sensitive micelles constituting elastin-like polypeptide (ELP) integrating seven tyrosine subunits conjugated with ^{131}I radionuclide to form an in situ hydrogel as a form of injectable brachytherapy were tested in athymic mice. ELP has a critical micelle temperature below a micelle coacervation transition temperature below body temperature. The tumor depot is created when soluble ELP micelles labeled with ^{131}I undergo a soluble to insoluble low critical solution temperature (LCST) transition phase in vivo. The viscous coacervate undergoes further stabilization into a hydrogel as ^{131}I emits high-energy beta particles [79].

Male athymic BALB/c nude mice were surgically injected into the right dorsolateral prostate lobe using PC-3 M-Luc-C6 cells (luciferase-expressing firefly luc). Potassium iodide in drinking water was provided to inhibit potential radioiodine uptake by the thyroid during the treatment as well. After cellular inoculation and 3 weeks for tumor volume to reach 90–120 mm^3, treatment was initiated. Prostate tumors were accessed via another survival surgery. Treatment consisted of ^{131}I-ELP or unlabeled ELP as a control administered intratumorally at an injection bolus volume of one-third of the tumor size. Tumor regression was noted within 9 days compared to the control group, and tumors were reduced to less than 5% of their original size within 26 days. At the end of the study after 60 days, four of eight ^{131}I-ELP treated mice remained tumor-free. No weight loss was observed either [79].

Disadvantages of brachytherapy consist of possible titanium "seed" migration to other organs in the body [80–82] or implanted "seeds" remaining permanently in the patient posttreatment [83, 84]. In this study, results suggested injectable ELP may provide an alternative to current titanium seed brachytherapy technology. It provided a nonpermanent substitute for a biodegradable treatment as well as diminishing seed migration. This model presented a 95% tumor regression with four mice remaining in full remission at the end of 60 days. The only limitation noted in certain circumstances was incomplete tumor coverage based on histological analysis [79].

As medicine advances, more discoveries tend to develop at a therapeutic level. New agents may be created to improve deficiencies noted with traditional therapy. For example, the ^{32}P-chromic phosphate-poly (L-lactide) (^{32}P-CP-PLLA) seed was explored for its anticancer effects against prostate cancer with local lymphatic metastasis. In prostate cancer, small primary tumors tend to metastasize to proximal and/or distant lymph nodes with a poor prognosis in early-stage cancer [85]. Once pelvic lymph node metastasis occurs, radical therapies fail to improve prognosis and may lead to side effects [86]. To evaluate the therapeutic effect of a sustained release, biodegradable ^{32}P-chromic phosphate-poly (L-lactide) seeds, male athymic BALB/c-nu/nu nude mice were injected into the ventral prostate with PC-3M human prostate cancer cells. The distribution, pathological morphological changes of the tumor and regional lymph nodes, and the toxic reaction of ^{32}P-CP-PLLA were evaluated [85].

Mice were anesthetized to perform surgery exposing the dorsal prostate for injection of PC-3M cells into the ventral prostate. After 4 weeks when the tumor mass reached a 1.0 cm diameter, ^{32}P-CP-PLLA seeds of various radioactive doses, 3.7, 7.4, 14.8, and 0 MBq (the nonradioactive control), were implanted through B-type ultrasonic guide. Seven and 14 days after implantation, mice received a static scan through single-photon emission computed tomography (SPECT) which revealed the seeds primarily gathered in the tumor and abdominal para-aortic lymph nodes of the nude mice. Local retention of the seeds was evidenced by lack of significant imaging in other organs or tissues. Additionally, part of the ^{32}P-CP could migrate through the lymphatic system into the abdominal aortic lymph nodes [85].

The findings of this study discovered inhibition rates and necrosis rate of the tumor cells were correlated with the radioactivity. Necrosis in the tumors and lymph node metastasis in groups with 7.4 MBq and 14.8 MBq activity of ^{32}P-CP-PLLA 14 days after implantation showed ^{32}P-CP-PLLA could kill cancer cells locally as well as in the nearby lymph nodes. Note that bone marrow suppression was seen after seed implantation in the first phase; however, the suppression could be restored to pretreatment levels after 28 days [85]. Additional studies will be required; however, ^{32}P-CP-PLLA is a promising agent for prostatic cancer patients with lymphatic metastasis.

Pancreatic Cancer

Pancreatic carcinoma is the fourth most cancer-related fatality in the United States [87]. Investigators in the field have attempted to improve outcomes of patients with pancreatic cancer through combination therapy such as radiotherapy with chemotherapy, applying antiangiogenesis drugs and/or epidermal growth factor receptor inhibitors [88]. The use of ^{32}P-chromic phosphate colloid (^{32}P-CP) was investigated as a potential treatment for pancreatic cancer. BALB/c-nu/nu nude mice were implanted subcutaneously with the pancreatic carcinoma cell line Pc-3 in the right axilla. After 10 days when tumors grew to 0.8–1.0 cm in size, treatment consisting of various radioactive doses and 0 MBq of ^{32}P-CP was administered intratumorally. The initial 2–3 days posttreatment resulted in slight appetite suppression; however, it resolved. The control group tumors grew in contrast to the ^{32}P-CP treated groups. Grossly, tumor growth was reduced with scattered ulceration and bleeding on the tumor surface within 5 days, but tumors shrunk in size and flattened [89].

It was found in this study that increased ^{32}P-CP dose caused greater concentration of radioactivity in the liver, spleen, and other organs causing unexpected toxicity to the liver and bone marrow, yet tumor volume decreased. Intratumoral injection of appropriate doses of ^{32}P-CP is the key for successful therapy. Through the use of various diagnostic techniques, the data suggested that intratumoral injections of ^{32}P-CP may lead to localized occlusion of vessels, inhibit angiogenesis, and suppress metastasis via blood vessels, thereby causing tumor cell death [89].

Some therapies have uses in a variety of cancer types. As previously mentioned, cyclopamine (CPA) which boosts tumor response to radiotherapy and was encapsulated in a liquid-lipid nanoparticle system (CPA-LLP) to enhance the response of tumor cells to lutetium-177 conjugated to core-cross-linked polymeric micelles (CCPM-^{177}Lu) was used for breast cancer, but it too was tested on pancreatic cancer [33].

Nu/Nu mice were subcutaneously injected with Miapaca-2 human pancreatic adenocarcinoma cells in the right flank. Mice were injected intratumorally approximately at 14 days when the tumor size reached 0.1 cm^3. Control mice were injected with saline three times over a 1-week period, one group received a single injection of CCPM-^{177}Lu, and one group received a combination of three injections of CPA-LLP IV over 1 week along with a single injection of CCPM-^{177}Lu when the first dose of CPA-LLP was administered. At the end of the study (day 120), as discussed in the breast cancer section, the group with the best survival rate was the combination therapy group compared to the other groups. All mice in the saline control group died within the first 3 weeks. The combination therapy killed cancer cells as well as delayed tumor growth. The CCPM-^{177}Lu therapy alone slowed tumor growth; however, the combination therapy slowed tumor growth rate by a greater difference [33].

The same thermally sensitive micelles constituting elastin-like polypeptide (ELP) integrating seven tyrosine subunits conjugated with ^{131}I radionuclide used for prostate cancer discussed above in athymic BALB/c nude mice were also utilized for pancreatic cancer. The orthotopic pancreatic model was created via surgery by cinching a portion of the pancreatic tissue with suture as an injection site for human BxPc3-luc2 pancreatic cells. A second survival surgery was performed approximately after day 28 when tumors reached approximately 90–120 mm^3 for treatment. Intratumoral injection of unlabeled ELP or ^{131}I-ELP was administered at a bolus volume of one of three of the tumor size. The response of the pancreatic BxPc3-luc tumors also exhibited tumor regression compared to the control mice which demonstrated significant tumor growth after 1 week. After 60 days, the ^{131}I-ELP treated tumors had four of six mice with tumors under 300 mm^3. Although pancreatic cancer is not typically treated with brachytherapy, the ^{131}I-ELP presents a potential novel therapy against the radiation-resistant BxPc3-luc2 pancreatic tumor [79].

Liver Cancer

Hepatocellular carcinoma (HCC) is the sixth most prevalent cancer and the third most frequent cause of cancer-related death. Surveillance with ultrasonography allows diagnosis at early stages when the tumor might be curable by resection, liver transplantation, or ablation, and 5-year survival higher than 50% can be achieved [90]. External beam radiation isn't useful due to the sensitivity of the normal liver which limits the dose that can be delivered [91]; therefore, additional therapies are needed for treatments for this cancer.

The effect of ^{131}I gelatin microspheres (^{131}I-GMSs) on human hepatocellular carcinoma cells (HepG2) in nude BALB/c male mice after intratumoral injection was explored. Selective internal radiotherapy (SIRT) using radioactive microspheres is becoming an established modality for treatment of patients with HCC [92]. When tumors of mice which were injected into the axillary region with HepG2 cells reached 1 cm in diameter, treatment was initiated. Treatment consisted of an intratumoral injection of 37 MBq ^{131}I-microspheres in a 0.1 ml 25% glucose solution (^{131}I-GMS) or a control of nonradioactive microspheres. Results indicated the ^{131}I-GMS group had statistically smaller tumors up to 8 weeks posttreatment injection; however, the tumors continued to grow at a slower rate when compared to the control group. At day 64 postinjection, survival was 73.3% of the mice in the ^{131}I-GMS group and 13.3% in the control group [92].

Radioactivity of the tumor was high throughout the study but also high in the lung which decreased. The thyroid also had high radioactivity; however, FT4 levels in serum were stable despite the relative high concentration in the thyroid. The uptake of radioactive iodine in the thyroid gland may be reduced in patients with oral administration of nonradioactive sodium iodine in advance of treatment. SPECT imaging demonstrated that the radioactive nuclide was concentrated in the tumor for the entire observation period. In addition, pathologic examination revealed the microspheres were concentrated at the injection site with large areas of necrotic foci surrounding the microsphere. By day 32, most of the microspheres had degraded to varying degrees, and by day 64, there was no visible microsphere in the treatment group [92]. Gelatin is a biodegradable material with good biocompatibility and low toxicity [93–95] which is a conceivable modality for treating hepatocellular carcinoma.

The choice among therapeutic options for hepatocellular carcinoma includes liver resection, liver transplantation, and locoregional and systemic treatments which must be individualized for each patient [96]. Despite better outcomes, recurrence after therapeutic treatments remains a problem and is reported as high as 70% at 5 years after resection. The best treatment of recurrent HCC remains unclear [97]. Additional therapies such as the ^{32}P BioSilicon have been used to investigate its efficacy against human hepatocellular tumors in nude mice.

Nude male mice (BALB/c) were injected subcutaneously into the right gluteal region with the human hepatocellular carcinoma cell line (HepG2). On day 15 when tumors reached approximately 1 cm in diameter, ^{32}P BioSilicon at various activity levels, 0.5, 1.0, and 2.0 MBq, was administered in the center of the tumor at a 4 mm depth as well as a control formulation of a microcrystalline cellulose and sodium carboxymethylcellulose. The results showed reduction in tumor volume across all three activity levels in comparison with the control at 10 weeks posttreatment. Complete response in 60% of the mice was confirmed by histopathology which indicated no viable tumor in the specimens with 2.0 MBq, but lower levels also had responded. For tumors which did not undergo complete response, histopathology revealed necrosis was the mode of cell death. This data suggests intratumoral radiotherapy may offer patients an option for unresectable hepatocellular carcinoma [98].

Rats too have been used for research involving liver cancer. Male Sprague-Dawley (SD) rats were utilized to examine ^{188}Re chelated with ethyl cysteinate dimer (ECD) in a lipiodol solution (^{188}Re-ECD/lipiodol) as therapeutics in a rodent hepatoma model. Lipiodol, a poppy seed oil, may serve as a carrier for radioisotopes. It is a clinically available embolic agent for hepatoma treatment as well as a carrier for radioisotopes [99, 100].

The SD rats were surgically inoculated with the N1-S1 rat hepatoma cells in the left or right liver lobe, under the liver capsule. On day 7 post-cellular inoculation, rats received a second laparotomy to confirm the presence of a liver tumor. At this point, treatment was initiated with a single intratumoral injection of ^{188}Re-ECD/lipiodol in the center of the tumor or normal saline. Micro-SPECT/CT imaging confirmed ^{188}Re-ECD/lipiodol was confined to the tumor site after 24 hours. Furthermore, on day 60, the end of the study, 52% of the treated rats had decreased tumor size by 10% or greater compared to pretreatment tumor volume and a survival rate of 62% compared to the control group. Some rats exhibited no tumor on day 60 but rather scarring at the former tumor site. ^{188}Re-ECD/lipiodol is a worthwhile agent to be investigated for treatment in human hepatomas [101].

Radiolabeled lipiodol employing rhenium-188 has been combined with other agents for treatment of hepatocellular carcinomas as well. Rhenium-188-N, N′-1,2-ethanediylbis-L-cysteine diethyl-ester dihydrochloride-Lipiodol (^{188}Re-EL) was blended with a hydrogel to create ^{188}Re-ELH (same as ^{188}Re-ECD-Lipiodol/hydrogel), a radioactive thermogelling emulsion. SD male rats were surgically implanted with N1-S1 cells into a liver lobe under the liver capsule. Seven days postinoculation, rats went under surgery again to confirm liver tumor growth. To evaluate a 60-day study endpoint, rats with N1-S1 tumor cells were treated intratumorally with ^{188}Re-ELH or ^{188}Re-EL or untreated. The ^{188}Re-ELH treated group had four of nine rats without residual tumors with one rat exhibiting an increased tumor volume. In comparison with the ^{188}Re-EL group, there was no difference statistically. Both groups had nine of ten rats survive to the study end. The ^{188}Re-EL rats did not have residual tumor cells in the liver upon microscopic examination. When analyzing the control group, only one of eight rats survived the full 60 days and one rat showed an increased tumor volume [102].

The experimental results indicated the therapeutic effect of ^{188}Re-EL in terms of hepatoma response was better; however, the therapeutic effect of ^{188}Re-El could be enhanced by the hydrogel. In addition, the radioactivity of ^{188}Re-ELH was approximately half of the ^{188}Re-EL group too. Furthermore, some radioactivity was noted in the lungs upon initial ^{188}Re-ELH administration which rapidly decreased to background levels [102]. Overall, additional validation in animal and/or clinical trials is warranted.

Miscellaneous Cancers

Head and Neck Cancer

Head and neck cancers are primarily squamous cell carcinomas which progress via local invasion of adjacent structures and locoregional lymph node metastasis [103]; therefore, interventional therapies are being explored. Elastin-like polypeptides (ELPs) are a class of genetically engineered peptide polymers that undergo phase separation in response to small temperature changes. These ELPs are soluble at room temperature but become viscous when warmed by body temperature. Thermally responsive ELP radiolabeled with ^{131}I and a tyrosine residue at the C-terminus (ELP-Tyr) that self-assembles into radionuclide seeds when intratumorally injected was experimented on mice with FaDu head and neck squamous cell carcinoma human xenografts [104].

Female nude mice (BALB/c, nu/nu) were injected subcutaneously in the right lower leg with FaDu carcinoma cells. To prevent thyroid accumulation of free radioiodine, 1% potassium iodide was added to the drinking water of all animals 1 week prior to treatment until the end of the radiotherapy experiment. Between days 7 and 9 when tumors reached approximately 170 mm^3, mice began treatment with ELPs of various molecular weights and an unlabeled ELP control. Intratumoral injections consisted of [^{131}I]ELP$_{120}$-Tyr$_1$, [^{131}I]ELP$_{120}$-TYR$_4$, and [^{131}I]ELP$_{120}$-Tyr$_7$. Results indicated ELP$_{120}$-Tyr$_1$ provided prolonged tumor retention while decreasing the amount of ELP required. Tyrosine content also affects the ELP viscosity. The higher the number of tyrosine residues, the higher the viscosity. The antitumor efficacy and survival time of mice correlated with tumor retention of the [^{131}I]ELP$_{120}$-Tyr$_7$ as the best therapeutics. By day 60, the end of the study, 10 of 12 mice survived while 8 of those 12 exhibited complete tumor regression. In comparison, the [^{131}I]ELP$_{120}$-Tyr$_1$, [^{131}I]ELP$_{120}$-TYR$_4$, and control groups required mice to be euthanized due to excessive tumor burden or weight loss at earlier time points. These nontoxic and biodegradable polymer seeds prolonged intratumoral retention, thus delaying tumor growth. Autoradiography of the tumor following [^{131}I]ELP$_{120}$-Tyr$_7$ injection showed

^{131}I activity was concentrated at the administration site of the single injection in the center of the tumor. In addition, the tumor necrosis noted on histopathology correlated with the ^{131}I distribution pattern [104].

This study demonstrated an alternative modality to conventional brachytherapy consisting of a biodegradable genetically engineered polypeptide conjugated to a radioisotope. Efficacy of the depot correlated with the number of tyrosines in the C-terminus tail, molecular weight, and solution concentration. Increasing the number of tyrosines, injection concentration, and molecular weight increased tumor retention. This seedlike depot of [^{131}I]ELP$_{120}$-Tyr$_7$ resulted in a 67% cure rate. Free ^{131}I was quickly cleared once released from the ELP into circulation. For better uniformity of coverage on larger tumors, it may be possible to provide multiple injections [104].

The use of drug-carrying lipid nanoparticle (liposomes) via convection-enhanced delivery has been used for head and neck cancer similar to the use in glioblastoma. Athymic male nude rats (rnu/rnu) were subcutaneously inoculated with human tongue cancer cells (SCC-4) over the scapula and infused intratumorally with liposomal ^{186}Re when tumors reached approximately 1.6 cm^3 on days 14–15 postinoculation. Control groups received either unlabeled liposomes, encapsulated ^{186}Re-perrhenate, or unencapsulated intermediate ^{186}Re-compound, a liposome-based preparation consisting of rhenium188 linked to the chelator N,N-bis (2-mercaptoethyl)-N′,N′-diethylethylenediamine (^{186}Re-BMEDA) [105].

The average volume in the ^{186}Re-liposome treated group decreased in comparison with all control groups. At the end of a 6-week study, 3 of 33 rats continued to display tumor regression; however, 2 of 33 had larger tumors which were slow growing compared to the control rats. There was no significant difference in the overall progression of the tumor growth between the three control groups. Body weight in the treated and control groups remained similar, but the ^{186}Re-liposome group appeared to tolerate treatment without observable systemic side effects. Histopathology of the ^{186}Re-liposome group showed necrotic tumor cells. These results indicated that intratumoral infusion of ^{186}Re as part of a liposome carrier has benefit with treating head and neck cancers [105].

Lung Cancer

Carrier-based radionuclide therapy is less toxic compared to chemotherapy and requires a shorter treatment period. By using the binding property of 17-Allylamino-17demethoxygeldanamycin (17-AAG), an HSP90 inhibitor, labeled with radioisotope ^{131}I (^{131}I-17-AAG), non-small cell lung carcinoma xenografts in mice were smaller when compared to controls. Heat shock protein 90 (HSP90) stabilizes proteins required for tumor growth; thus, by inhibiting HSP90, conceivable tumor growth will be repressed [106].

BALB/c female nude mice were implanted subcutaneously with H460 human non-small cell lung carcinoma (NSCULC) into the right flank. When tumors reached 8–10 mm in diameter, intratumoral or intravenous treatment was initiated.

Mice were provided 1% potassium perchlorate water solution 3 days prior to any injections to inhibit potential radioiodine uptake by the thyroid. Treatment consisted of one or two injections of ^{131}I-17-AAG of various radioactive doses compared to untreated mice. All treatment groups had a degree of tumor growth suppression; however, the effects were greater in the intratumoral group than the intravenous group. When comparing the intratumoral groups, the optimal inhibitive ratio was noted in the group which received ^{131}I-17-AAG twice 8 days apart at 5.5 MBq in a 16-day study. Histopathologic exam revealed distinct damage of individual tumor cells with no evidence of treatment-induced abnormalities in major organs [106].

Increased expression of HSP90 at higher levels than normal tissue is a common feature of most human cancers [107]. These results verified that ^{131}I-17-AAG may contribute to the inhibition of HSP90 in H460 NSCLC, thereby having a target-specific role in lung cancer treatment [108].

Large Animal and Rodent Diagnostic and Therapeutic Use

Before radioactive agents can be safely used for treatment purposes, it should be determined if the agent will target the area and tissues that need to be treated and there will be minimal damage to surrounding tissues to eliminate systemic effects. Studies conducted in the 1980s looked at isotopes of radium and plutonium in rats and dogs to determine comparative doses, exposure routes, and bone cancer induction rates in humans who had been injected with plutonium in the 1940s [109, 110].

Molecular imaging is often tested using animal models prior to being translated and used in human medicine. Several molecular imaging modalities exist and have their own advantages and disadvantages. One advantage that all imaging provides is the ability to repeat imaging in the same animal, conduct uniform imaging, and perform noninvasive imaging. This can lead to reduction in the use of animals and refinement of current practices. Of the four popular imaging techniques used, only SPECT or PET uses radioisotopes. The least costly option for imaging is the ultrasound. In 2013, less than 1% of drugs in development have been approved by the FDA. Molecular imaging and the use of biomarkers can help establish earlier humane endpoints. This could hopefully speed the translation from animal models to clinical use [21]. The common types of imaging is listed in Table 9.3.

Dogs were used in studies to determine the distribution in tissues for ligand DMPE [1,2-bis(di-methylphosphino)ethane] combined with either ^{99m}Tc or ^{186}Re. The goal was to determine which would be good heart imaging agents when combined with either ^{99m}Tc or ^{186}Re. The standard in this study was the Tc, and Re was an analog with the hope of being more lesion specific. Depending on the outcome of the study, a therapeutic radiation dose may be delivered without negative effects on normal tissue. One dog was given doses of $^{99m}Tc(DMPE)_2$ followed by $^{186}Re(DMPE)_2$. Blood clearance and scintigraphic measurements were taken up to

4 hours after each intravenous injection. Blood clearance is similar for both agent combinations. There is less reduction of ^{186}Re in vivo, so it appears to be a better agent for myocardial imaging [111, 112].

Animal models allow studies to be performed in a controlled environment. Animal models for the study of tumor uptake of radionuclide should have the following three qualities:

- Rapid and reproducible tumor growth
- Tumor growth that doesn't exceed acceptable humane endpoints too rapidly
- Tumor that replicates the angiogenesis commonly observed in natural tumor formation [113]

Tissue distribution of radionuclides is often the first step when designing new drugs for diagnostic or therapeutic purposes. Hypericin (Hyp) has an affinity for necrotic tissue and is known as a necrosis-avid compound. It can be labeled with ^{131}I. ^{131}I-Hyp was injected intravenously in three 8-year-old male neutered beagle dogs, and a biodistribution study was conducted. Free radioiodine uptake was blocked by first giving the dogs potassium iodide capsules. Most of the labeled hypericin was found in the liver, lungs, and heart. The dogs exhibited mild gastrointestinal clinical signs that resolved within 48 hours. Hyp is excreted primarily in the hepatobiliary pathway. The gastrointestinal system has rapidly dividing cells and is vulnerable to radiation exposure which may be the dose-limiting factor in its administration. Clearance from all organs occurred within 7 days [114].

Some of the common non-rodent animal models that are used for radionuclide therapy testing are listed in Table 9.4. The canine transmissible venereal tumor (CTVT) can be implanted in many locations including the brain to study various treatments.

Table 9.3 Common types of imaging

Type of imaging	Type of signal	Type of probe	Advantages	Disadvantages
Ultrasound	Sound waves	Microbubbles	Real time, low cost, good translation	Limited molecular applications
MRI	Radio waves	Gadolinium	Good spatial resolution and tissue contrast, good translation	Low molecular sensitivity, can be costly, may have extended scanning time
Nuclear (SPECT/PET)	Gamma rays	Radioisotopes	Good molecular sensitivity, good translation, several probes available	Limited anatomical resolution, specialty equipment may be required, can be costly
Optical	Light or near infrared	Luciferin, coelenterazine, fluorophore	High molecular sensitivity, many probes available	Limited anatomical resolution, limited translation capability, poor tissue penetration

Table 9.4 Common hamster and non-rodent animal models of cancer

Model	Origin	Host species	Tumor site(s)	References
Melanoma	Spontaneous flank	Syrian hamster	Subcutaneous	Haynie [113], Greene [115]
Melanoma	Human bile	Hamster	Subcutaneous	Haynie [113]
Melanoma	Spontaneous	Hamster	Cheek pouch	Haynie [113]
Carcinoma-VX2	Spontaneous/virally induced	Rabbit	Intramedullary	Haynie [113]
Brown-Pearce	Scar of syphilitic lesion from rabbit scrotum	Dutch rabbit	Intrahepatic	Haynie [113]
Sarcoma	Human calf	Syrian hamster	Cheek pouch	Haynie [113], Toolan [116]
Adenovirus-SA7	Spontaneous, African green monkey	Hamster	Intracranial, subcutaneous	Haynie [113], Levenbook [117]
Choriocarcinoma	Human transplant	Syrian hamster	Cheek pouch	Haynie [113], Quinones [118]
Mammary tumor	Spontaneous	Dog	Breast	
Colonic tumor-GW-39	Human transplant	Syrian hamster	Subcutaneous, cheek pouch	Haynie [113], Blumenthal [119]
Canine transmissible venereal tumor	Spontaneous	Dog	Multiple implantable locations	Chuang [120]
DPC-1	Canine prostate carcinoma cell line	Dog	Prostate	Anidjar [121]

Imaging Using Radiolabeled Antibodies

Early studies looking at radioimmunodetection of tumors utilized Syrian hamsters implanted with the GW-39 human colonic carcinoma tumor in the thigh and cheek pouches. GW-39 produces carcinoembryonic antigen (CEA). Antibodies to CEA were labeled with ^{131}I or ^{125}I. The antigens used were carcinoembryonic antigen and colon-specific antigen-p antibody and injected intracardially. Prior to injection of labeled antibody, the hamsters were given Lugol's solution in the drinking water to reduce thyroid uptake of free radioiodine. The hamsters were photoscanned 4–5 days after administration of the radiolabeled antibody, and blood and tissues were measured using a scintillation counter. Photoscans showed accumulation of the isotope-labeled colon-specific antigen-p antibody in the tumors. The mixture of both of the antibodies indicated a more effective radioimmunodetection than one given alone [122, 123].

Sharkey et al. performed a similar study using hamsters implanted with GW-39 in both rear legs, and both ^{131}I-labeled anti-CEA antibody and ^{125}I-labeled anti-goat

IgG were injected intraperitoneally. This method reduced the level of radioactivity in blood by a factor of 4 reducing the need to use computer-assisted subtraction techniques [124]. This group also created a human colon cancer metastasis model in hamsters by injecting GW-39 tumor suspension directly into the liver. Lesions were present in the lungs within a week after liver injections of GW-39 in hamsters. These hamsters were also given injections of a mixture of ^{131}I-labled anti-CEA antibody and ^{125}I-labeled IgG, and liver and cheek tumors were visualized using scintigraphy without subtraction techniques. The lung tumors were not detected via scintigraphy but were detected using whole-body autoradiography and ^{125}I-labeled anti-CEA antibody 7 days after the original implantation in the liver. Another group did similar work using the same liver injected metastatic model and was able to visualize the lung tumors using ^{131}I-labeled anti-CEA antibody [125, 126].

Radionuclide imaging has been used for diagnostic purposes in hamsters. Hyperplastic goiter (enlargement of the thyroid gland) was suspected in a closed breeding colony of Syrian hamsters. The prevalence of goiter in this colony was 45% and typical prevalence is 6–7%. To diagnose goiter in these hamsters, they were given ^{123}I intraperitoneally and in 4 hours performed whole-body gamma counts using a scintillation camera. Imaging was able to diagnose that 8 of the 18 hamsters had goiter. The original cause of the goiter was attributed to genetics. The clinical signs for hyper- and hypothyroidism were absent from this colony. These hamsters were considered euthyroid [127].

One common imaging target for many tumors is the blood vessels that develop to nurture them. Endoglin (CD105) is a marker for neovascularization. The monoclonal antibody, MAEND3, was used to target CD105 for imaging purposes. In this study, a 6-year-old female beagle and an 8-year-old mixed-breed dog with spontaneous ductal mammary adenocarcinomas were injected intravenously with MAEND3 labeled with ^{125}I and imaged with a gamma camera after 8 hours. Both dogs were given iodine tablets 8 days before the injection of the monoclonal antibody labeled with ^{125}I. The spontaneous tumors were imaged and visible using a gamma camera. The tumors were removed 10 days after the injection. Neither dog exhibited side effects up to 3 months after the imaging [128].

Copper-64 has been used to label monoclonal antibodies for the purpose of imaging. Initially, biodistribution studies were conducted in golden Syrian hamster implanted with GW39 human colon cancer cell lines in the right thigh. The ^{64}Cu-benzyl-TETA-1A3-F(ab')$_2$ was found and retained at higher levels in the implanted tumor compared to the kidney, blood, and liver. It was determined that the kidney was the primary route of excretion. In addition, a male baboon was serially imaged using PET to determine the biodistribution of ^{64}Cu-benzyl-TETA-1A3-F(ab')$_2$, and the same baboon was serially imaged after being injected with ^{64}Cu-F(ab')$_2$. The values obtained for the baboon study are considered predictive for the pharmacokinetics in humans. Distribution in baboons appeared to be in the blood and liver and higher amounts in the kidneys. The high kidney uptake may be a problem but may be alleviated through purification. There is value in the ability to use PET imaging to visualize the ^{64}Cu-labeled monoclonal antibody [129, 130].

Thyroid Tumor Diagnostic

Thyroid tumors that are undifferentiated often lose the ability to update iodine. These tumors still have the ability to express thyrotropin receptors. Well-differentiated thyroid tumors retain the ability to be stimulated by thyrotropin, and metastases take up radioiodine through the sodium iodide symporter (NIS) and synthesize and release thyroglobulin. Differentiated thyroid tumors (10–15%) can lose the ability to express NIS and uptake iodine. New diagnostic tools were needed for the undifferentiated for staging and follow-up evaluations. Because the undifferentiated thyroid tumors still produce thyrotropin receptor (rhTSH), an analog of rhTSH (TR1401) was labeled with Technetium-99m (^{99m}Tc) using the chelator succinimidyl-6-hydrazinonicotinate hydrochloride (HYNIC) and administered to a neutered dachshund with a spontaneous undifferentiated thyroid tumor. The dog was imaged using SPECT/CT 3 hours after injection of the radiopharmaceutical ^{99m}Tc-HYNIC-TR1401. Imaging resulted in high uptake of the probe in the thyroid lobe with the tumor. After imaging, the tumor was surgically removed [131].

Prostate Cancer Therapeutics

As previously mentioned, prostate cancer is the second leading cause of cancer death in the United States for men. Gene therapy is being explored as a treatment for metastatic prostate cancer. The system used is based on the processes performed naturally by the thyroid gland utilizing the sodium-iodide symporter (NIS) which transports and concentrates iodide. The study performed in male beagle dogs showed that NIS could be locally expressed in the prostate gland with no toxicity. Dogs were injected directly in the prostate with virus (Ad5/CMV/NS) followed by ^{123}I (3 mCi) administrated intravenously. The dogs were then given therapeutic doses of ^{131}I (116 mCi/m^2) and observed for 7 days. There were localized NIS expression in the prostate gland and no vector-related toxicity. There was acceptably low radiation in all organs except the target organ, the prostate. This study served as a precursor to a Phase I trial using an adenovirus vector to transfer the NIS gene into prostate cancer. This system has led to delay of tumor growth and increased survival in patients with cancer [132, 133].

Animal models have proven to be useful for translation into human medicine. DPC-1 is an epithelial cell line from a prostatic adenocarcinoma from a Doberman pinscher. Spontaneous dog prostatic adenocarcinoma behaves similarly to that in humans with a predisposition toward benign hyperplasia and malignant transformation. Dogs with spontaneous prostate cancer are often diagnosed when the cancer is at end stage and often metastasizes to the iliac lymph nodes, lung, and bone. This tumor still lacks a prostate-specific biochemical marker which differentiates this tumor from the human equivalent. The tumor was grown in nude mice and in a dog that was immunosuppressed with cyclosporin. Immunoscintigraphy was performed using ^{131}I-labeled human PSMA monoclonal antibody in mice and dogs and allowed the tumor to be easily visualized [121].

There are occasions where tumors are unresectable and require intravenous administration of radiotherapy to target neoplasias. In this study, an oxidized derivative of avidin (AvidinOX) is used as a receptor for a radioactive biotin (^{68}Ga-ST2210). Domestic female pigs that were 4-months-old were given AvidinOX either in the tongue or in the urinary bladder. Twenty-four hours later, the pigs were scanned using a PET/CT and given ^{68}Ga-ST2210 intravenously. The bladder and tongue lesions were observed by PET 1 hour after ^{68}Ga-ST2210 administration. Rabbits were injected in the tongue with AvidinOX and 24 hours later given Gd-ST2210 intravenously. A similar study was performed in dogs where AvidinOX was injected into the prostate in two beagles and immunohistochemistry was performed. The AvidinOX was found to localize in the dog prostate as predicted. Similar studies have been conducted in humans with AvidinOX followed by ^{177}Lu-ST2210. These studies support the concept that radioactive biotin can be injected intravenously to target on neoplastic lesions after AvidinOX is injected into tissues and organs that may be harboring primary or secondary tumors that cannot be removed through surgical means [134].

Palliative Treatment of Bone Cancer

One of the major challenges in selecting agents to palliatively treat metastatic bone cancer is to deliver an adequate dose of ionizing radiation while minimizing bone marrow suppression [135]. Palliative treatment is aimed at alleviating a problem without necessarily addressing the underlying cause. In the case of metastatic bone cancer, the treatment is focused primarily on pain relief.

Prior to use in humans or animals, testing must occur to ensure safety, targeting of the appropriate tissue, and efficacy. ^{186}Re-1-hydroxy-ethylidene-diphosphonate (^{186}Re-HEDP) and ^{153}Sm-ethylene-diamine-tetramethylene-phosphonate (^{153}Sm-EDTMP) were selected as potential palliative treatments for metastatic bone cancer. Although ^{89}Sr has been tested in clinical trials for palliative treatment for metastatic bone cancer, its half-life of over 50 days may prevent its use for multiple doses. ^{131}I has also been used clinically and has an even shorter half-life than ^{89}Sr. It still may be desirable to seek radionuclide treatments with even shorter half-lives. Dogs and rabbits have been used to study the distribution of ^{153}Sm-EDTMP after injection. After refining the ^{186}Re-HEDP, human patients with metastatic bone cancer were treated with this agent, and it localized to the bone lesions. A clinical study using 20 dogs with spontaneous osteosarcoma injected intravenously with ^{153}Sm-EDTMP was performed. A majority of the treated dogs had positive responses such as reduction of pain, extended survival times, or tumor regression [136].

Animals have benefitted from radionuclide therapy. In Norway, 15 dogs were given radionuclide therapy with ^{153}Sm-ethylene-diamine-tetramethylene-phosphonate (EDTMP) to treat spontaneous osteosarcoma. Most of the tumors were located in the extremities. The prognosis is poor due to a high rate of metastases and an average survival time of 19 weeks. The 2-year survival rate is only 2%. The dogs were treated intravenously. Although none of the dogs were cured, 9 of 15 dogs did experience pain relief. There also appeared to be delay in growth of the primary tumor itself. Ultimately, this treatment with ^{153}Sm-EDTMP may prolong the lifespan and postpone metastases in dogs [137].

One area of animal research that appears to making headway into translational medicine using animal models is that of palliative treatment of bone metastasis. There are many clinical signs associated with primary and metastatic bone cancer, some of which affect both humans and animals. These clinical signs range from skeletal pain, decreased mobility, depression, neurological deficits, and other symptoms. Palliative radionuclide therapy has been successful in improving quality of life in both animal and human patients. A study was conducted using ^{177}Lu-ethylene-diamine-tetramethylene-phosphonate (EDTMP). ^{177}Lu was selected due to its being a moderate beta emitter and having a relatively short half-life and due to the feasibility of large-scale production. This agent was tested in Wistar rats, NZW rabbits, and dogs after intravenous injection. Using serial scintigraphic imaging, it was determined that the ^{177}Lu- EDTMP accumulates in the skeleton with little activity in other organs and in the circulating blood [135].

Conclusion

As indicated, animal models are necessary in science when exploring viable options that lead to translational research. Radiotherapy is an effective cancer treatment modality. The utilization of radionuclides locally as a therapeutic provides a mechanism to target specific organs or tissues while reducing the distribution to other organs, thus resulting in less damage to surrounding tissues, more rapid recovery, and reduction of pain for the patient. Various techniques including external beam, locoregional, intravenous, or a combination of these modalities provide greater application options for the various clinical indications. As described in this chapter, there are multiple formulations using radionuclides which have different uses including as diagnostic and therapeutic or a combination of the two, theranostic. Many of the studies discussed in this chapter demonstrated promising choices of therapy for the numerous types of cancers.

References

1. Luna Pais H, Alho I, Vendrell I, Mansinho A, Costa L. Radionuclides in oncology clinical practice - review of the literature. Dalton Trans. 2017;46(42):14475–87.
2. de Jong M, Mather S, Maina T. Preclinical in vivo cancer, straightway to patients? Q J Nucl Med Mol Imaging. 2017;61(2):145–52.
3. Harrison JD, Muirhead CR. Quantitative comparisons of cancer induction in humans by internally deposited radionuclides and external radiation. Int J Radiat Biol. 2003;79(1):1–13.

4. Moore K. The radium girls : they paid with their lives, their final fight was for justice. London: Simon & Schuster; 2016. xiii, 465 pages.
5. Wilson DA, Diel JH, Hoel DG. Lung fibrosis and lung cancer incidence in beagle dogs that inhaled 238PuO2 or 239PuO2. Health Phys. 2009;96(4):493–503.
6. Wilson DA, Mohr LC, Frey GD, Lackland D, Hoel DG. Lung, liver and bone cancer mortality after plutonium exposure in beagle dogs and nuclear workers. Health Phys. 2010;98(1):42–52.
7. Raabe OG. Comparison of the carcinogenicity of radium and bone-seeking actinides. Health Phys. 1984;46(6):1241–58.
8. Raabe OG. Concerning the health effects of internally deposited radionuclides. Health Phys. 2010;98(3):515–36.
9. Hahn FF, Muggenburg BA, Menache MG, Guilmette RA, Boecker BB. Comparative stochastic effects of inhaled alpha- and beta-particle-emitting radionuclides in beagle dogs. Radiat Res. 1999;152(6 Suppl):S19–22.
10. Lloyd RD, Miller SC, Taylor GN, Bruenger FW, Angus W, Jee WS. Comparison of internal emitter radiobiology in animals and humans. Health Phys. 1997;72(1):100–10.
11. Taylor GN, Lloyd RD, Mays CW, Shabestari L, Miller SC. Promotion of radiation-induced liver neoplasia by ethanol. Health Phys. 1992;62(2):178–82.
12. Lloyd RD, Taylor GN, Miller SC. Does body size contribute to sensitivity of bone tumor induction by radionuclide exposure? Health Phys. 2000;79(2):199–202.
13. Taylor GN, Lloyd RD, Mays CW, Miller SC, Jee WS, Mori S, et al. Relationship of natural incidence and radiosensitivity for bone cancer in dogs. Health Phys. 1997;73(4):679–83.
14. Lloyd RD, Bruenger FW, Angus W, Taylor GN, Miller SC. Mammary tumor occurrence in beagles given 239Pu. Health Phys. 1995;69(3):385–90.
15. Lloyd RD, Fisher DR, Schlenker RA, Miller SC. Some problems in the skeletal dosimetry of bone-seeking radionuclides. Health Phys. 1999;76(4):402–12.
16. Lloyd RD, Taylor GN, Miller SC. Does soft tissue cancer affect the development of radionuclide-induced skeletal malignancy? Health Phys. 2003;84(1):111–4.
17. Muggenburg BA, Boecker BB, Hahn FF, McClellan RO. Lung lavage therapy to lessen the biological effects of inhaled 144Ce in dogs. Radiat Res. 1990;124(2):147–55.
18. Tanderup K, Menard C, Polgar C, Lindegaard JC, Kirisits C, Potter R. Advancements in brachytherapy. Adv Drug Deliv Rev. 2017;109:15–25.
19. Perera M, Krishnananthan N, Lindner U, Lawrentschuk N. An update on focal therapy for prostate cancer. Nat Rev Urol. 2016;13(11):641–53.
20. Fernandes RS, de Aguiar Ferreira C, Soares DCF, Maffione AM, Townsend DM, Rubello D, et al. The role of radionuclide probes for monitoring anti-tumor drugs efficacy: a brief review. Biomed Pharmacother. 2017;95:469–76.
21. Kalimuthu S, Jeong JH, Oh JM, Ahn BC. Drug discovery by molecular imaging and monitoring therapy response in lymphoma. Int J Mol Sci. 2017;18(8):1639.
22. Qiao W, Zhao L, Wu S, Liu C, Guo L, Xing Y, et al. SPECT imaging and radionuclide therapy of glioma using (131)I labeled Buthus martensii Karsch chlorotoxin. J Neuro-Oncol. 2017;133(2):287–95.
23. Park JB, Kwak HJ, Lee SH. Role of hyaluronan in glioma invasion. Cell Adhes Migr. 2008;2(3):202–7.
24. Girard N, Courel MN, Vera P, Delpech B. Therapeutic efficacy of intralesional 131I-labelled hyaluronectin in grafted human glioblastoma. Acta Oncol. 2000;39(1):81–7.
25. Mi Y, Shao Z, Vang J, Kaidar-Person O, Wang AZ. Application of nanotechnology to cancer radiotherapy. Cancer Nanotechnol. 2016;7(1):11.
26. Cikankowitz A, Clavreul A, Tetaud C, Lemaire L, Rousseau A, Lepareur N, et al. Characterization of the distribution, retention, and efficacy of internal radiation of (188) Re-lipid nanocapsules in an immunocompromised human glioblastoma model. J Neuro-Oncol. 2017;131(1):49–58.
27. Chatterjee S, Behnam Azad B, Nimmagadda S. The intricate role of CXCR4 in cancer. Adv Cancer Res. 2014;124:31–82.

28. Sehedic D, Chourpa I, Tetaud C, Griveau A, Loussouarn C, Avril S, et al. Locoregional confinement and major clinical benefit of (188)Re-loaded CXCR4-targeted nanocarriers in an orthotopic human to mouse model of glioblastoma. Theranostics. 2017;7(18):4517–36.
29. Jannetti SA, Carlucci G, Carney B, Kossatz S, Shenker L, Carter LM, et al. PARP-1-targeted radiotherapy in mouse models of glioblastoma. J Nucl Med. 2018;59(8):1225–33.
30. Badie B, Goh CS, Klaver J, Herweijer H, Boothman DA. Combined radiation and p53 gene therapy of malignant glioma cells. Cancer Gene Ther. 1999;6(2):155–62.
31. Pulaski BA, Ostrand-Rosenberg S. Mouse 4T1 breast tumor model. Curr Protoc Immunol. 2001;Chapter 20:Unit 20 2.
32. Cancer AIf. Worldwide cancer data, global cancer statistics for the most common cancers 2018. Available from: https://www.wcrf.org/dietandcancer/cancer-trends/worldwide-cancer-data.
33. You J, Zhao J, Wen X, Wu C, Huang Q, Guan F, et al. Chemoradiation therapy using cyclopamine-loaded liquid-lipid nanoparticles and lutetium-177-labeled core-crosslinked polymeric micelles. J Control Release. 2015;202:40–8.
34. Clarke M, Collins R, Darby S, Davies C, Elphinstone P, Evans V, et al. Effects of radiotherapy and of differences in the extent of surgery for early breast cancer on local recurrence and 15-year survival: an overview of the randomised trials. Lancet. 2005;366(9503):2087–106.
35. Melancon MP, Zhou M, Li C. Cancer theranostics with near-infrared light-activatable multimodal nanoparticles. Acc Chem Res. 2011;44(10):947–56.
36. Li J, Hu Y, Yang J, Wei P, Sun W, Shen M, et al. Hyaluronic acid-modified Fe3O4@Au core/shell nanostars for multimodal imaging and photothermal therapy of tumors. Biomaterials. 2015;38:10–21.
37. Zhou M, Zhao J, Tian M, Song S, Zhang R, Gupta S, et al. Radio-photothermal therapy mediated by a single compartment nanoplatform depletes tumor initiating cells and reduces lung metastasis in the orthotopic 4T1 breast tumor model. Nanoscale. 2015;7(46):19438–47.
38. Haume K, Rosa S, Grellet S, Smialek MA, Butterworth KT, Solov'yov AV, et al. Gold nanoparticles for cancer radiotherapy: a review. Cancer Nanotechnol. 2016;7(1):8.
39. Molina MA, Codony-Servat J, Albanell J, Rojo F, Arribas J, Baselga J. Trastuzumab (herceptin), a humanized anti-Her2 receptor monoclonal antibody, inhibits basal and activated Her2 ectodomain cleavage in breast cancer cells. Cancer Res. 2001;61(12):4744–9.
40. Cai Z, Yook S, Lu Y, Bergstrom D, Winnik MA, Pignol JP, et al. Local radiation treatment of HER2-positive breast cancer using Trastuzumab-modified gold nanoparticles labeled with (177)Lu. Pharm Res. 2017;34(3):579–90.
41. Alexis F, Pridgen E, Molnar LK, Farokhzad OC. Factors affecting the clearance and biodistribution of polymeric nanoparticles. Mol Pharm. 2008;5(4):505–15.
42. Cai Z, Chattopadhyay N, Yang K, Kwon YL, Yook S, Pignol JP, et al. (111)In-labeled trastuzumab-modified gold nanoparticles are cytotoxic in vitro to HER2-positive breast cancer cells and arrest tumor growth in vivo in athymic mice after intratumoral injection. Nucl Med Biol. 2016;43(12):818–26.
43. Li CC, Chi JL, Ma Y, Li JH, Xia CQ, Li L, et al. Interventional therapy for human breast cancer in nude mice with 131I gelatin microspheres ((1)(3)(1)I-GMSs) following intratumoral injection. Radiat Oncol. 2014;9:144.
44. Yu P, Wang X, Fu YX. Enhanced local delivery with reduced systemic toxicity: delivery, delivery, and delivery. Gene Ther. 2006;13(15):1131–2.
45. Wenig BL, Werner JA, Castro DJ, Sridhar KS, Garewal HS, Kehrl W, et al. The role of intratumoral therapy with cisplatin/epinephrine injectable gel in the management of advanced squamous cell carcinoma of the head and neck. Arch Otolaryngol Head Neck Surg. 2002;128(8):880–5.
46. Tomita T. Interstitial chemotherapy for brain tumors: review. J Neuro-Oncol. 1991;10(1):57–74.
47. Wang Y, Hu JK, Krol A, Li YP, Li CY, Yuan F. Systemic dissemination of viral vectors during intratumoral injection. Mol Cancer Ther. 2003;2(11):1233–42.
48. Bier J, Benders P, Wenzel M, Bitter K. Kinetics of 57Co-bleomycin in mice after intravenous, subcutaneous and intratumoral injection. Cancer. 1979;44(4):1194–200.

49. Begg AC, Bartelink H, Stewart FA, Brown DM, Luck EE. Improvement of differential toxicity between tumor and normal tissues using intratumoral injection with or without a slow-drug-release matrix system. NCI Monogr. 1988;(6):133–6.
50. Liu W, MacKay JA, Dreher MR, Chen M, McDaniel JR, Simnick AJ, et al. Injectable intratumoral depot of thermally responsive polypeptide-radionuclide conjugates delays tumor progression in a mouse model. J Control Release. 2010;144(1):2–9.
51. Liu T, Soong SJ. Epidemiology of malignant melanoma. Surg Clin North Am. 1996;76(6):1205–22.
52. de Braud F, Khayat D, Kroon BB, Valdagni R, Bruzzi P, Cascinelli N. Malignant melanoma. Crit Rev Oncol Hematol. 2003;47(1):35–63.
53. Barranco SC, Romsdahl MM, Humphrey RM. The radiation response of human malignant melanoma cells grown in vitro. Cancer Res. 1971;31(6):830–3.
54. Doss LL, Memula N. The radioresponsiveness of melanoma. Int J Radiat Oncol Biol Phys. 1982;8(7):1131–4.
55. Hall EJ and Giaccia AJ: Radiobiology for the Radiologist, Lippimcott Williams and Wilkins 2006.
56. Cooks T, Tal M, Raab S, Efrati M, Reitkopf S, Lazarov E, et al. Intratumoral 224Ra-loaded wires spread alpha-emitters inside solid human tumors in athymic mice achieving tumor control. Anticancer Res. 2012;32(12):5315–21.
57. Allen BJ, Rizvi SM, Tian Z. Preclinical targeted alpha therapy for subcutaneous melanoma. Melanoma Res. 2001;11(2):175–82.
58. Morgan AC Jr, Wang KM, Woodhouse CS, SchroffK RW, Foon A, Oldham RK. Preclinical and clinical evaluation of a monoclonal antibody to a human melanoma-associated antigen. Sci Direct. 1985;32:773–7.
59. Bumol TF, Reisfeld RA. Unique glycoprotein-proteoglycan complex defined by monoclonal antibody on human melanoma cells. Proc Natl Acad Sci U S A. 1982;79(4):1245–9.
60. Morgan AC Jr, Galloway DR, Reisfeld RA. Production and characterization of monoclonal antibody to a melanoma specific glycoprotein. Hybridoma. 1981;1(1):27–36.
61. Schroff RW, Woodhouse CS, Foon KA, Oldham RK, Farrell MM, Klein RA, et al. Intratumor localization of monoclonal antibody in patients with melanoma treated with antibody to a 250,000-dalton melanoma-associated antigen. J Natl Cancer Inst. 1985;74(2):299–306.
62. McCready VR, Cornes P. The potential of intratumoural unsealed radioactive source therapy. Eur J Nucl Med. 2001;28(5):567–9.
63. Lee JD, Yang WI, Lee MG, Ryu YH, Park JH, Shin KH, et al. Effective local control of malignant melanoma by intratumoural injection of a beta-emitting radionuclide. Eur J Nucl Med Mol Imaging. 2002;29(2):221–30.
64. Haniffa M, Gunawan M, Jardine L. Human skin dendritic cells in health and disease. J Dermatol Sci. 2015;77(2):85–92.
65. Lee TH, Cho YH, Lee JD, Yang WI, Shin JL, Lee MG. Enhanced antitumor effect of dendritic cell based immunotherapy after intratumoral injection of radionuclide Ho-166 against B16 melanoma. Immunol Lett. 2006;106(1):19–26.
66. Slastnikova TA, Rosenkranz AA, Zalutsky MR, Sobolev AS. Modular nanotransporters for targeted intracellular delivery of drugs: folate receptors as potential targets. Curr Pharm Des. 2015;21(9):1227–38.
67. Slastnikova TA, Rosenkranz AA, Morozova NB, Vorontsova MS, Petriev VM, Lupanova TN, et al. Preparation, cytotoxicity, and in vivo antitumor efficacy of (111)in-labeled modular nanotransporters. Int J Nanomedicine. 2017;12:395–410.
68. Wasson JH, Cushman CC, Bruskewitz RC, Littenberg B, Mulley AG Jr, Wennberg JE. A structured literature review of treatment for localized prostate cancer. Prostate Disease Patient Outcome Research Team. Arch Fam Med. 1993;2(5):487–93.
69. Li Y, Tian Z, Rizvi SM, Bander NH, Allen BJ. In vitro and preclinical targeted alpha therapy of human prostate cancer with Bi-213 labeled J591 antibody against the prostate specific membrane antigen. Prostate Cancer Prostatic Dis. 2002;5(1):36–46.

70. Horoszewicz JS, Leong SS, Kawinski E, Karr JP, Rosenthal H, Chu TM, et al. LNCaP model of human prostatic carcinoma. Cancer Res. 1983;43(4):1809–18.
71. Montgomery BT, Young CY, Bilhartz DL, Andrews PE, Prescott JL, Thompson NF, et al. Hormonal regulation of prostate-specific antigen (PSA) glycoprotein in the human prostatic adenocarcinoma cell line, LNCaP. Prostate. 1992;21(1):63–73.
72. Israeli RS, Powell CT, Corr JG, Fair WR, Heston WD. Expression of the prostate-specific membrane antigen. Cancer Res. 1994;54(7):1807–11.
73. Veldscholte J, Ris-Stalpers C, Kuiper GG, Jenster G, Berrevoets C, Claassen E, et al. A mutation in the ligand binding domain of the androgen receptor of human LNCaP cells affects steroid binding characteristics and response to anti-androgens. Biochem Biophys Res Commun. 1990;173(2):534–40.
74. Lim DJ, Liu XL, Sutkowski DM, Braun EJ, Lee C, Kozlowski JM. Growth of an androgen-sensitive human prostate cancer cell line, LNCaP, in nude mice. Prostate. 1993;22(2):109–18.
75. Kleinman HK. Role of basement membrane and laminin in metasteses and tumour growth. Proc Am Assoc Cancer Res. 1990;31:490–1.
76. Hruby M, Pouckova P, Zadinova M, Kucka J, Lebeda O. Thermoresponsive polymeric radionuclide delivery system--an injectable brachytherapy. Eur J Pharm Sci. 2011;42(5):484–8.
77. Sano K, Kanada Y, Kanazaki K, Ding N, Ono M, Saji H. Brachytherapy with intratumoral injections of Radiometal-labeled polymers that thermoresponsively self-aggregate in tumor tissues. J Nucl Med. 2017;58(9):1380–5.
78. Kwak C, Hong SK, Seong SK, Ryu JM, Park MS, Lee SE. Effective local control of prostate cancer by intratumoral injection of (166)Ho-chitosan complex (DW-166HC) in rats. Eur J Nucl Med Mol Imaging. 2005;32(12):1400–5.
79. Schaal JL, Li X, Mastria E, Bhattacharyya J, Zalutsky MR, Chilkoti A, et al. Injectable polypeptide micelles that form radiation crosslinked hydrogels in situ for intratumoral radiotherapy. J Control Release. 2016;228:58–66.
80. Merrick GS, Butler WM, Dorsey AT, Lief JH, Benson ML. Seed fixity in the prostate/periprostatic region following brachytherapy. Int J Radiat Oncol Biol Phys. 2000;46(1):215–20.
81. Hathout L, Donath D, Moumdjian C, Tetreault-Laflamme A, Larouche R, Beliveau-Nadeau D, et al. Analysis of seed loss and pulmonary seed migration in patients treated with virtual needle guidance and robotic seed delivery. Am J Clin Oncol. 2011;34(5):449–53.
82. Stutz M, Petrikas J, Raslowsky M, Lee P, Gurel M, Moran B. Seed loss through the urinary tract after prostate brachytherapy: examining the role of cystoscopy and urine straining post implant. Med Phys. 2003;30(10):2695–8.
83. Stock RG, Kao J, Stone NN. Penile erectile function after permanent radioactive seed implantation for treatment of prostate cancer. J Urol. 2001;165(2):436–9.
84. Potters L, Torre T, Fearn PA, Leibel SA, Kattan MW. Potency after permanent prostate brachytherapy for localized prostate cancer. Int J Radiat Oncol Biol Phys. 2001;50(5):1235–42.
85. He X, Jia R, Xu L, Liang K, Wang Z, Shao G, et al. (3)(2)P-chromic phosphate-Poly(L-Lactide) seeds of sustained release and their brachytherapy for prostate cancer with lymphatic metastasis. Cancer Biother Radiopharm. 2012;27(7):446–51.
86. Rongs LH, Mao QZ. Significance of laparoscopic pelvic lymph node sampling in the staging of prostate cancer. Chin J Urol. 2004;25:408.
87. Pancreatic cancer: statistics. 2018. https://www.cancer.net/cancer-types/pancreatic-cancer/statistics. Accessed 12/27/2018.
88. Pierantoni C, Pagliacci A, Scartozzi M, Berardi R, Bianconi M, Cascinu S. Pancreatic cancer: progress in cancer therapy. Crit Rev Oncol Hematol. 2008;67(1):27–38.
89. Gao W, Liu L, Liu ZY, Wang Y, Jiang B, Liu XN. Intratumoral injection of 32P-chromic phosphate in the treatment of implanted pancreatic carcinoma. Cancer Biother Radiopharm. 2010;25(2):215–24.
90. Forner A, Llovet JM, Bruix J. Hepatocellular carcinoma. Lancet. 2012;379(9822):1245–55.
91. Nowak AK, Chow PK, Findlay M. Systemic therapy for advanced hepatocellular carcinoma: a review. Eur J Cancer. 2004;40(10):1474–84.

92. Chi JL, Li CC, Xia CQ, Li L, Ma Y, Li JH, et al. Effect of (131)I gelatin microspheres on hepatocellular carcinoma in nude mice and its distribution after intratumoral injection. Radiat Res. 2014;181(4):416–24.
93. Djagny VB, Wang Z, Xu S. Gelatin: a valuable protein for food and pharmaceutical industries: review. Crit Rev Food Sci Nutr. 2001;41(6):481–92.
94. Choi SSRJ. Physicochemical and sensory characteristics of fish gelatin. J Food Sci. 2000;65:194–9.
95. Esposito E, Cortesi R, Nastruzzi C. Gelatin microspheres: influence of preparation parameters and thermal treatment on chemico-physical and biopharmaceutical properties. Biomaterials. 1996;17(20):2009–20.
96. Tabrizian P, Roayaie S, Schwartz ME. Current management of hepatocellular carcinoma. World J Gastroenterol. 2014;20(30):10223–37.
97. Llovet JM, Fuster J, Bruix J. Intention-to-treat analysis of surgical treatment for early hepatocellular carcinoma: resection versus transplantation. Hepatology. 1999;30(6):1434–40.
98. Zhang K, Loong SL, Connor S, Yu SW, Tan SY, Ng RT, et al. Complete tumor response following intratumoral 32P BioSilicon on human hepatocellular and pancreatic carcinoma xenografts in nude mice. Clin Cancer Res. 2005;11(20):7532–7.
99. Park CH, Suh JH, Yoo HS, Lee JT, Kim DI. Evaluation of intrahepatic I-131 ethiodol on a patient with hepatocellular carcinoma. Therapeutic feasibility study. Clin Nucl Med. 1986;11(7):514–7.
100. Ohishi H, Uchida H, Yoshimura H, Ohue S, Ueda J, Katsuragi M, et al. Hepatocellular carcinoma detected by iodized oil. Use of anticancer agents. Radiology. 1985;154(1):25–9.
101. Luo TY, Shih YH, Chen CY, Tang IC, Wu YL, Kung HC, et al. Evaluating the potential of (188)Re-ECD/lipiodol as a therapeutic radiopharmaceutical by intratumoral injection for hepatoma treatment. Cancer Biother Radiopharm. 2009;24(5):535–41.
102. Shih YH, Lin XZ, Yeh CH, Peng CL, Shieh MJ, Lin WJ, et al. Preparation and therapeutic evaluation of (188)Re-thermogelling emulsion in rat model of hepatocellular carcinoma. Int J Nanomedicine. 2014;9:4191–201.
103. Chandu A, Adams G, Smith AC. Factors affecting survival in patients with oral cancer: an Australian perspective. Int J Oral Maxillofac Surg. 2005;34(5):514–20.
104. Liu W, McDaniel J, Li X, Asai D, Quiroz FG, Schaal J, et al. Brachytherapy using injectable seeds that are self-assembled from genetically encoded polypeptides in situ. Cancer Res. 2012;72(22):5956–65.
105. French JT, Goins B, Saenz M, Li S, Garcia-Rojas X, Phillips WT, et al. Interventional therapy of head and neck cancer with lipid nanoparticle-carried rhenium 186 radionuclide. J Vasc Interv Radiol. 2010;21(8):1271–9.
106. Sun J, Liu L, Jiang X, Chen D, Huang Y. Therapeutic effects of radiolabeled 17-allylamino-17-demethoxygeldanamycin on human H460 nonsmall-cell lung carcinoma xenografts in mice. Cancer Biother Radiopharm. 2010;25(2):155–64.
107. Whitesell L, Lindquist SL. HSP90 and the chaperoning of cancer. Nat Rev Cancer. 2005;5(10):761–72.
108. Connett JM, Anderson CJ, Guo LW, Schwarz SW, Zinn KR, Rogers BE, et al. Radioimmunotherapy with a 64Cu-labeled monoclonal antibody: a comparison with 67Cu. Proc Natl Acad Sci U S A. 1996;93(13):6814–8.
109. DuMouchel W, Groer PG. A Bayesian methodology for scaling radiation studies from animals to man. Health Phys. 1989;57(Suppl 1):411–8.
110. Rowland RE, Durbin PW. Survival, causes of death, and estimated tissue doses in a group of human beings injected with plutonium. United States, 1975.
111. Deutsch E, Libson K, Vanderheyden JL, Ketring AR, Maxon HR. The chemistry of rhenium and technetium as related to the use of isotopes of these elements in therapeutic and diagnostic nuclear medicine. Int J Rad Appl Instrum B. 1986;13(4):465–77.
112. Argyrou M, Valassi A, Andreou M, Lyra M. Dosimetry and therapeutic ratios for Rhenium-186 HEDP. ISRN Mol Imaging. 2013;2013:1–6.

113. Haynie TP, Konikowski T, Glenn HJ. Experimental models for evaluation of radioactive tumor-localizing agents. Semin Nucl Med. 1976;6(4):347–69.
114. Abma E, Peremans K, De Vos F, Bosmans T, Kitshoff AM, Daminet S, et al. Biodistribution and tolerance of intravenous iodine-131-labelled hypericin in healthy dogs. Vet Comp Oncol. 2018;16:318.
115. Greene HS. A spontaneous melanoma in the hamster with a propensity for amelanotic alteration and sarcomatous transformation during transplantation. Cancer Res. 1958;18(4):422–5.
116. Toolan HW. Transplantable human neoplasms maintained in cortisone-treated laboratory animals: H.S. No. 1; H.Ep. No. 1; H.Ep. No. 2; H.Ep. No. 3; and H.Emb.Rh. No. 1. Cancer Res. 1954;14(9):660–6.
117. Levenbook IS, Chigirinsky AE, Tsetlin EM, Dodonova NN, Altstein AD. Morphology of tumors induced in hamsters by simian adenoviruses. Int J Cancer. 1968;3(6):712–9.
118. Quinones J, Mizejewski G, Beierwaltes WH. Choriocarcinoma scanning using radiolabeled anti-body to chorionic gonadotrophin. J Nucl Med. 1971;12(2):69–75.
119. Blumenthal RD, Sharkey RM, Kashi R, Natale AM, Goldenberg DM. Influence of animal host and tumor implantation site on radio-antibody uptake in the GW-39 human colonic cancer xenograft. Int J Cancer. 1989;44(6):1041–7.
120. Chuang TF, Lee SC, Liao KW, Hsiao YW, Lo CH, Chiang BL, et al. Electroporation-mediated IL-12 gene therapy in a transplantable canine cancer model. Int J Cancer. 2009;125(3):698–707.
121. Anidjar M, Villette JM, Devauchelle P, Delisle F, Cotard JP, Billotey C, et al. In vivo model mimicking natural history of dog prostate cancer using DPC-1, a new canine prostate carcinoma cell line. Prostate. 2001;46(1):2–10.
122. Gaffar SA, Pant KD, Shochat D, Bennett SJ, Goldenberg DM. Experimental studies of tumor radioimmunodetection using antibody mixtures against carcinoembryonic antigen (CEA) and colon-specific antigen-p (CSAp). Int J Cancer. 1981;27(1):101–5.
123. Wahl RL, Philpott G, Parker CW. Monoclonal antibody radioimmunodetection of human-derived colon cancer. Investig Radiol. 1983;18(1):58–62.
124. Sharkey RM, Primus FJ, Goldenberg DM. Second antibody clearance of radiolabeled antibody in cancer radioimmunodetection. Proc Natl Acad Sci U S A. 1984;81(9):2843–6.
125. Sharkey RM, Filion D, Fand I, Primus FJ, Goldenberg DM. A human colon cancer metastasis model for radioimmunodetection. Cancer Res. 1986;46(7):3677–83.
126. Fand I, Sharkey RM, Goldenberg DM. Use of whole-body autoradiography in cancer targeting with radiolabeled antibodies. Cancer Res. 1990;50(3 Suppl):885s–91s.
127. Livingston RS, Franklin CL, Lattimer JC, Dixon RS, Riley LK, Hook RR Jr, et al. Evaluation of hyperplastic goiter in a colony of Syrian hamsters (Mesocricetus auratus). Lab Anim Sci. 1997;47(4):346–50.
128. Fonsatti E, Jekunen AP, Kairemo KJ, Coral S, Snellman M, Nicotra MR, et al. Endoglin is a suitable target for efficient imaging of solid tumors: in vivo evidence in a canine mammary carcinoma model. Clin Cancer Res. 2000;6(5):2037–43.
129. Anderson CJ, Schwarz SW, Connett JM, Cutler PD, Guo LW, Germain CJ, et al. Preparation, biodistribution and dosimetry of copper-64-labeled anti-colorectal carcinoma monoclonal antibody fragments 1A3-F(ab')2. J Nucl Med. 1995;36(5):850–8.
130. Anderson CJ, Connett JM, Schwarz SW, Rocque PA, Guo LW, Philpott GW, et al. Copper-64-labeled antibodies for PET imaging. J Nucl Med. 1992;33(9):1685–91.
131. Galli F, Manni I, Piaggio G, Balogh L, Weintraub BD, Szkudlinski MW, et al. (99m) Tc-labeled-rhTSH analogue (TR1401) for imaging poorly differentiated metastatic thyroid cancer. Thyroid. 2014;24(8):1297–308.
132. Ahmed KA, Davis BJ, Wilson TM, Wiseman GA, Federspiel MJ, Morris JC. Progress in gene therapy for prostate cancer. Front Oncol. 2012;2:172.
133. Dwyer RM, Schatz SM, Bergert ER, Myers RM, Harvey ME, Classic KL, et al. A preclinical large animal model of adenovirus-mediated expression of the sodium-iodide sym-

porter for radioiodide imaging and therapy of locally recurrent prostate cancer. Mol Ther. 2005;12(5):835–41.
134. Albertoni C, Leoni B, Rosi A, D'Alessio V, Carollo V, Spagnoli LG, et al. Radionuclide therapy of Unresectable tumors with AvidinOX and (90)Y-biotinDOTA: tongue cancer paradigm. Cancer Biother Radiopharm. 2015;30(7):291–8.
135. Chakraborty S, Das T, Banerjee S, Balogh L, Chaudhari PR, Sarma HD, et al. 177Lu-EDTMP: a viable bone pain palliative in skeletal metastasis. Cancer Biother Radiopharm. 2008;23(2):202–13.
136. Ketring AR. 153Sm-EDTMP and 186Re-HEDP as bone therapeutic radiopharmaceuticals. Int J Rad Appl Instrum B. 1987;14(3):223–32.
137. Aas M, Moe L, Gamlem H, Skretting A, Ottesen N, Bruland OS. Internal radionuclide therapy of primary osteosarcoma in dogs, using 153Sm-ethylene-diamino-tetramethylene-phosphonate (EDTMP). Clin Cancer Res. 1999;5(10 Suppl):3148s–52s.

Chapter 10
An Overview of the Regulations of Radiopharmaceuticals

Dao Le

Introduction

According to the American Board of Nuclear Medicine, "nuclear medicine is the medical specialty that uses tracer principle, most often with radiopharmaceuticals, to evaluate molecular, metabolic, physiologic, and pathologic conditions of the body for the purposes of diagnosis, therapy and research" [1]. Additionally, radiopharmaceuticals are defined as substances that contain both a drug component and a radioactive element used to diagnose and treat disease. In the USA, radiopharmaceuticals are considered a special group of medicines bound by complex regulatory elements. According to the Society of Nuclear Medicine and Molecular Imaging (SNMMI), nuclear medicine has faced tremendous regulatory scrutiny since its entrance into the realm of medicine [2].

Radiopharmaceuticals, as compounds that contain a drug labeled with a radioactive isotope, are primarily under the regulatory control of two federal central agencies: the Nuclear Regulatory Commission (NRC) and the Food and Drug Administration (FDA). The principal role of the FDA is to regulate the safety and efficacy of the radioactive drugs as they are used in medical practice, whereas the mission of the NRC is to "ensure the safe use of radioactive materials for beneficial civilian purposes while protecting people and the environment" [3]. Beyond these two federal agencies, oversight of the production, preparation, handling, transport, and use of radiopharmaceuticals is also governed by other regulatory authorities such as the Environmental Protection Agency (EPA), the Occupational Safety and Health Administration (OSHA), and the Department of Transportation (DOT).

The regulations set forth by these federal agencies may be administered at the state level. For example, the State Boards of Pharmacy governs the practice of pharmacy; the State Department of Health Services may oversee matters relating to

D. Le (✉)
The University of Texas, MD Anderson Cancer Center, Houston, TX, USA
e-mail: DBLE@mdanderson.org

F. C. L. Wong (ed.), *Locoregional Radionuclide Cancer Therapy*,
https://doi.org/10.1007/978-3-030-56267-0_10

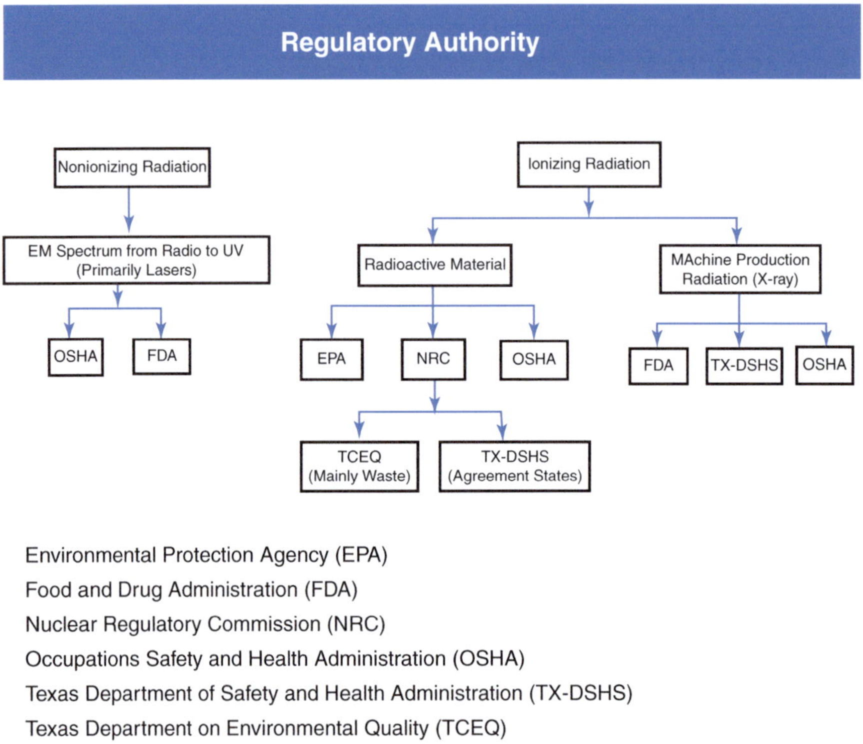

Fig. 10.1 Regulatory authority over radioactive material (RAM) use for Texas

radiation exposure to the public; and the State Department of Environmental Quality manages the radioactive waste programs. Figure 10.1 depicts a typical paradigm of regulatory authority over radioactive material use for a specific state like Texas. Additionally, for most large hospitals, there also exists an additional internal or local regulatory layer to ensure compliance with appropriate federal and state regulations. For instance, hospitals that use radioactive materials often have a radiation safety (RS) group to oversee the institution's radiation program, facilities, and procedures. Typically, the RS group works with the institutional Radiation Safety Committee (RSC), in compliance with federal/state regulations, to oversee all uses of radioactive material, as permitted by the radioactive material (RAM) license, in the institution. Consequently, no one may order, possess, receive, or administer RAM until he/she has been approved as an authorized user by the local RSC.

The purpose of this chapter is to offer a basic understanding of the regulations that govern the preparation, handling, and use of radiopharmaceuticals in a hospital nuclear medicine department. The aim is to assist healthcare providers to better navigate the steadily increasing regulatory oversight over the use of radioactive materials. There is a high level of expectation from these oversight organizations, and full compliance is mandatory in order to continue the necessary nuclear medicine procedures. This chapter provides an overview of the regulations related to the use of both FDA-approved radiopharmaceuticals and investigational radiopharmaceuticals in a clinical nuclear medicine practice. It is important to note that detailed discussion on all regulations pertaining to radiopharmaceuticals is beyond the scope of this chapter. This chapter cannot be a substitute for an in-depth understanding of specific regulations. It is advised that healthcare providers always obtain up-to-date information regarding federal, state, and local regulations pertaining to your specific practice.

Historical Background on Regulatory Authority of Radiopharmaceuticals

Nuclear Regulatory Commission

Because radioactive pharmaceuticals are comprised of ionizing radiation, there are legal restrictions as to who is permitted to transport, obtain, handle, and use these agents. At the federal level, the NRC was created by Congress to protect the patients, public, and workers from unnecessary exposure to radiation. The mission of the NRC is as follows:

> The NRC licenses and regulates the Nation's civilian use of radioactive materials to provide reasonable assurance of adequate protection of public health and safety and to promote the common defense and security and to protect the environment [3].

The US government's history of nuclear regulation dates back to 1946, with the congressional passage of the Atomic Energy Act, which created a five-member Atomic Energy Commission (AEC). The priority of the federal government was to maintain strict control over atomic technology. At the same time, in order to encourage use, the government was working to convince the people that the atomic age can bring benefits and not just threats of nuclear war. The purpose of the AEC is to promote and regulate atomic research and development. Thus, procurement of radionuclides for medical use required submission of an application to a special Subcommittee of Human Applications. According to the NRC historian, "the 1946 law created a virtual Government monopoly of the technology" [4]. The 1946 law was replaced by the Atomic Energy Act of 1954, where Congress gave the AEC power to promote and regulate civilian nuclear power. Because of the inherent conflict between promoting and regulating atomic energy, the result was the passage of the Energy Reorganization Act of 1974 which splits the AEC in order to avoid the conflicting obligations of both promoting and regulating nuclear power. As a result of the Act of 1954, the NRC was established as a stand-alone agency specializing in reactor safety [5].

Today's NRC is still very focused on reactor licensing and safety, but the agency also has oversight over radioactive materials licensing for a variety of purposes, including medical use of radioisotopes. NRC issues specific licenses to medical, industrial, and academic centers for possession and use of by-product, source, and special nuclear materials. Once issued, the radioactive materials (RAM) license can be changed during renewal or by submission of an amendment. Many facilities are in a constant state of amendment submissions in order to stay current with both authorized users listed and radionuclides being used [6].

Additionally, the NRC also regulates both high- and low-level radioactive waste. High-level radioactive wastes are a by-product of reactions that occur inside nuclear reactors, whereas low-level waste typically consists of low energy producing radionuclides with long half-lives such as carbon-14. Generally, most hospitals do not fall in the low-level waste category because nuclear medicine clinics predominately administer short-lived isotopes (i.e., isotopes with <120 days half-life) that are allowed to be decayed in storage and then disposed of in normal waste streams as regular biohazard waste for blood products or regular landfill trash for gloves and paper products. In situations where the institution may have low-level waste (i.e., academic and research hospitals), low-level waste can be stored on-site until acceptable decay level is achieved (if allowed by the radioactive materials license), or it can be shipped to an NRC-approved low-level waste disposal site [7].

As previously mentioned, due to the radioactive nature of radiopharmaceuticals, the NRC has oversight over the safe use of these agents. However, the NRC can also transfer its authority to regulate the use of radioactive material to individual states. In such instances, the NRC enters into "agreements" with the state, and this gives the state the authority to license and inspect most radioactive material within its borders. The states that have entered into this agreement with the NRC are called Agreement States. It is important to note that the NRC requires Agreement States to adopt equivalent, or more stringent, regulations for each NRC rule issued. As a result, rules regarding radiation are often consistent from state to state. Figure 10.2, obtained from the NRC website, illustrates the 38 Agreement States, 11 Non-Agreement States, and 1 State that is pursing agreement with the NRC [8].

The NRC and the Agreement States regulate nuclear medicine through the Code of Federal Regulations (CFR), particularly CFR 10. The CFR is a codification of the general and permanent rules and regulations published in the Federal Register by the federal government [9]. The CFR is composed of 50 titles covering different areas under federal oversight. There are five relevant codes for the regulation of radioactive materials. Table 10.1 lists applicable Code of Regulations for radioactive materials.

Food and Drug Administration

Historically, the use of radioactive materials was solely under the auspice of the AEC/NRC. It was not until 1975 that the Food and Drug Administration (FDA) assumed authority over the approval and licensing of radiopharmaceuticals.

It is well established that the FDA regulates radiopharmaceutical's use in terms of their chemical toxicity and efficacy. A summary of the mission of the FDA is as follows:

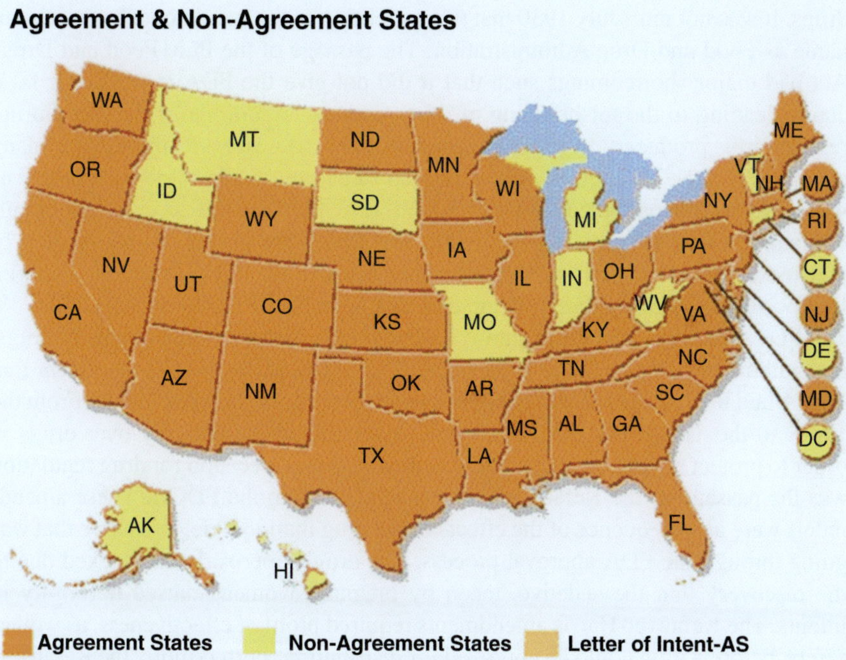

Fig. 10.2 Agreement States. States that have entered into agreement with the NRC is called "Agreement States." As of 2019, there are currently 38 Agreement States and 1 state that has filed a petition to the NRC. This map was obtained from the NRC 2019 website

Table 10.1 Applicable Code of Federal Regulations for radioactive materials (RAM)

Radiation regulations			
Applicable Code of Federal Regulations (CFRs)			
CFR	Title	Type	Federal agency
10	Energy	RAM	Nuclear Regulatory Commission (NRC)
21	Food and Drug	X-ray *RAM	Food and Drug Administration (FDA) *For drug and device trials
29	Labor	RAM X-ray	Occupational Safety and Health Administration (OSHA)
40	Protection of Environment	RAM	Environmental Protection Agency (EPA)
49	Transportation	RAM	Department of Transportation (DOT)

> The Food and Drug Administration is responsible for protecting the public health by ensuring the safety, efficacy, and security of human and veterinary drugs, biological products, and medical devices; and by ensuring the safety of our nation's food supply, cosmetics, and products that emit radiation [10].

The regulatory jurisdiction of the US government, under the auspice of the Bureau of Chemistry, over drugs began with the Pure Food and Drugs Act of 1906, a law that prohibited interstate commerce of adulterated and misbranded food and drugs. It was not until July 1930 that this governing entity was known by its present name as Food and Drug Administration. The passage of the Pure Food and Drugs Act had major shortcomings such that it did not give the FDA control over false claims leading to the misbranding of drug products. Additionally, the Act did not require drug producers to provide proof of safety. As a result, there were many examples of false drug cures that often lead to painful deaths. One such case was when over 100 people died, many of whom were children, due to ingestion of sulfanilamide elixir which was produced using diethylene glycol, a toxic analog of antifreeze. As a result of this catastrophic disaster of 1937, President Franklin D. Roosevelt signed the Food, Drug, and Cosmetic Act (FDCA) on June 25, 1938. The FDCA required that drugs show proof of safety, outlawed false claims of drugs, and authorized inspections of drug manufacturing facilities [11]. It is evident that FDCA laid the foundation and continues to be the basis of drug regulation. From the 1940s to the 1960s, the FDA continued to strengthen its authority over drugs in order to protect the public consumer. Another landmark decision for drug regulation was the passage of the Kefauver-Harris amendments to the FDCA. These amendments were a consequence of the effects of the drug thalidomide, a sedative that was going through the FDA approval process. The drug's approval was blocked due to the discovery that the sedative, taken by pregnant women, caused deformity in infants. The Kefauver-Harris amendments required proof of effectiveness, as well as safety, before a drug could be approved for distribution. Furthermore, the Kefauver-Harris amendments the FDA control over investigations, authority to regulate advertising of prescription drugs, and established good manufacturing practices. The amendments also laid the groundwork for the clinical trials process [12]. Here lies the concept and infrastructure of Investigational New Drug (IND) and new drug application (NDA) process. This history provides a framework for understanding the regulatory powers of the FDA today. Working knowledge of these regulations is critical to ensuring regulatory compliance of radiopharmaceutical use in both the clinical and research realm in nuclear medicine.

Other Pertinent Regulatory Agencies

For the five relevant federal codes for the regulation of radioactive materials, there are five regulatory agencies that have direct regulatory authority over radiopharmaceuticals at the federal level. Beyond the first two, NRC and FDA, which have been discussed, the list also includes the Occupational Safety and Health Administration (OSHA), the Environmental Protection Agency (EPA), and the Department of Transportation (DOT).

OSHA is an agency under the US Department of Labor with the charge to ensure the safe and healthy working conditions for working individuals [13]. OSHA enforces standards that focus on worker safety by monitoring and limiting exposure to workers. To comply with set regulations, radiation workers are required to wear radiation dosimeters in order to monitor radiation exposure. Radiation dosimeters are issued based on the worker's use of radioactive materials. For instance, personnel monitoring for radiation exposure is required for personnel who have the potential to reach 10% of the applicable limits: Annual deep-dose equivalent (DDE) limit is 5000 mrem (50 mSv) per year to a radiation worker and 100 mrem (1 mSV) per year to a member of the public. An annual report of radiation exposure must be provided by the employee to any radiation worker who received a measure exposure of 100 mrem (1 mSv) or greater during the previous calendar year [14].

On the other hand, the EPA is an independent agency with a mandate from the federal government to protect human health and the environment [15]. In regard to radiation, the EPA has regulations governing the levels of radioactive materials in the general environment and outside of the boundaries that are under the control of persons possessing or using radioactive materials under a RAM license such as a nuclear medicine clinic or a nuclear pharmacy. Examples of outside boundaries include radioactive materials released into the air or into the water supply. It is important to point out that the EPA does not regulate radioactive material that enters the environment from patients. Therefore, patient release of radiation after administration of a radioactive agent via urination or defecation into public sewer systems does not count toward effluent release into the environment. Conversely, in an academic research hospital setting, besides patient release, there can be release of radioactive material down the drain. Generally, the hospital radiation safety group or the radiation safety officer (RSO) works to ensure that the amount of radioactive material released into the water is within regulatory limits by performing an annual calculation. The easiest way to demonstrate compliance is by calculation that assumes worst-case scenario: If the hospital were to dump all radioactive material allowed on the RAM license down the sewer, divide that total by the number of gallons of water used. The result needs to be below set levels. This number is often documented in an annual report and presented to the NRC or State Radiation Inspector. Keep in mind that individual states may set more stringent effluent release standards. The way in which the EPA operates is that Congress often writes the environmental law which is then implemented by the EPA through the creation of regulations. Frequently, the EPA is seen as an agency that sets national standards, and individual states aspire to meet these standards by issuing their own guidelines and rules [15].

An NRC or State Radiation Inspector could also inquire about the training documents for shippers and transporters of radiopharmaceuticals. The NRC and DOT share responsibilities of regulating radioactive transport. The transfer and shipment of packages that contain radioactive materials are considered hazardous material (hazmat) shipments and are governed by the US Department of Transportation (USDOT/DOT). The DOT issues most of the regulations regarding transportation in Title 49: 49CFR Part 107-Hazardous Materials Program Procedures and 49CFR Parts 171-180, 390-397-Hazardous Materials Regulations-Department of Transportation. In the same way, the NRC regulations relating to the transport of hazmat are found in 10CFR Part 30.34(c) and Part 30.41-Nuclear Regulatory Commission (NRC) and 10CFR Part 71-Nuclear Regulatory Commission-Packaging and Transportation of Radioactive Material. The NRC is most concerned with high-level quantities of radiation and advises licensees in 10CFR 71.5 to comply with DOT regulations when NRC regulations do not apply [16]. In a hospital nuclear medicine department, typically the foremost concern is the documentation and maintenance of training documents.

The US DOT under 49CFR. 172.700 stipulates general training in the safe handling of hazmat for all employees who prepare packages of hazmat for shipment, operate a vehicle to transport hazmat, and are responsible for the safety of transporting hazmat. In a nuclear medicine department, where radiopharmaceuticals are supplied by an outside nuclear pharmacy vendor, nuclear medicine technologists (NMT) are responsible for preparing return shipments, of either unused doses or used doses with residual activity, to the pharmacy vendor. Therefore, according to 49CFR 172.404, a RAM licensee must provide certificate of training for all employees involved with packaging, marking, labeling, measuring, loading, transporting, and storage of packages containing RAM. This training must be completed within 90 days of employment and every 3 years thereafter [17]. The DOT training must address the following topics:

- General awareness and knowledge of radioactive materials
- Function-specific training on tasks that the employee will perform such as packaging or labeling
- Safety considerations of radioactive materials
- Security awareness training

The DOT requires that the employee is tested in the four topic areas and successful completion is usually in the form of a certificate. Many hospitals either have an in-house DOT training program or subscribe to outside vendors for either live or web-based DOT training.

State Regulatory Control

Federal regulatory agencies generally have a memorandum of understanding with different state agencies and give states the right to ensure compliance through enforcement of laws governing the use of radioactive materials.

For a clinical NM practice, the day-to-day regulatory scrutiny is experienced more at state and local level. In a nuclear medicine clinic, the inspectors that come through the facility are often from either the local State Health Radiation Control group (if the state is an Agreement State) or the State Boards of Pharmacy (if the hospital has a nuclear pharmacy operation). Additionally, the State Medical Board would handle issues related to physicians' use of radiopharmaceuticals, but an inspection of the facility from the State Medical Board is not common.

Although not tied to either federal or state regulatory agencies, accreditation organizations have surveyors to evaluate hospital compliance to set standards which are reflective of federal and state regulations. Generally, the difference between a regulatory agency inspection and an accreditation assessment is that the regulator focuses on exactly what is in the regulations, whereas the accreditation inspector looks at the institution's overall standard of operation. One such organization is The Joint Commission, an independent, not-for-profit group that accredits and certifies healthcare organizations [18].

For state inspections, well-established laws and regulations are enforceable, and if violated, civil and criminal enforcement is warranted. More often than not, the result is an issuance of monetary penalties, but in extreme cases, the right to use RAM can be revoked. However, in the case of an accreditation body such as TJC, standards issued by accrediting bodies do not have a force of law but carry a symbol of quality. Typically, accreditation is voluntary but is often tied to monetary reimbursement for the institution or program. Another example of an accreditation body is the American College of Radiology (ACR) where accreditation is a recognition that the facility operates at a high level in medical imaging [19].

NRC/State Health Radiation Control: RAM Inspection

As noted previously, there are currently 38 states that have entered into agreement with the NRC. Commonly, the Agreement States have their own equivalent regulations to the NRC regulations found in Title 10 CFR. Texas is an example of an Agreement State, and Fig. 10.3 illustrates a comparison of the NRC Title 10 CFR and Texas Title 25 of Texas Administrative Code. For the State of Texas, the rules and regulations that govern the use of RAM are enforced by the Texas Department of State Health Services (TXDSHS), Radiation Control Program. The mission of the TXDSHS, Radiation Control Program, is to "protect and promote the physical and environmental health of the people of Texas. The goal of the program is to prevent unnecessary radiation exposure to the public through licensing, registration, inspection, enforcement, and managing emergency response" [20]. For hospitals

Radiation Regulations- Radioactive Material

- **NRC regulations found in Title 10 CFR**
  - Part 19 – Notices, instructions and reports to workers: inspection and investigations
  - Part 20 – Standards for Protection Against Radiation
  - Part 30 – General Provisions for Byproduct Material
  - Part 33 – Specific domestic licenses of broad scope for byproduct material
  - Part 35 – Medical Use
- **Texas equivalent regs found in Title 25 of Texas Administrative Code**
  - §289.203 – Notices, Instructions, and Reports To Workers; Inspections
  - §289.202 – Standards for Protection Against Radiation
  - §289.201 – General Licensing of Byproduct Material
  - §289.252 – Licensing of Radioactive Material
  - §289.256 – Medical Use

Fig. 10.3 Comparison of the NRC Title 10 CFR and Texas Title 25 of the Texas Administrative Code

Compliances Tips

How to Avoid Compliance Problems Relating to Radioactive Material Licenses

1. READ YOUR LICENSE

2. Know what radioactive material your license authorizes you to use. The license specifies the isotope, curie quantity, make and model of the device and its use.

3. Verify that your license is correct, that what you requested on your application, amendment request or renewal is what you received. Or, that you understand why your request was not granted.

4. Specific variances or exemptions from Department of State Health Services (DSHS) regulations must be requested in writing with compelling evidence as to why it should be granted.

5. You are responsible for compliance with the sections of the DSHS regulations listed on your license unless specifically exempted.

6. Read and be familiar with your operating, safety and emergency procedures.

7. You will be inspected for compliance with your operating, safety and emergency procedures submitted with your application, as well as DSHS reoulations and other correspondence listed in the last condition of your license.

8. Requests for changes to your Radioactive Material license should be sent to the attention of the specific licensing program. (i.e. Industrial Licensing, Medical Licensing, General License Acknowledgment)

9. You must request an amendment to your license when something on the license has changed. (i.e. company name, address, new storage location, termination of storage location, etc.)

10. You may not designate a new individual as the radiation safety officer or change a storage location without PRIOR approval from the Agency.

11. Your license does not automatically terminate on the expiration date. However, the authorization to use radioactive material does expire.

12. Failure to pay your license fee DOES NOT terminate your license. You must request termination of your license in writing or license fees, which you will be responsible for, will continue to accrue. Continued failure to pay license fees may result in collection by the Texas Attorney General's Office.

13. Payment of the license fee DOES NOT renew your license.

14. Do not hesitate to contact the Radiation Control Program concerning your Radioactive Material License or a compliance matter. Really...we are here to help you.

15. READ YOUR LICENSE

Last updated January 28, 2016

Texas Department of State Health Services-Radiation Control Program, Compliance tips for successful site RAM inspection. https://dshs.texas.gov/radiaton/ram/compliance-tips.aspx.

Fig. 10.4 Texas Department of State Health Services, Radiation Control Program, compliance tips. Texas Department of State Health Services, Radiation Control Program, compliance tips for successful site RAM inspection. https://dshs.texas.gov/radiaton/ram/compliance-tips.aspx

with broad-scope RAM licenses in Texas, RAM inspections are performed at least every 2 years. The number 1 compliance tip offered by the State is to read the RAM license carefully and know what the license authorizes in terms of isotope, quantity (millicurie vs. Curie levels), make/model of devices, and their use. Figure 10.4 is a list of compliance tips issued by the TXDSHS, Radiation Control Program. This list can be found on their website to help RAM licensees with RAM inspections [21].

State Boards of Pharmacy: Pharmacy Inspection

Not all regulatory agencies have set inspection schedules. For hospitals that have an in-house nuclear pharmacy or a hot lab listed under the hospital pharmacy department, BOP inspections can be expected. Depending on your state, inspections can occur on an annual or biennial schedule. However, if the nuclear medicine department uses a centralized commercial nuclear pharmacy for all their radiopharmaceutical products, then hospital BOP inspections are typically an uncommon occurrence. There are only a small number of hospitals or imaging centers that have their own nuclear pharmacies to prepare and dispense radiopharmaceuticals for on-site use. In general, only academic hospitals have on-site nuclear pharmacies.

Nuclear pharmacies are responsible for preparing and dispensing radiopharmaceutical prescriptions under the auspice of the practice of pharmacy thus regulated by the BOP. Radiopharmaceuticals are not dispensed directly to the patient but rather to healthcare professionals licensed to handle and administer the radioactive drug. There are a few radiopharmaceuticals that are available as ready-to-use which thus can be appropriately labeled and delivered to the nuclear medicine clinics. However, most radiopharmaceuticals must be prepared on an as-needed basis. The preparation of the radioactive drug often consists of reconstituting cold drug kits (lyophilizate in a vial) with a radioactive solution, typically technetium Tc-99m sodium pertechnetate. In this case, both the cold drug kit and the technetium Tc-99m generator are commercially available as FDA-approved drugs. Technetium Tc-99m pertechnetate, along with other similar radionuclide products, are used for single photon emission computed tomography (SPECT) imaging, hence termed SPECT radiopharmaceuticals. See Table 10.2 for common single photon emission computed tomography radionuclides. By and large, the preparation of these products is done according to the manufacturer's package insert therefore falls under the jurisdication of the BOP. On the other hand, positron-emission tomography (PET) radiopharmaceuticals generally require a cyclotron or special PET generators such as gallium Ga-68 for preparation. The radionuclide components of PET drugs are generally short-lived positron-emitting isotopes obtained from the cyclotron, which are a type of particle accelerator [22]. Table 10.3 contains a list of common positron emission tomography radionuclides. In the case of PET radiopharmaceuticals requiring the use of a cyclotron, the FDA asserts that production does not fall under the practice of medicine or practice of pharmacy but rather the act of manufacturing. Moreover, manufacturing regulations are under the jurisdiction of the FDA [23]. Nuclear pharmacies that provide both SPECT and PET drug and are involved in the compounding and dispensing of investigational research radiopharmaceuticals do so under the authority of the local State BOP and the FDA.

Table 10.2 Commonly used SPECT radionuclides

Single photon-emitting isotopes	
Nuclide	Half-life
^{67}Ga	78.3 h
^{111}In	67.9 h
^{123}I	13 h
^{131}I	8.05 days
^{99m}Tc	6.07 h
^{201}Tl	73 h

Table 10.3 Commonly used PET radionuclides

Positron-emitting isotopes	
Nuclide	Half-life
^{15}O	2 min
^{13}N	10 min
^{11}C	20 min
^{18}F	110 min
*^{82}Rb	72 s
*^{68}Ga	68 min

*PET isotopes produced from a generator

State Boards of Pharmacy are responsible for establishing regulations for pharmacy practice. In an inspection, the inspector could ask for a variety of documentation to ensure compliance to set regulations such as licensing and registration, appropriate training documents for pharmacy personnel, and prescription files. Additionally, State BOP expect pharmacies to have policies and procedures that adhere to guidelines that apply to their unique practice settings. The US Pharmacopeia (USP) is a nonprofit organization that sets standards for drug quality, thus influencing medicine and pharmacy practice. USP General Chapter <797> Pharmaceutical Compounding-Sterile Preparations (USP<797>) is a general chapter that provides guidance on the preparation of compounded sterile preparations (CSPs), including radiopharmaceuticals [24]. These standards were put into place in January 2004, but radiopharmaceuticals were not specifically mentioned. It was not until the first revision of USP <797> in 2008 that radiopharmaceuticals were included as CSPs. Since nuclear pharmacy practice includes the preparation of sterile radiopharmaceuticals, incorporation of these standards into daily practice is an expectation. However, it is important to note that USP is a nongovernmental, nonprofit organization and standards issued are only legally enforceable when a regulatory agency, such as State BOP or FDA, with authority requires compliance. According to the USP, almost all states have laws governing pharmaceutical compounding. In August of 2016, the National Association of Boards of Pharmacy (NABP) adopted the Model State Pharmacy Act and Model Rules which provide guidance to State BOP on developing state rules which incorporate USP <797> [25]. Moreover, in the NABP Survey of Pharmacy Law conducted in 2016, at least 87 percent of boards of pharmacy require full compliance or have incorporated aspects of USP<797> into their state regulations [26]. Besides State BOP, the FDA has included provisions of USP standards into the FDCA, mandating USP standards for compounding sterile products. For instance, under Section 503A of the FDCA, pharmacists and physicians are qualified for an exemption of the requirements of a new drug application (NDA) if they observe USP guidance on pharmacy compounding using bulk drug substances and ingredients that comply with the standards of USP or National Formulary (NF) monographs [23]. USP<797> contains quality standards for many areas of compounding such as training of personnel, cleaning and disinfecting of compounding area, preparation of release checks, and determining beyond-use dates [27]. In a nuclear pharmacy, a BOP inspector may ask for a demonstration of gowning and garbing procedures or documentation on validation of personnel aseptic technique training. Moreover, these standards apply not only to pharmacists practicing in a nuclear pharmacy but also to anyone manipulating CSPs, including nuclear pharmacy technicians and nuclear medicine physicians and technologists. The SNMMI published a very informative document addressing general questions about USP<797> containing examples of the influence of USP <797> in a clinical nuclear medicine practice. For instance, compliance with USP <797> is necessary in the case of addition of normal saline to a patient dose [28]. If the radiopharmaceutical dose is administered within 1 h after manipulation, then it would fall under the immediate use provision and does not require conditions outlined in USP <797> for low-, medium-, or high-risk-level CSPs. However, if the dose is not administered within the 1-h window, then the manipulation of the dose (i.e., addition of saline) must be performed under conditions outlined in USP <797> for low-risk-level CSPs such as an ISO Class 5 biological safety cabinet located in an ISO Class 7 environment [27]. Another prime example of how USP <797> guidelines affect NM clinical operation is in the autologous red blood cell labeling for localization of GI bleeds. Technetium Tc-99m pertechnetate is ordered from the nuclear pharmacy for RBC labeling, using an Ultratag™ RBC kit. This labeling is often done on an open bench, in the hot lab of a nuclear medicine department, requiring at least three punctures into the septum of the vial [29]. Under the USP <797> immediate use provision, which allows for exemption from requirements of low-risk-level CSP conditions, there can only be two entries into any one container (i.e., vial) [27]. As a consequence, this labeling procedure is noncompliant with USP <797> immediate use provision.

As previously mentioned, radiopharmaceuticals as CSPs were not mentioned in the original USP<797> sterile compounding guidelines and were subsequently included in the first revision. However, there were still many questions due to the special issues related to compounding of radiopharmaceuticals. In 2015, USP published a proposed revision of <797> and included a slightly expanded section on "Radiopharmaceuticals as CSPs" published in the Pharmaceutical Forum for public comment. However, the proposed revision still lacked sufficient details to fully elucidate vital differences for this unique class of drugs. Accordingly, USP received over more than 8000 comments by 2016. The consensus of the nuclear medicine and nuclear pharmacy community was that Section 17, Radiopharmaceuticals as CSPs, was inadequate as a guidance document. As a result, in May 2017, USP staff agreed on the development of a new chapter: General Chapter <825>. The scope and rational of this chapter is to provide clear and effective guidance for compounded sterile radiopharmacetuicals [30]. In short, this chapter is an expansion of the <797> section on compounding radiopharmaceuticals, tailoring to the specific needs of radiopharmaceutical preparations. After the publication of <825> on June 1, 2019, with an anticipated official date of December 1, 2019; USP received an appeal to the General Chapter <825>. After careful review, USP denied the appeal and established a new offical date of December 1, 2020 [31].

Accreditation Organizations: The Joint Commission Inspection

USP works closely with state legislatures, State Boards of Pharmacy, and different accrediting organizations, such as TJC, to ensure quality compounding of drugs for patients. Although accreditation bodies do not have a force of law, hospitals strive to establish compliance with accreditation standards to demonstrate commitment to providing the highest quality of patient care. Moreover, hospitals are required to be in compliance with the federal requirements stated in the Medicare Conditions of Participation (CoP), set forth in 42 CFR Part 482, in order to receive reimbursement from the Centers for Medicare and Medicaid Services (CMS) [32]. CMS acknowledges that the standards of certain accrediting organizations meet or exceeds CMS's expectations and therefore will accept the certification from these accreditation organizations. For hospitals, achieving certification status from CMS-accepted accreditation organizations ensures that the facility also meets CMS standards. Keep in mind that in order to validate an organization's accreditation process, CMS can come and perform a validation survey, and typically these validation surveys can be performed shortly after an accreditation visit [33].

In a hospital nuclear medicine setting, a common accreditation organization encountered is The Joint Commission. A compliance checklist for diagnostic imaging can be found on the TJC website [34]. Additionally, TJC defines medication as any product designated by the FDA as a drug; therefore, this ensures that radiopharmaceuticals have the same level of supervision as other medications in terms of prescribing, dispensing, storage, security, administration, and monitoring of adverse events. For a nuclear medicine clinic and hospital nuclear pharmacy, the primary difference between a NRC and a BOP inspection is that the regulatory agencies focus exactly on their regulations, whereas the accreditation inspection is all-encompassing, covering all aspects that may affect the quality of healthcare. Questions from TJH auditors can include radiation safety (similar to NRC) matters and encompass the preparation of a radiopharmaceutical (similar to BOP).

Regulatory Overlap of the FDA and BOP

FDA's mission is to ensure safety and efficacy of drugs and medical devices, and it is under that encompassing umbrella that FDA steps into the boundaries of the practice of medicine or practice of pharmacy.

For hospital nuclear pharmacies that provide SPECT drugs and PET drug and are involved in the compounding and dispensing of investigational research radiopharmaceuticals, the BOP and NRC/Agreement State are not the sole regulators of this practice.

The path toward development of a suitable regulatory framework for PET drugs has been challenging for the nuclear medicine community. Prior to the FDA Modernization Act which was passed in 1997, the preparation of PET drugs was under the practice of medicine and pharmacy and regulated by the respective Boards. Under the provisions of the Durham-Humphrey amendments to the FDCA, facilities preparing radiopharmaceuticals are able to do so *without* registering with the FDA as a drug manufacturing facility. Also, in 1984 the FDA adopted the "Nuclear Pharmacy Guideline: Criteria for Determining when to Register as a Drug Establishment," which firmly establishes the preparation of all radiopharmaceuticals under the practice of pharmacy and medicine [35]. However, this all changed in 1997 with the adoption of the FDA Moderation Act which established current good manufacturing practice (cGMP) for all PET drugs. It took the FDA many years to establish new manufacturing guidelines for PET drugs. By 2009, the FDA finalized these guidelines and issued a mandate that all PET-producing facilities had until December 2012 to reach full compliance with the new regulations [36]. Moving forward, hospital nuclear pharmacies that produce and dispense PET radiopharmaceuticals such as fluorine F-18 FDG to the nuclear medicine clinic are subjected to FDA audits and inspections. The job of the FDA inspectors is to confirm compliance of the PET facility to established cGMP regulations and to ensure that the facility honors all commitments made to the agency. Typically, FDA performs inspections of PET producers on an annual basis. However, FDA will not typically have routine inspections of facilities that produce PET drugs for investigational drug research [37].

In 1975, FDA issued a final rule that placed all radiopharmaceuticals, both established radioactive drugs and investigational radioactive drugs, under the regulatory authority of the FDA. The FDA would regulate radiopharmaceuticals the same way as traditional pharmaceuticals. According to the agency, there are three pathways for conducting research studies involving an investigational new radioactive drug or biological product.

1. Under an approved Investigational New Drug (IND) application
2. Exempt from IND requirements (i.e., protocol involving placebo)
3. Under the authority of an FDA-approved Radioactive Research Committee (RDRC) [38]

For new drugs, the FDA regulatory process comes into effect when the drug has proven to be safe and effective in preclinical studies (animal data) and now is ready to be tested on human patients. At this point, the researcher would determine whether the research study now involving human patients require an IND application to the FDA. The IND, among serving other functions, is also an exemption from the FDA allowing for the shipment of drugs across state lines. Recall that FDA requires that only drugs that have submitted a NDA and obtained approval can be transported across state lines. Since investigational drugs have not gained NDA approval status, the only way for distribution is by obtaining IND approval. The IND application must contain three main components:

1. Animal pharmacology and toxicology studies to show safety
2. Manufacturing information ensuring that the new drug will be available for the study
3. Clinical protocol which contains details of the study [39]

There are three types of IND applications:

- *Investigator IND*, also known as physician-sponsored IND, is when a physician who is conducting the study submits the application. Under this type of IND, the physician is held responsible for all aspects of the study including preparation, dispensing, and administration of the drug.
- *Emergency Use IND* can be used when a physician determines that the use of the experimental agent is needed for urgent medical conditions to benefit the patient. Due to the time sensitivity, the physician was unable to go through the traditional submission and approval process. Further, this type of IND can also be used in circumstances where the patient does not meet the requirements for existing studies or if an approved study protocol does not exist.
- *Treatment IND*, also known as expanded access protocols, is submitted when an experimental agent has shown to be safe and effective and, while it is being reviewed by the FDA, the experimental agent can be used for treatment of patients with immediate life-threatening conditions or serious diseases where there is no alternative therapy.

Once the IND has been submitted, the investigator must wait 30 calendar days before initiating the clinical study [39]. While the FDA is reviewing the application, the FDA may contact the sponsor for additional information or further clarification. Importantly, for most institutions, there exists an internal or local regulatory pathway for research protocols prior to the actual submission of the IND to the FDA. In this way, hospitals add an extra layer of oversight to ensure full compliance with various federal and state regulatory agencies. For example, all clinical studies must be approved by the hospital's Institutional Review Board (IRB) to ensure the protection of the research patients. Internal/local regulatory pathways will be discussed later in the chapter.

Once the study has been initiated, the FDA has the right to conduct both announced and unannounced inspections of facilities that conduct clinical studies. The primary goal of the inspection is to determine if the clinical investigators are conducting the study in accordance to the approved IND application. In an FDA IND audit, the FDA inspector could go through study documents and standard operating procedures (SOPs) related to the study and conduct interviews with individuals involved with the study, as listed on the IND [40].

Local/Internal Regulatory Authority

Radioactive Drug Research Committee

Another route for conducting human research involving a radioactive drug is through the approval of a local Radioactive Drug Research Committee (RDRC). The committee allows investigators to conduct research studies using radiotracers in human subjects to establish feasibility prior to committing to the significant expense and effort of filing IND application.

This arrangement is similar to the agreement between NRC and Agreement States. Here, the FDA is allowing the RDRC to approve radioactive drug research studies if, and only if, the RDRC commits to upholding FDA regulations.

FDA regulations (21 CFR Sec. 361.1) allow for the research use, in human subjects, of radioactive drugs that are not currently under an FDA-accepted IND or NDA application, provided that certain specified conditions outlined in 21 CFR Sec. 361.1 are met:

- The research is considered basic science research and is done for the purpose of advancing scientific knowledge. This type of research is:
  - Intended to obtain basic information regarding the *metabolism* (including kinetics, distribution, dosimetry, and localization) of a radioactive drug or regarding *human physiology, pathophysiology, or biochemistry*
  - *Not* intended for immediate therapeutic, diagnostic, or similar purposes (e.g., preventive benefit to the study subject from the research)
  - *Not* intended to determine the safety and effectiveness of a radioactive drug in humans
- The research study is approved by an FDA-approved RDRC based on the following requirements:
  - Qualified study investigators
  - Properly licensed medical facility to possess and handle radioactive materials
  - Appropriate selection and consent of research subjects
  - Appropriate quality assurance of radioactive drug administered
  - Sound research protocol design
  - Reporting of adverse events by the investigator to the RDRC
  - Approval by an appropriate Institutional Review Board (IRB)
- The pharmacologic dose of the radioactive drug to be administered is known not to cause any clinically detectable pharmacologic effect in humans.
- The radiation dose to be administered is justified by the quality of the study being undertaken and the importance of the information it seeks to obtain and is within the limits specified [41].

The RDRC, established under such authority and in accordance with the stated regulations, serves to initially and continually review such research investigations to ensure compliance with the provisions of FDA guidelines. RDRC operating procedures outlining responsibilities, approval of research studies, continual oversight of approved protocols, committee meeting documentation, and the committee membership shall be carefully established to ensure compliance with the provisions of 21 CFR Sec. 361.1. RDRC members require specialized expertise in radiopharmaceuticals. Consequently, FDA regulations permit the RDRC to be comprised of a minimum of five members to include representation from each of the following required areas of specialization:

- Nuclear medicine physician
- Radioactive drug preparation/formulation/quality control (e.g., a nuclear pharmacist or radiochemist)
- Radiation safety/radiation dosimetry [42]

Moreover, the committee's review of submitted protocols may involve consultants from other medical disciplines, if, in the committee's opinion, additional expertise is required to sufficiently review the scientific merit or technical aspects of a submitted research study. For instance, protocols involving pediatric subjects will require involvement of a reviewer with pediatric medicine expertise and experience.

FDA regulations require that the RDRC work together with hospital's Institutional Review Board (IRB). The function of the IRB is to protect the rights and welfare of human research. Typically, the names and credentials of all core RDRC members and potential consultants shall be submitted to the IRB for approval prior to the formation of the committee.

Furthermore, all protocols approved by RDRC must also be approved by the IRB. With the proposed structure of the RDRC, competitive advances in radioactive drug research studies can be performed while remaining within the continual purview of the IRB [42]. Once the study has been approved, the RDRC requires submission of reports by the study principal investigator. The RDRC also audits studies to ensure compliance to all set rules.

Although the FDA has given the RDRC authority over these types of research, the agency has continuous oversight over these studies through mandated scheduled report submission on all approved RDRC studies to the FDA. The FDA will also perform inspections of all RDRCs. The Office of Regulatory Affairs (ORA) field investigators handle these types of inspections and will generate an inspection report [43]. If the report indicates failure of the Institutional RDRC to comply with FDA regulations, then the FDA could withdraw approval of the RDRC. Some examples of violations include failure to assure the quality of the radioactive drug, reviewing and approving research studies when meeting quorum was not met, failure to assure that investigators reported adverse events in a timely manner, and/or allowing studies to proceed without approval by the IRB. In most cases, the FDA will place a clinical hold on all RDRC studies and allow the Institution to notify the FDA, in writing, actions taken to correct and prevent the reoccurrence of such violations. To ensure that the RDRC commits to the corrective actions, the FDA would conduct follow-up inspections.

Investigational Research Board

The protection of human research patients is addressed in 45 CFR 46. Here contains the provisions for the requirement and establishment of an Institutional Review Board (IRB) which is an administrative body established to protect the rights and welfare of human research subjects recruited to participate in research activities conducted under the auspices of the institution with which it is affiliated [44].

The IRB is charged with the responsibility to review and have oversight of all research involving human participants. The function of the IRB is to protect the welfare, rights, and privacy of human subjects. The IRB has the authority to approve, disapprove, and monitor all research activities that fall within its jurisdiction as specified by both the federal regulations and institutional policy. In addition, for many hospitals, the Clinical Research Committee (CRC) is another committee that works with the IRB. The CRC is charged with the responsibility of overseeing all aspects of the scientific research that is in the protocol such as the methods used to validate the scientific questions, the relevance of the biostatistical analysis, and the pertinence of the proposed procedures.

Many hospitals have an elaborate research infrastructure, built around the charge of the IRB, in order to maintain high ethical standards and ensure strict compliance with all regulatory policies. In instances where hospital research programs are disbanded, the cause is often due to regulatory deficiencies. When there is research conducted at the hospital, the FDA holds the sponsor-investigators (i.e., hospital) to the same standards as industry (i.e., large pharmaceutical companies). The responsibility, the liability, and the funding are immense; thus, it is vital that the hospital has a clinical research infrastructure that is robust.

For research studies that involve a radiopharmaceutical, there is an extra layer of oversight due to the risks associated with radiation. This chapter focuses primarily on issues related to the regulation of radiopharmaceuticals; thus, the focus will be on radiopharmaceutical research in an academic hospital setting. The rules and

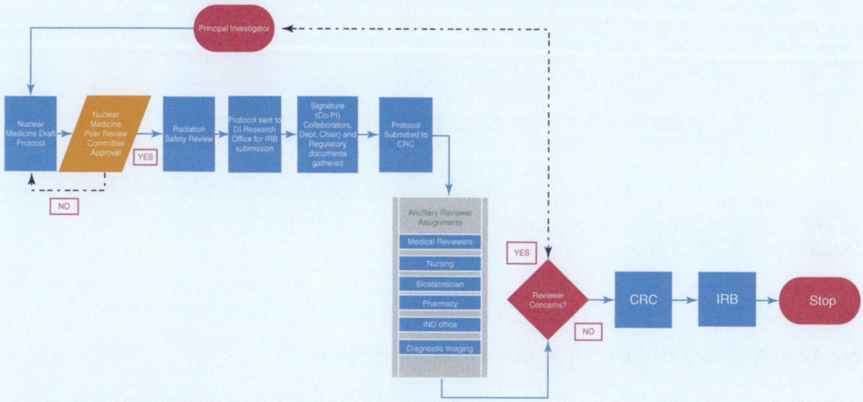

Fig. 10.5 Illustration of one research pathway involving RAM use

regulations surrounding human research of each academic hospital vary, but the end goal is the same: to maintain high ethical standards and full compliance with all regulatory agencies. Figure 10.5 is an illustration of one internal research infrastructure and is the basis for the following discussion.

In this research pathway, most of the steps are applicable to all research protocols. However, there are a two review committees that are specific to studies that involve radiopharmaceuticals: the Nuclear Peer Review Committee (NMPRC) and the Radiation Safety Committee (RSC). At this Institution, the purpose of the NMPRC is to allow for the review of all aspects related to nuclear medicine by the experts in this field. The members of the NMPRC would typically include NM physicians, health physicists, and nuclear pharmacists. Similar to the RDRC, the NMPRC allows for additional subject matter experts when warranted. The committee members evaluate the clinical protocol on matters to include, but not limited to, need and feasibility of the study, eligibility criteria, imaging parameters, safety and

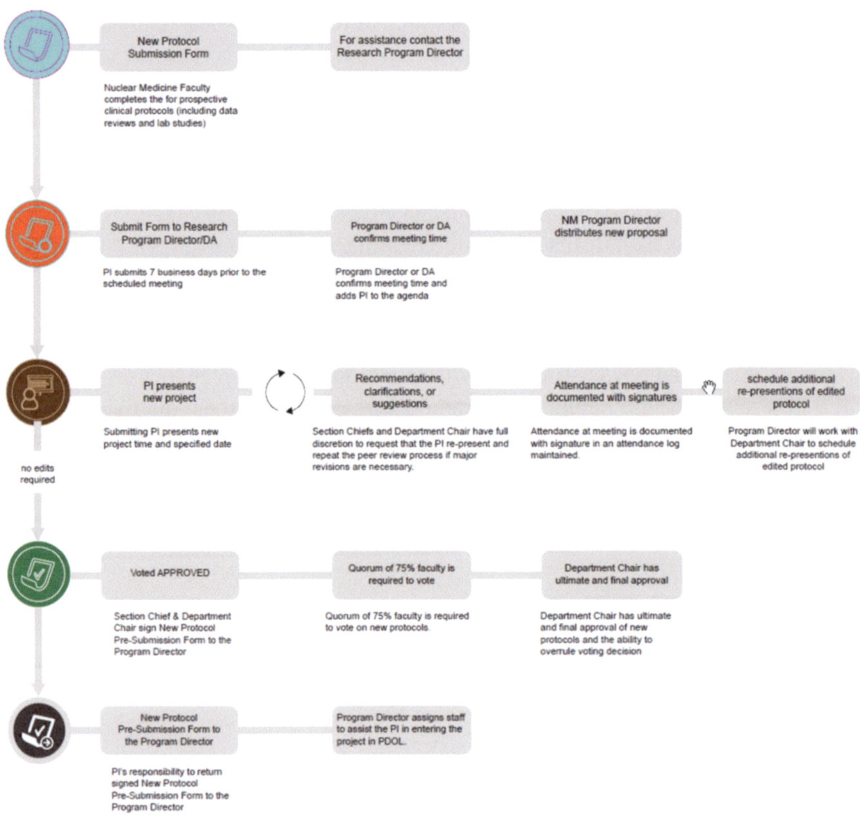

Fig. 10.6 Nuclear Medicine Peer Review Committee pathway

safety monitoring plans, and procurement of the investigational radiopharmaceutical. Once the clinical study has been approved by the NMPRC, it will then proceed to the next review committee which is the radiation safety committee. Figure 10.6 is an example of the standard of operation for a NMPRC.

The RSC, as discussed previously, will review and approve all aspects related to the radioisotopes involved in the clinical study. The RSC grants the researcher AU status for the investigational radioisotope, and this allows the investigator to use the isotope for the clinical study. Furthermore, before the hospital can order and receive the isotope, it must be on the hospital RAM license. If the isotope is not on the RAM license, the RS group will submit an amendment to the NRC/Agreement State to add the isotope. A typical amendment would include an outline of the use, user qualification, maximum amount, storage, preparation details, and waste disposal. When the amendment is approved, the hospital must put processes and procedures in place that adhere strictly to the commitments made to the NRC/State regarding the isotope.

Regulatory Outlook of Radiopharmaceuticals

For those practicing clinical NM, dealing with regulations can be a daunting task. A common challenge is to comply with the regulations and not have the regulations dictate the practice. For a hospital NM clinical practice, the rules and regulations of internal committees act as a safeguard or a checkpoint of compliance for users. Ideally, all violations can be identified at the local level before progression into state and federal infractions.

The future of radiopharmaceuticals is promising. Many believe that nuclear medicine has experienced an exponential resurgence of interest. In the last 7 years, there have been unprecedented numbers of new FDA-approved radiopharmaceuticals. The excitement is beyond individual diagnostic imaging or single therapeutic agents but rather theranostic radionuclides that offer low-dose imaging followed by high-dose therapy such as the agents used for neuroendocrine tumors (NETS): gallium Ga-68 dotatate and lutetium Lu-177 dotatate. With tremendous growth in the use of radiopharmaceuticals, governing agencies will have increased involvement in the regulation of nuclear medicine. However, due of the complexity of the regulations, there is many published guidance available to assist with implementing programs that will comply with all the different regulations. As nuclear medicine professionals, it is our responsibility to provide the most safe and effective care to our patients. To honor this obligation, we must continually work to increase our knowledge of the regulations and find ways for seamless integration into our daily practice.

References

1. The American Board of Nuclear Medicine. History. https://www.abnm.org/index.php/sample-page-2/history/. Accessed Dec 2018.
2. Society of Nuclear Medicine and Molecular Imaging. A framework for the regulations of nuclear medicine. July, 29 1998. http://snmmi.files.cms-plus.com/docs/framework.pdf. Accessed Dec 2018.
3. United States Nuclear Regulatory Commission. About NRC. https://www.nrc.gov/about-nrc.html. Accessed Nov 2018.
4. Walker JS, Wellock TR. A short history of nuclear regulation, 1946–2009. https://www.nrc.gov/docs/ML1029/ML102980443.pdf. Accessed Nov 2018.
5. United States Nuclear Regulatory Commission. History. https://www.nrc.gov/about-nrc/history.html. Accessed Nov 2018.
6. United States Nuclear Regulatory Commission. Licensing. https://www.nrc.gov/about-nrc/regulatory/licensing.html. Accessed Nov 2018.
7. United States Nuclear Regulatory Commission. Radioactive waste. https://www.nrc.gov/waste.html. Accessed Nov 2018.
8. United States Nuclear Regulatory Commission. Office of Nuclear Material Safety and Safeguards. https://scp.nrc.gov/. Accessed Feb 2019.
9. National Archives. About the code of federal regulations. https://www.archives.gov/federal-register/cfr/about.html. Accessed Nov 2018.
10. United States Food & Drug Administration. What we do. https://www.fda.gov/aboutfda/whatwedo/. Accessed Nov 2018.
11. United States Food & Drug Administration. FDA's origin. https://www.fda.gov/AboutFDA/History/Forgshistory/evolvingpowers/ucm124403.htm. Accessed Nov 2018.
12. Green JA, Podolsky SH. Reform regulation, and pharmaceuticals-the Kefauver-Harris amendments at 50. N Engl J Med. 2012;367(16):1481–3.
13. United States Department of Labor. About OSHA. https://www.osha.gov/about.html. Accessed Jan 2019.
14. 25 Texas Administrative Code §289.256. Medical and veterinary use of radioactive material. Texas regulations for control of radiation. September 24, 2018.
15. United Stated Environmental Protection Agency. Our mission and what we do. https://www.epa.gov/aboutepa/our-mission-and-what-we-do. January 2019.
16. United State Nuclear Regulatory Commission. Transportation of radioactive material. https://www.nrc.gov/reading-rm/basic-ref/students/for-educators/11.pdf. Accessed Jan 2019.
17. Electronic Code of Federal Regulations e-CFR. Title 49-Transportation. https://ecfr.io/Title-49/.
18. The Joint Commission. About the Joint Commission. https://www.jointcommission.org/about_us/about_the_joint_commission_main.aspx. Accessed Jan 2019.
19. American College of Radiology. The gold standard in accreditation. https://www.acr.org/Clinical-Resources/Accreditation. Accessed Jan 2019.
20. Texas Department of State Health Services. Radioactive Materials Licensing and Radiation Control Program. Radioactive Materials Program Authorization and Scope. https://www.dshs.texas.gov/radiation/ram/. Accessed Nov 2018.
21. Texas Department of State Health Services. Radiation Control Program. How to avoid compliance problems relating to radioactive materials licenses. https://www.dshs.texas.gov/radiation/ram/compliance-tips.aspx. Accessed Nov 2018.
22. Moerlein SM. Radiopharmaceutical chemistry: PET agents. In: Kowalsky RJ, Fallen SW, editors. Radiopharmaceuticals in nuclear pharmacy and nuclear medicine. Washington, DC: American Pharmacist Association; 2011. p. 229–54.
23. United States Food and Drug Administration. Guidance: PET drugs-current good manufacturing practice (CGMP). https://www.fda.gov/downloads/drugs/guidancecomplianceregulatoryinformation/guidances/ucm266640.pdf. Accessed Nov 2018.
24. United States Pharmacopeia. General chapter <797> pharmaceutical compounding-sterile preparations. http://www.usp.org/compounding/general-chapter-797. Accessed Nov 2018.

25. National Association of Boards of Pharmacy. Model Pharmacy Act/Rules. https://nabp.pharmacy/publications-reports/resource-documents/model-pharmacy-act-rules/. Accessed Feb 2019.
26. United States Pharmacopeia. Recognition of USP compounding standards. http://www.usp.org/compounding/legal-considerations. Accessed Jan 2019.
27. <797> Pharmaceutical compounding—sterile preparations. In: The United States Pharmacopeia 40th ed and National Formulary, 35th ed. Rockville: United States Pharmacopeial Convention, Inc; 2017.
28. Society of Nuclear Medicine and Molecular Imaging. General questions about USP <797>. http://www.snmmi.org/issuesadvocacy/content.aspx?ItemNumber=4901. Accessed Feb 2019.
29. Ultratag RBC. {Package insert}. St. Louis: Mallinckrodt Inc; 2015.
30. United States Pharmacopeia. <825> Compounding—radiopharmaceuticals. https://www.uspnf.com/notices/825-compounding-radiopharmaceuticals. Accessed Dec 2019.
31. United States Pharmacopeia. Developing USP general chapter <825>. http://www.usp.org/chemical-medicines/general-chapter-825. Accessed Feb 2019.
32. Centers for Medicare & Medicaid Services. Conditions for Coverage (CfCs) & Conditions of Participations (CoPs). https://www.cms.gov/Regulations-and-Guidance/Legislation/CFCsAndCoPs/index.html?redirect=/CFCsAndCoPs/16_ASC.asp. Accessed Dec 2018.
33. Centers for Medicare & Medicaid Services. CMS to strengthen oversight of Medicare's Accreditation Organizations. https://www.cms.gov/newsroom/press-releases/cms-strengthen-oversight-medicares-accreditation-organizations. Accessed Feb 2019.
34. The Joint Commission. Compliance checklist: diagnostic imaging. https://www.jointcommission.org/assets/1/18/imaging_checklist-June-2016.pdf.
35. United States Food and Drug Administration. Nuclear pharmacy: criteria for determining when to register as a drug establishment. Rockville: Division of Drug Labeling Compliance, Center for Drugs and Biologics, Food and Drug Administration; 1984.
36. United States Food and Drug Administration. Guidance PET drugs—current good manufacturing practice (CGMP). https://www.fda.gov/downloads/drugs/guidancecomplianceregulatoryinformation/guidances/ucm266640.pdf. Accessed Dec 2018.
37. United States Food and Drug Administration. Positron emission tomography (PET): questions and answers about CGMP regulations for PET drugs. https://www.fda.gov/drugs/developmentapprovalprocess/manufacturing/ucm193476.htm. Accessed Dec 2018.
38. United States Food and Drug Administration. Guidance for industry and researchers: the Radioactive Drug Research Committee: human research without an investigational new drug application. August 2010. https://www.fda.gov/downloads/Drugs/Guidances/UCM163892.pdf. Accessed Jan 2019.
39. United States Food and Drug Administration. Investigational New Drug (IND) application. https://www.fda.gov/drugs/developmentapprovalprocess/howdrugsaredevelopedandapproved/approvalapplications/investigationalnewdrugindapplication/default.htm. Accessed Jan 2019.
40. United States Food and Drug Administration. Information Sheet Guidance for IRBs, Clinical Investigators, and Sponsors FDA Inspections of Clinical Investigators. https://www.fda.gov/downloads/regulatoryinformation/guidances/ucm126553.pdf. Accessed Jan 2019.
41. United States Federal Food and Drug Administration. CFR-Code of Federal Regulations Title 21. https://www.accessdata.fda.gov/scripts/cdrh/cfdocs/cfcfr/CFRSearch.cfm?FR=361.1. Accessed Dec 2018.
42. United States Federal Food and Drug Administration. Radioactive Drug Research Committee (RDRC) Program. https://www.fda.gov/drugs/scienceresearch/ucm574871.htm. Accessed Dec 2018.
43. United States Federal Food and Drug Administration. Compliance Program. https://www.fda.gov/downloads/ICECI/ComplianceManuals/ComplianceProgramManual/UCM244484.pdf. Accessed Jan 2019.
44. United States Department of Health & Human Services. 45 CFR 46. https://www.hhs.gov/ohrp/regulations-and-policy/guidance/faq/45-cfr-46/index.html. Accessed Feb 2019.

Chapter 11
Locoregional Radionuclide Cancer Therapy (LRCT) Using Sealed and Unsealed Radionuclides

Franklin C. L. Wong

Treatment of Human Cancer Using Radionuclides

The state of the arts of radionuclide therapy, regulation, dispensing, administration, dosimetry, and efficacy correlations have been reviewed in previous chapters. As illustrated by the treatment of residual thyroid cancer after thyroidectomy, a diagnostic scan using orally administered I-123 sodium iodide is performed, and the whole-body scan typically reveals thyroidal remnant uptake of <2% in 24 hours. A typical dose of 100 mCi of I-131 is administered orally. For patients with subtotal thyroidectomy or residual uptake over 2%, higher oral dose (>100 mCi) will render better outcome than those treated with 30–50 mCi [1]. A similarly low concentration of radiopharmaceutical in the target tumor should be noted of radiolabeled monoclonal anti-CD20 antibody treatment of lymphoma using intravenous injection of a maximum of 32 mCi Y-90-labeled Zevalin [2] or about 100 mCi of I-131-labeled Bexxar [3]. Typically, lymphomas take up <0.01%/g of injected radiolabeled monoclonal antibodies, i.e., <0.0032 mCi/g of Y-90 or 0.01 mCi/g of I-131. Based on an effective established systemic cancer therapy using systemic radiopharmaceuticals, suppression and eradication of tumor can be accomplished if there is a relatively low radioactivity dose (e.g., 1–5 mCi) inside the tumor for sufficiently long duration to allow deposition of radiation-absorbed doses (RAD) from radiation decays. As illustrated in the dosimetry chapters (Chaps. 6 and 7), RAD is a product of residence time multiplied by the fractional radiation absorption rate (S value) which is a function of all radiation emissions and of the volume of the injectate. One of the major hurdles in dosimetry estimate is that the volume of the uptake cannot be determined

F. C. L. Wong (✉)
Department of Nuclear Medicine, University of Texas, M. D. Anderson Cancer Center, Houston, TX, USA
e-mail: fwong@mdanderson.org

F. C. L. Wong (ed.), *Locoregional Radionuclide Cancer Therapy*,
https://doi.org/10.1007/978-3-030-56267-0_11

because of the instrumentation limits. However, progresses have been made by an ongoing research to using a combination of calibrating sources of different volume and different contrast along with multiple threshold settings to de-convolute the injectate volumes.

As illustrated by I-131 sodium iodide therapy of thyroid cancers and Y-90 Zevalin and I-131 Bexxar treatment of lymphoma, locoregional retention of 1–5 mCi/g I-131 or Y-90 is able to treat tumors as the standard of care. Therefore, the extension from systemic radionuclide cancer therapy to locoregional radionuclide cancer therapy can be achieved by interventional radiologic techniques to deliver radiopharmaceuticals to the target tumor and maneuvers to assure retention of radioactivities (as in Chap. 8). Radiation dosimetry models (Chap. 6) will allow choices of radionuclides and radiopharmaceuticals. Accurate image quantification and image-guided radiation dosimetry (Chap. 7) will enable monitoring and refinement of radionuclide therapies. Understanding of the regulatory requirements at the national, state, and institutional levels as well as compliance with radiopharmacy practice (Chap. 10) will assure seamless translation from the laboratory to the clinics in the practice of locoregional radionuclide cancer therapy. This chapter examines the practical aspects of locoregional use of radionuclide cancer therapy in humans.

Regulatory approval of therapeutic radiopharmaceuticals is typically through two pathways: investigational device exemption (IDE) and investigation of new drug (IND) pathways by the Food and Drug Administration in the United States. The IDE pathway allows a faster entry to the market but restricts application to the specifically stated clinical indication (e.g., inoperable hepatocellular carcinoma for Y-90 TheraSpheres) only. Devices under this pathway could not be used for other disease or tumor types without additional approval. Meticulous manufacture of "devices" (and hence high production costs) is required to assure that the radionuclide is not released into the surrounding tissue or systemic circulation to assure safety and efficacy. Great efforts are made to assure the device under IDE is unaltered, as illustrated by immobilization of I-125 brachytherapy seeds stranded on strings [4], containment of I-125 Iotrex solution [5] enclosed inside an intracavitary balloon catheter of GliaSite [6], and neutron activation of precursor element inside microscopic polymers to produce Y-90 TheraSpheres [7], Y-90 SIR-Spheres [8], and P-32 OncoSil [9].

Compared with the IDE pathway, regulatory approval of radiopharmaceuticals under the investigation of new drug (IND) pathway requires a more comprehensive description of manufacturing processes and submission of more evidence for safety and efficacy and hence more extensive testing and reporting and longer duration to reach the market. On the other hand, upon regulatory approval, radiopharmaceutical approved by IND processes would be readily applied to treat different cancers as long as justification can be made that the rationale of treatment is under a similar scope. Manufacturers' choice of IDE or IND approval pathways for a therapeutic radiopharmaceutical is a strategic one, not necessarily dictated by molecular properties or physical forms of solution or particles. Instead, whether the study radiopharmaceutical is sealed (contained) or unsealed (not contained) has directed the choice of regulatory pathways to IDE or IND pathway, respectively. Because of the less onerous regulatory requirement, more radiopharmaceuticals (including Ho-166 seeds, GliaSite, I-125 Iotrex, etc.) are pursued under the IDE than the IND phase I, II, or III studies for cancer therapy.

There have been increasingly extensive applications of radiopharmaceuticals in the treatment of human cancers. Theoretical modeling as in Chap. 6 and preclinical studies as in Chap. 8 have provided important platforms for IRCT to reach the clinical arena. Nevertheless, extension of preclinical studies to treat human cancer inevitably requires validation in clinical trials. The design of LRCT will require consideration of logistic and practical issues as illustrated by the following approaches of LRCT.

LRCT Using Sealed Device/Radiopharmaceuticals

The classical use of sealed radiopharmaceuticals in locoregional treatment of human cancer is the use of I-125 seeds in brachytherapy involving multiple seeds lined up in strings (or needles) to implant into prostate cancers [4]. The manufacturing of these seeds on strings mandated that I-125 will not diffuse outside of the seeds into the target tumor tissues. Seeds of I-125 emit multiple electrons and photons of lower energies to reach only millimeters of tissue. It has a half-life of 59.5 days. Diffusion or physical movement within or outside the tumor bed would result in decreased efficacy and increased toxicity but is prevented by tight binding to the metal and surface coating with polymers. The use of the strings/needles is to ensure that the seeds remain in the target tissue without moving away because of either interstitial fluid flow or tumor/tissue shrinkage. I-125 seeds may or may not be removed at the end of the treatment session over months.

Another example is intracavitary implantation of GliaSite balloon catheter filled with I-125 iodohydroxybenzene sulfonate (Iotrex) solution [10] after resection of brain tumor in the range of 300–700 mCi (Fig. 11.1). Upon completion of a prescribed duration (4–5 days) to deliver 60–100 Gys to the tumor bed within 1 cm from the balloon surface, the balloon would be deflated to retrieve I-125 Iotrex for disposal and surgically removed. Iotrex solution is a proprietary compound designed to be rapidly eliminated by the kidneys from the body in case of leakage into the body [5]. Similarly, implantation of double-lumen balloon catheters within the postsurgical cavity after removal of breast cancer and insertion of an affixed Ir-192 radiation source for a prescribed duration (of hours) can be performed to deliver prescribed radiation-absorbed dose to the tumor bed [11]. Both GliaSite and double-lumen balloon catheters require surgical implantation and removal of the radiation source (devices) after the prescribed duration of exposure, thereby increasing the technical and logistic complexities.

The intra-arterial use of yttrium-90-labeled microparticles Y-90 TheraSpheres [7] and Y-90 SIR-Spheres [8] to treat unresectable hepatocellular tumors and colorectal metastasis depends on the radiolabeled microparticles to embolize selected tumor capillaries and arterioles and to ablate them until complete radiation decay.

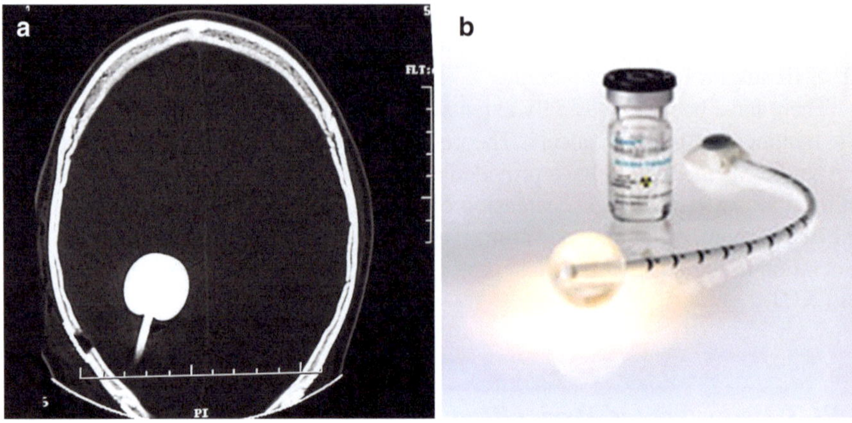

Fig. 11.1 A patient underwent implantation of a balloon catheter GliaSite after surgical removal of a brain metastasis. The balloon integrity was confirmed by brain CT after injection of contrast (**a**). This patient underwent intracavitary irradiation with 540 mCi of I-125 Iotrex (**b**) for 96 hours before deflation and then surgical removal of the balloon catheter

Retrieval of these latter microparticles (devices) is not required, therefore involving less morbidity and less cost.

Therapeutic Use of Unsealed Radiopharmaceuticals

Parenteral unsealed soluble radiopharmaceuticals with tumor affinity The first use of I-131 sodium iodide (NaI) to treat human disease was reported in 1947 [12]. I-131 is concentrated in thyroid tissues and most thyroid cancers via the sodium-iodide symporter and tyrosine peroxidase mechanisms. Since then, a single-dose oral administration of I-131 NaI has been utilized as the standard of care treatment of primary hypothyroidism (Graves' disease with up to 20 mCi) [13] and residual thyroid cancer remnants (up to 250 mCi). The published radiation dosimetry after oral administration of I-131 NaI indicates acceptably low radiation exposure to the vital organs with the critical organs being red bone marrow and urinary bladder [14].

As illustrated in Chap. 7, accurate quantification and imaging logistics are required to derive reliable image-based radiation dosimetry from internal radionuclides, whether with planar imaging or tomographic imaging. Although radiation dosimetry is not routinely available to many facilities nor mandated for radionuclide therapies in humans, it nevertheless provides invaluable guidance, especially for critical considerations of bone-marrow exposure from repeated treatment or for treatment of lesions nearby vital structures [15].

Additional therapeutic insights are demonstrated by a dosimetry session acquiring serial whole-body images over 4 days after an oral dose of 5 mCi of I-131

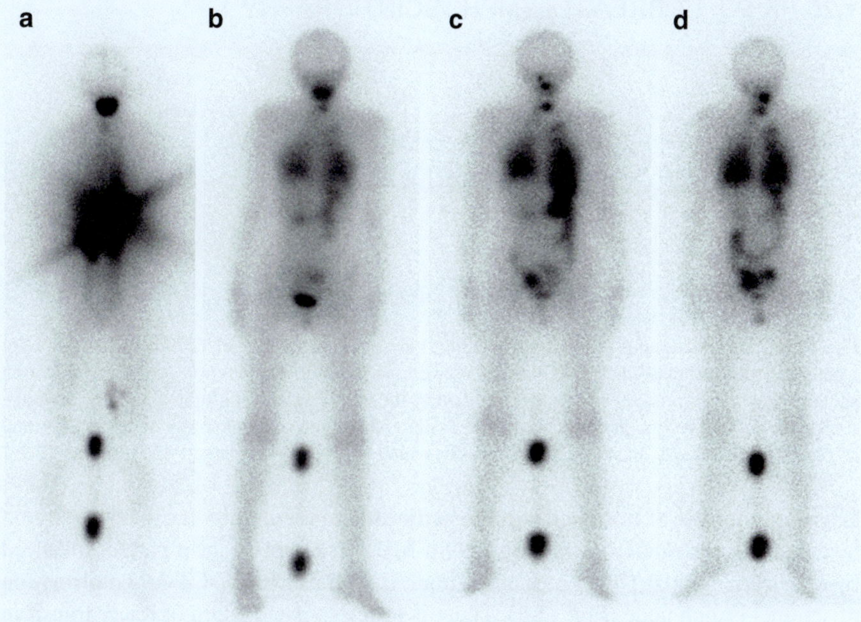

Fig. 11.2 For radioiodide ablation planning, a post-thyroidectomy thyroid cancer patient underwent serial whole-body imaging immediately (10 minutes) (**a**), at 22 hours (**b**), 42 hours (**c**), and 67 hours (**d**) after ingestion of 5 mCi of oral I-131 NaI. There is progressive transit of I-131 to the body and elimination from normal organs with residual I-13 uptake in the thyroidectomy bed and in lung metastases. Standards are placed between the legs for quantification reference. Images and image-based dosimetry provide guidance for the dosing radioactivity with consideration of radiation-absorbed doses to critical organs (lungs, bladder, and red marrow)

NaI. There was a progressive distribution of I-131 from the stomach to major organs, increasing concentration of I-131 by pulmonary thyroid cancer metastases and continuing washout of I-131 from the rest of the body (Fig. 11.2). While the rest of the body received lower levels of radiation exposure, the target metastases retained <2% of I-131 at 24 hours, or less than 4 mCi (from an intended oral dose of 200 mCi) which was able to suppress and/or eliminate tumors for long durations (typically recurrence-free for 5 years).

Locoregional unsealed particulate radiopharmaceuticals without tumor affinity Locoregional applications of unsealed particulate radiopharmaceuticals without tumor affinity can be illustrated by breast lymphoscintigraphy to identify sentinel lymph nodes with multiple planar imaging after peritumoral injection of 0.5–2.5 mCi of Tc99m-sulfur colloid (Fig. 11.3). Typically only minute amounts (<1%) of sulfur colloid microparticles travel through the lymphatic channels to reach the sentinel lymph node, while the majority of the tracer remain indefinitely in the injection site until complete decay. This is a moot issue for patients scheduled for breast cancer resection.

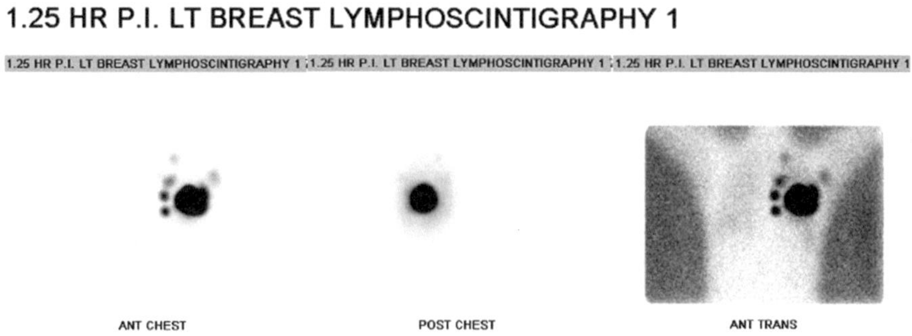

Fig. 11.3 After 80 minutes following peritumoral injection of 0.5 mCi of Tc99m-sulfur colloid in a patient with left breast cancer, static images were acquired in the anterior, posterior projection and also with a transmission background to identify the body contour. Multiple lymphatic drainage sites are identified to lymph nodes in the left axilla and left internal mammary stations. The total amount of radioactivity left in the injection site is <1%

Locoregional use of unsealed soluble radiopharmaceuticals It can be illustrated by a case of interstitial injection of Tc99m-MDP in a breast cancer patient followed by planar imaging at 10 minutes and 1 hour as well as SPECT-CT for confirmation of sentinel lymph node (Fig. 11.4). There is prompt visualization of tracer transit in the lymphatic channel to reach the sentinel lymph node, followed by gradual tracer uptake by the skeleton which is the ultimate target organ of the tracer. While this study illustrated the transit of locoregionally administered soluble radiopharmaceuticals, it also demonstrated the orderly transit from the injection site via dual pathways, lymphatic drainage, and venous return which reaches the general circulation before final deposition into the target organ. In contrast to particulate radiopharmaceuticals as in Fig. 11.3 with <1% exit, a substantially larger amount (>50%) of soluble radiopharmaceuticals exited the injection site to reach the target organ, bones.

Preclinical studies (Chap. 8) showed upon intratumoral injection of a soluble tumor-seeking agent F-18 FDG into rat tumor xenograft, serial PET imaging revealed prolonged retention in the injection site when compared with F-18 sodium fluoride injection. These findings confirm that intratumoral injection of tumor-seeking soluble radiopharmaceuticals will increase residence time and radiation-absorbed dose to the tumor when compared to similar use of radiopharmaceuticals without tumor-seeking ability. The radionuclide residence time in the tumor and other organs can be quantified from scintigraphic or tomographic images as in Chap. 7 to correlate with efficacy. Fractional radiation-absorbed doses (S values) from theoretic modeling (as in Chap. 6) together with residence times determined from imaging (Chap. 7) would provide sufficient dosimetry data to determine whether a particular radiopharmaceutical could be efficacious and safe in locoregional/intratumoral injection. This approach of image-derived radiation dosimetry of LRCT may be readily applied in clinical studies.

Locoregional soluble radiopharmaceuticals with tumor affinity Although inadvertent infiltration at the injection site occurs infrequently (<0.5% in our PET clinic), a patient study revealed substantial extravasation in the injection site and

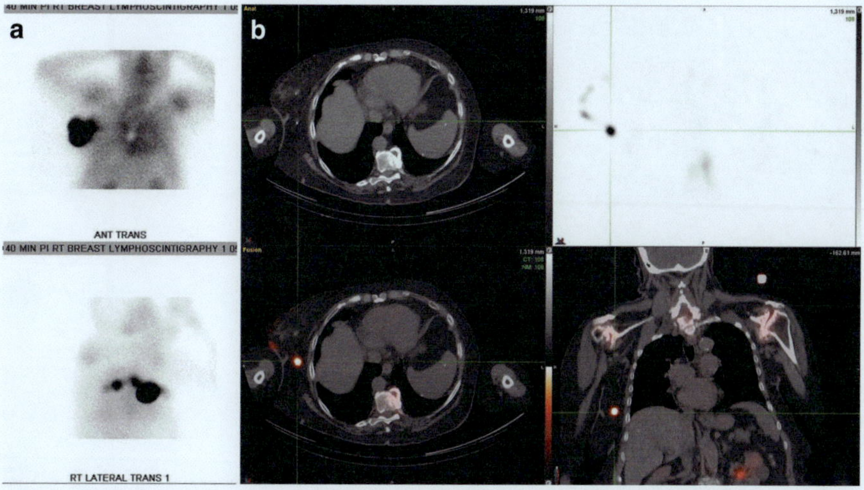

Fig. 11.4 Static images at 40 minutes and SPECT-CT at 1 hour of a patient inadvertently injected with 20 mCi of Tc99m-MDP (a bone tracer) in her right breast. There is prompt visualization of a right lymphatic drainage channel and of a right axillary lymph node on the static images (**a**). SPECT-CT images aptly identified the right axillary lymph node (**b**). There was also a continuous systemic return of tracer, presumably through the local capillary and venous network, resulting in visualization of the skeleton. This case again demonstrates dual drainage (lymphatics and venous) after interstitial injection of soluble radiopharmaceuticals

provided invaluable physiologic insights after the study was repeated the following day. A large portion of the injected radiopharmaceutical remained in the right antecubital fossa (the standard uptake value SUV is 189, versus expected value of less than 1) and lymphatics, and two right axillary lymph nodes were visualized (Fig. 11.5a). The repeated scan without extravasation the following day showed no abnormal uptake in the injection site (Fig. 11.5b). Two right axillary lymph nodes with high FDG uptakes were visualized and presumed to be metastasis.

This study suggests that interstitial injection of F-18 FDG or other radiopharmaceuticals with tumor affinity may be also useful in identifying lymph nodes involved with metastasis via interstitial or peritumoral injection. The direct identification of metastatic lymph nodes by lymphoscintigraphy using soluble radiopharmaceuticals with tumor affinity will be a welcome advance for cancer care. Further studies will be necessary to confirm such utility.

LCRT: Sealed Versus Unsealed Radiopharmaceuticals

The contrast between locoregional use of sealed radionuclides and locoregional use of unsealed radiopharmaceuticals can be illustrated by a recently published ongoing multicenter US clinical trial of P-32-labeled OncoSil (production of P-32 from neutron activation of silicon-containing microparticles) to treat inoperable pancreatic

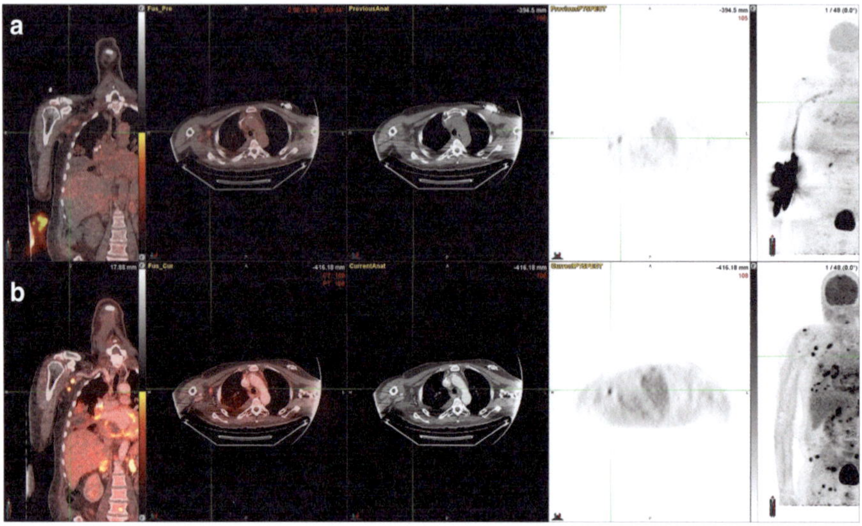

Fig. 11.5 Inadvertent infiltration of injection site in the right antecubital fossa with 8 mCi of F-18 FDG in a cancer patient (who had no complaint of discomfort) was discovered by the PET-CT acquired 1 hour later. (**a**, top row) F-18 FDG PET-CT revealed extravasation in the right antecubital fossa and right axilla. The SUV in the injection site was 189 indicating high amount of retention. Nevertheless, there is visualization of metastatic right axillary lymph nodes that were subsequently confirmed by the repeated F-18 FDG PET-CT. (**b**, bottom row) Repeated F-18 FDG PET-CT showed multiple metastasis in right axillary lymph nodes, lungs and body

cancer [16]. In fact, no acute toxicity was observed in the entire study group of nine patients [17]. In a MDACC cohort of four patients who received intratumoral injection of a prescribed radioactivity of P-32 OncoSil under endoscopic ultrasound guidance, no acute toxicity was observed up to 2 weeks of initial observation. Additional analysis revealed retention of radioactivity as measured by planar scintigraphy over 7 days varies from 72% to 0%. Tumor regression on CT was observed with the patient having 72% retention at 2 weeks along with normalization of biomarker at 6 months, while patients with lower retention of P-32 in the pancreas at 7 days had earlier recurrence.

Although these microparticles were manufactured to contain the radionuclide and limit its diffusion away from the target, there was still significant departure of radioactivity from the tumor indicating significant departure of the microparticles before complete decay of the radionuclide. Radioactivity (presumably embedded inside the microparticles) that exited from the pancreatic cancer could not be located, likely because of their small sizes that are below spatial resolution of detection. Nevertheless, no adverse effect based on symptom nor blood tests was identified. Furthermore, preliminary results showed that retention of radioactivity as

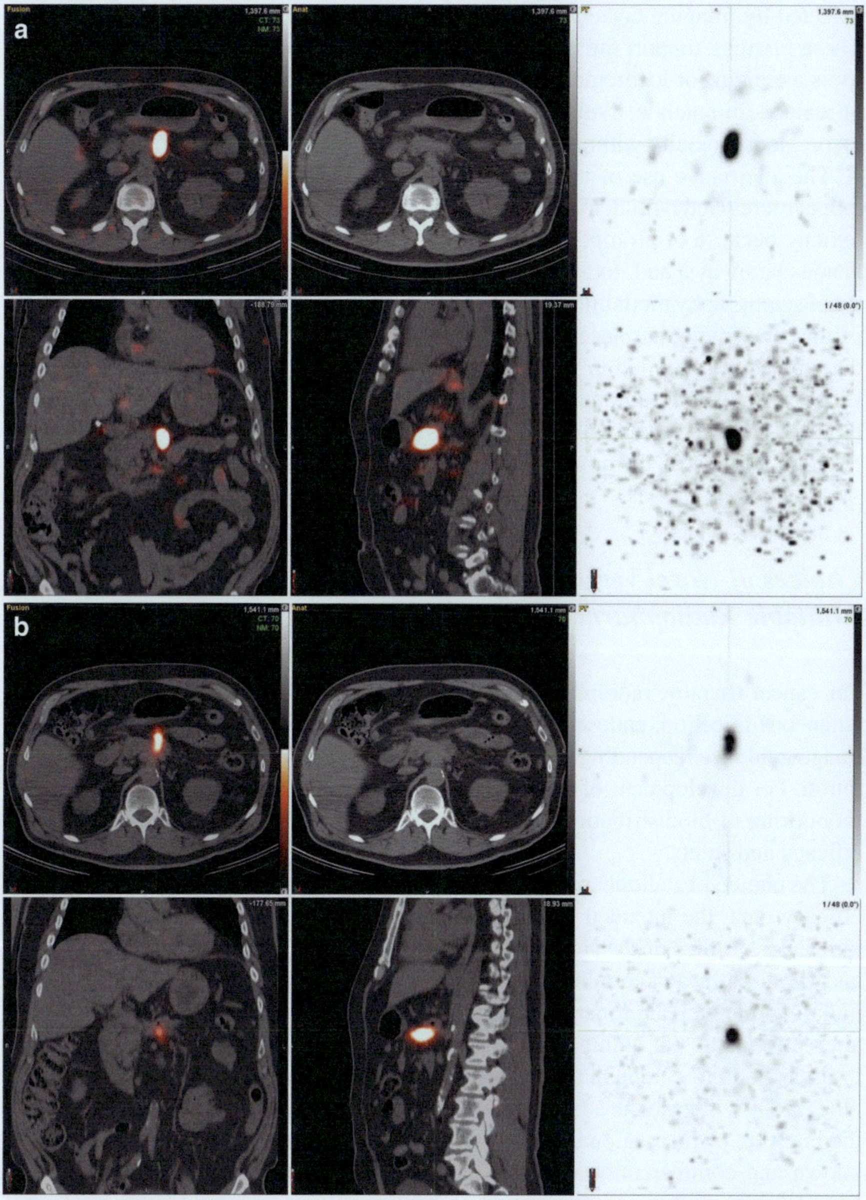

Fig. 11.6 Following injection of P-32 OncoSil (microparticles) under endoscopic ultrasound guidance, Bremsstrahlung SPECT-CT at 2 hours (**a**) and 7 days (**b**) revealed persistent retention in the injection site, pancreatic cancer [17]

detected by imaging correlates with efficacy in this small sample of four patients. These findings support the contention that retention (residence time) of radioactivity is essential for locoregional radionuclide cancer therapy. Unintended departure of sealed radionuclide, likely by leakage, did not amount to significant systemic nor locoregional toxicity within the dose range administered.

The alternative use of unsealed radiopharmaceuticals administered via locoregional routes (interstitial, intratumoral, or intrathecal) will have even less unintended toxicity because of prompt local diffusion, rapid return to systemic circulation via venous pathways, and, to a lesser extent, lymphatic channels. With the state of the art of scintigraphy modalities including PET-CT and SPECT-CT, the biodistribution of unsealed radiopharmaceuticals may be monitored and the radiation dosimetry determined for estimation of efficacy and potential toxicity. In comparison with LRCT using sealed radionuclides in clinical trials via the IDE regulatory pathways, the use of unsealed radiopharmaceuticals in LRCT trials will almost certainly be required to undergo the more onerous IND regulatory pathways.

Choices of Novel Versus Commercially Available Radiopharmaceuticals

For cancer therapy, radiopharmaceuticals can be delivered locoregionally by percutaneous injection, endoscopic injection, or intrathecal injection, with or without image guidance, depending on the availability of interventional radiologic collaboration. For development of LRCT using sealed or unsealed radiopharmaceuticals, monitoring of biodistribution and radiation dosimetry is essential to correlate with efficacy and safety.

The choice of radiopharmaceuticals requires consideration of known safety and efficacy data, the intended treatment duration (in contrast to residence time), and molecular profiles of the study radiopharmaceuticals. While studying novel agents and novel pathways certainly is intellectually stimulating and conducive to accumulating intellectual properties, studying known agents and known pathways using alternative routes of administration may have less regulatory and logistic hurdles to initiate and to complete the study. The use of known radiopharmaceuticals from other INDs will have the advantage of adapting known systemic toxicity data, while the question of locoregional toxicity or efficacy is the subject of study. The use of known and commercially available radiopharmaceuticals may be costly, but will have logistic advantage of having the agent available on demand and in clinical grade. The vast possible combinations of known and available radionuclides and radiopharmaceuticals indeed will enable LRCT studies that are limited only by imagination and available resources.

All the above issues and factors need to be deliberated before the design of clinical trials of LRCT. Guidance from dosimetric modeling (Chap. 6), image-derived dosimetry (Chap. 7), and preclinical trials (Chap. 8) is indispensable. Certainly, high-quality radiopharmaceutical supply (Chap. 10), meticulous interventional radiologic support (Chap. 5), and patient screening and monitoring are also critical for a successful LRCT. Nevertheless, pharmacokinetic advantages (because of high initial delivery) and the available imaging modalities to directly monitor radiopharmaceutical biodistribution are the major advantages of LRCT. With the recent novel development of therapeutic radiopharmaceuticals and in scintigraphic imaging devices, LRCT will serve as important therapeutic tools to alleviate suffering by cancer patients.

The Future of LRCT: What More Can Be Achieved

Following the rising applications of cancer therapies using radiopharmaceuticals by systemic administration, the prospect of LRCT is indeed promising to help alleviating human suffering. The following are opportunities that may help accelerating LRCT into the clinical arena:

Better instruments for detection and monitoring Firstly, more LRCT are becoming clinical realities because more advanced scanners are available to monitor, localize, and quantify radiopharmaceuticals and more radiopharmaceuticals are available for systemic therapy. Several parallel scientific developments would help accelerating LRCT clinical trials, such as recent advances of whole-body PET-CT scanners which would enable prompt, accurate quantification and localization of radiopharmaceuticals [18]. Secondly, Cherenkov light imaging may be applied to study the biodistribution of radiopharmaceuticals after LRCT of superficial lesions (animal or humans) using radiopharmaceuticals such as F-18 FDG (Chap. 8).

Better integration with radiation science The high signal-to-noise ratios of radiopharmaceutical distribution during LRCT also provide unique opportunities to explore in vivo interactions of radiation with soft tissues and tumors. The potential for targeted remote delivery of substrates to target organs [19] as well as monitoring of interaction between radiation and biomaterials may be further explored.

Combination with other therapeutic modalities Rational combination between LRCT and systemic therapy (including immunotherapy) may provide synergistic benefits while minimizing adverse effects from individual treatment modalities. Combination with conventional external beam radiation therapy and/or proton therapy may harness the advantages of both the high-dose-rate ablation and the low-dose-rate ablation of cancer.

Potential use as a means to induce cancer immunity LRCT as a potential means for tumor recurrence prevention (as NuTuVIS in Chap. 8) should be further explored. If successful LRCT can be confirmed to prevent the growth of subsequent tumors grafting in humans, as reported in rat experiments and as in the cTVT canine tumor models, this added advantage will be another worthwhile goal of human LRCT.

Potential variations and alternatives to current clinical trials LRCT methodologies allow in vivo monitoring and serial quantification of radionuclides injected into tissues (tumors). With many commercially available therapeutic radiopharmaceuticals, LRCT certainly can serve as parallel protocols or alternatives to current locoregional radiotherapy trials such as those testing the abscopal effects and immune responses [20, 21].

More creative alternatives may involve intratumoral injection of admixtures (by coprecipitation or adsorption) of radiopharmaceuticals with radiation-enhancing nanoparticles such as hafnium oxide, or NBTXR3 as in European trials [22]. After intratumoral injection of milligrams of these agents, the intratumoral radiation dosimetry of external beam radiation can be increased up to nine times [23]. Accurate quantification of the injectate over time allows for accurate dosimetry of enhancement of radiation therapy. Conversely, radiation enhancers providing multifold enhancement of radiation dosimetry from the selected radiopharmaceuticals may be sufficient to deliver intratumoral radiation dose so as to even eliminate the need of the external beam.

Locoregional radionuclide monitoring from LRCT may also be applied to augment neutron capture therapy (NCT) [24] which utilizes thermal neutron beam to activate boron (B-10 for intratumoral proton production) or gadolinium (Gd-155 or Gd-157 for intratumoral photon production). F-18-labeled boron radiopharmaceuticals have been produced to monitor boron uptake in tumors in NCT [25]. While higher efficacy can be achieved by intratumoral injection to avoid systemic toxicity, quantification of retained boron in the tumor will allow more exact prescription of the neutron beam. Gd contents may be quantified in NCT, because Gd-153 is a gamma-emitter. When admixed with Gd-155 and Gd-157 (natural abundance of 15% and 16%, respectively) in producing intratumoral neutron-activating injectate, Gd-153 can be imaged and quantified with derived calculations for Gd-155 and Gd-157. The localization and retention of intratumoral gadolinium can then be determined to allow accurate dosimetry for precise neutron beam prescription. Additionally, intratumoral injection of admixtures of Gd-153 (radioactive) with naturally occurring Gd compounds with radioenhancers will be another worthwhile venture to make use of intense intratumoral gamma emissions (from abundant Gd-155 and Gd-157) upon thermal neutron capturing.

Each of the above exciting possibilities can be studied using the current state of the art in radiopharmaceuticals, existing dosimetry modeling, and available scanners and imaging algorithms. More therapeutic radiopharmaceuticals are arriving the clinical stage; better dosimetry models and easier imaging algorithms are being developed. Newer generations of scanners for humans and for animals are being commercialized. While the regulatory paths remain rigid between sealed and unsealed radionuclides, such distinction is becoming more blurred in animal experiments and in clinical practice. This is a wonderful time to study locoregional radionuclide dispersion and retention in tumors and in normal tissues. Findings from further explorations will provide invaluable input to further develop LRCT and other oncologic disciplines to better alleviate human sufferings from cancer.

References

1. Andresen NS, Buatti JM, Tewfik HH, Pagedar NA, Anderson CM, Watkins JM. Radioiodine ablation following thyroidectomy for differentiated thyroid cancer: literature review of utility, dose, and toxicity. Eur Thyroid J. 2017;6(4):187–96.
2. Wiseman GA, White CA, Stabin M, Dunn WL, Erwin W, Dahlbom M, et al. Phase I/II 90Y-Zevalin (yttrium-90 ibritumomab tiuxetan, IDEC-Y2B8) radioimmunotherapy dosimetry results in relapsed or refractory non-Hodgkin's lymphoma. Eur J Nucl Med. 2000;27(7):766–77.
3. Boucek JA, Turner JH. Validation of prospective whole-body bone marrow dosimetry by SPECT/CT multimodality imaging in (131)I-anti-CD20 rituximab radioimmunotherapy of non-Hodgkin's lymphoma. Eur J Nucl Med Mol Imaging. 2005;32(4):458–69.
4. Delouya G, Bahary P, Carrier JF, Larouche RX, Hervieux Y, Beliveau-Nadeau D, et al. Refining prostate seed brachytherapy: comparing high-, intermediate-, and low-activity seeds for I-125 permanent seed prostate brachytherapy. Brachytherapy. 2015;14(3):329–33.
5. Stubbs JB, Strickland AD, Frank RK, Simon J, McMillan K, Williams JA. Biodistribution and dosimetry of an aqueous solution containing sodium 3-(125I)iodo-4-hydroxybenzenesulfonate (Iotrex) for brachytherapy of resected malignant brain tumors. Cancer Biother Radiopharm. 2000;15(6):645–56.
6. Wernicke AG, Sherr DL, Schwartz TH, Pannullo SC, Stieg PE, Boockvar JA, et al. Feasibility and safety of GliaSite brachytherapy in treatment of CNS tumors following neurosurgical resection. J Cancer Res Ther. 2010;6(1):65–74.
7. Arnold CA, Pezhouh MK, Lam-Himlin D, Pittman ME, VandenBussche C, Voltaggio L. 90Y-TheraSpheres: the new look of Yttrium-90. Am J Surg Pathol. 2019;43(5):688–94.
8. Aranda E, Aparicio J, Bilbao JI, Garcia-Alfonso P, Maurel J, Rodriguez J, et al. Recommendations for SIR-Spheres Y-90 resin microspheres in chemotherapy-refractory/intolerant colorectal liver metastases. Future Oncol. 2017;13(23):2065–82.
9. Javed S, Bhutani MS. Endoscopic ultrasound-guided radiation therapy in pancreatic cancer. Minerva Gastroenterol Dietol. 2013;59(4):377–86.
10. Gobitti C, Borsatti E, Arcicasa M, Roncadin M, Franchin G, Minatel E, et al. Treatment of recurrent high-grade gliomas with GliaSite brachytherapy: a prospective mono-institutional Italian experience. Tumori. 2011;97(5):614–9.
11. de Campos TP, Nogueira LB, Trindade B, Cuperschmid EM. Dosimetric intercomparison of permanent Ho-166 seed's implants and HDR Ir-192 brachytherapy in breast cancer. Rep Pract Oncol Radiother. 2016;21(3):240–9.
12. Marinelli LD, Trunnell JB, et al. Factors involved in the experimental therapy of metastatic thyroid cancer with I131; a preliminary report. Radiology. 1948;51(4):553–7.
13. Soley MH, Miller ER, Foreman N. Graves' disease; treatment with radioiodine (I131). Miss Valley Med J. 1949;71(4):131–4.
14. Marinelli LD, Hill RF. Radiation dosimetry in the treatment of functional thyroid carcinoma with I131. Radiology. 1950;55(4):494–501.
15. Sparks RB, Crowe EA, Wong FC, Toohey RE, Siegel JA. Radiation dose distributions in normal tissue adjacent to tumors containing (131)I or (90)Y: the potential for toxicity. J Nucl Med. 2002;43(8):1110–4.
16. Gholami YH, Wilson N, James D, Kuncic Z. Toward personalized dosimetry with (32) P microparticle therapy for advanced pancreatic cancer. Int J Radiat Oncol Biol Phys. 2017;99(4):1029–38.
17. Bhutani MS, Cazacu IM, Luzuriaga Chavez AA, Singh BS, Wong FCL, Erwin WD, et al. Novel EUS-guided brachytherapy treatment of pancreatic cancer with phosphorus-32 microparticles: first United States experience. VideoGIE. 2019;4(5):223–5.
18. Reardon S. Whole-body PET scanner produces 3D images in seconds. Nature. 2019;570(7761):285–6.
19. Wong FC, Boja J, Ho B, Kuhar MJ, Wong DF. Affinity labeling of membrane receptors using tissue-penetrating radiations. Biomed Res Int. 2013;2013:503095.

20. Bellia SR, Feliciani G, Duca MD, Monti M, Turri V, Sarnelli A, et al. Clinical evidence of abscopal effect in cutaneous squamous cell carcinoma treated with diffusing alpha emitters radiation therapy: a case report. J Contemp Brachytherapy. 2019;11(5):449–57.
21. Brix N, Tiefenthaller A, Anders H, Belka C, Lauber K. Abscopal, immunological effects of radiotherapy: narrowing the gap between clinical and preclinical experiences. Immunol Rev. 2017;280(1):249–79.
22. Bonvalot S, Rutkowski PL, Thariat J, Carrere S, Ducassou A, Sunyach MP, et al. NBTXR3, a first-in-class radioenhancer hafnium oxide nanoparticle, plus radiotherapy versus radiotherapy alone in patients with locally advanced soft-tissue sarcoma (Act.In.Sarc): a multicentre, phase 2–3, randomised, controlled trial. Lancet Oncol. 2019;20(8):1148–59.
23. Pottier A, Borghi E, Levy L. New use of metals as nanosized radioenhancers. Anticancer Res. 2014;34(1):443–53.
24. Deagostino A, Protti N, Alberti D, Boggio P, Bortolussi S, Altieri S, et al. Insights into the use of gadolinium and gadolinium/boron-based agents in imaging-guided neutron capture therapy applications. Future Med Chem. 2016;8(8):899–917.
25. Yeh CN, Chang CW, Chung YH, Tien SW, Chen YR, Chen TW, et al. Synthesis and characterization of boron fenbufen and its F-18 labeled homolog for boron neutron capture therapy of COX-2 overexpressed cholangiocarcinoma. Eur J Pharm Sci. 2017;107:217–29.

Index

A
Adenosine triphosphate (ATP), 10
Afterloader, 56
17-Allylamino-17demethoxygeldanamycin
(17-AAG), 209, 210
Alpha emitters, 65–67
LET, 64
American College of Radiology (ACR), 233
Animal tumor models
biodistribution studies, 190
B16-OVA tumor in C57BL/6 mice, 169
breast cancer in F344 rat
differential intramuscular retention, 161
GIMA, 164
HSA, 163
indium-111 DTPA, 164–166
intervention schemes, 162
nonradioactive deoxyglucose, 164
oral Lugol solution, 164
radiopharmaceuticals, 161
residence time, 161
serial images, 161
tumor growth suppression, 161
yttrium-90 chloride, 166, 169
cTVT tumors in dogs, 169–171, 174
diagnostic and therapeutic use, 210, 211
bone cancer, 215, 216
CTVT, 212
imaging types, 210, 211
prostate cancer, 214, 215
qualities, 211
radiolabeled antibodies, 213, 214
thyroid tumors, 214
tissue distribution, 212
early studies, 190
image guidance, 182
immune system activation, 177, 180
interventional schemes, 182
intratumoural injections, 160
molecular properties, 182
optical imaging, 174–177
radioisotopes, 191
radiopharmaceuticals, 182
rats and mice experiments, 160, 161
rodent models
brain cancer, 191–194
breast cancer, 194–197
colorectal cancer, 210
head and neck cancers, 208, 209
liver cancer, 206–208
lung cancer, 209, 210
malignant melanoma, 198–201
pancreatic cancer, 204–206
prostate cancer, 201–204
sample sizes estimation, 161
treatment strategy, 190
Antibody-drug conjugates (ADC), 28
Atomic Energy Commission (AEC), 227
Attenuation correction (AC), 137
Authorized User (AU), 226

B
Background compensation (BC)
method, 140
Barcelona Clinic Liver Cancer (BCLC)
staging, 94
Bladder cancer, epidemiology, 5
Bone cancer, rodent animal models, 215, 216
Brachytherapy, 54–56
BRAF V600 mutations, 27
Brain cancer, rodent animal models, 191–194

F. C. L. Wong (ed.), *Locoregional Radionuclide Cancer Therapy*,
https://doi.org/10.1007/978-3-030-56267-0

Breast cancer
  detection, 11
  epidemiology, 2, 3
  rodent animal models, 194–197
Buthus martensii Karsch chlorotoxin (BMK CT), 192

C
Cancer treatment
  locoregional treatment modalities
    interventional radiology, 23, 24
    radiation therapy, 22, 23
    surgery, 18–21
  multimodal approach, 17, 18
  systemic treatments
    cytotoxic chemotherapy, 25, 26
    drug development, 24
    hormonal therapy, 26, 27
    immunotherapy, 29–32
    normal/vital structures, 24
    targeted therapy, 27–29
Canine transmissible tumor model, 117, 118
Canine transmissible venereal tumor (CTVT), 169–171, 174, 212
Centers for Medicare and Medicaid Services (CMS), 238
Cervical cancer, epidemiology, 4
Chimeric-antigen receptor T (CART), 29
Clinical Research Committee (CRC), 243
Clinical target volume, 45
Clinical tumor volumes (CTV), 119
Code of Federal Regulations (CFR), 228
Collimator-detector response (CDR), 137
Colon cancer, detection, 11
Colorectal cancer
  epidemiology, 3, 4
  rodent animal models, 210
Complete response (CR) rate, 78
Compounded sterile preparations (CSPs), 236
Conditions of Participation (CoP), 238
Cryoablation (CYA), 97
Current good manufacturing practice (cGMP), 239
Cyclopamine (CPA), 194

D
Defense strategies, 11–13
Dendritic cells (DCs), 199, 200
Department of Transportation (DOT), 231, 232
Depth dosimetry (DD)
  biodistribution, 119, 120
  estimation, 117
  interpolation and extrapolation, 117
  micrometastases, 119
  nonspherical masses, 119
  peripheral distribution model, 116
  ranges, 117
  target tumor volumes, 119
  uniform distribution model, 114, 115
  variations, 117
Differential toxicity, 11–13
Differentiated thyroid cancers (DTC), 72, 73
  epidemiology, 5
Dimethyl sulfoxide (DMSO), 202
Disability-adjusted life years (DALY), 2
Drug-eluting beads (DEB-TACE), 92

E
Effective source scatter estimation (ESSE), 137
Elastin-like polypeptides (ELPs), 208
Environmental Protection Agency (EPA), 231
Expanded access protocols, 240
External beam radiation therapy (EBRT)
  breathing cycle, 45
  CTV, 45
  electron therapy
    skin ailments, 43
    steep dose falloff, 43
    superficial lesions, 43
  GTV, 45
  IMRT, 47, 49, 50
  ITV, 45
  OAR, 45, 46
  overview, 43
  proton therapy, 53, 54
  SBRT, 51–53
  2D radiation, 44, 45
  3D conformal radiation, 45
  4D-CT capturing, 45

F
Female nude mice, 208
Filtered backprojection (FBP) method, 137
5-Fluorouracil (5-FU), 26
Food and Drug Administration (FDA), 228–230, 238, 239
Food, Drug and Cosmetic Act (FDCA), 230

G
Gallium iron macroaggregates (GIMA), 117, 118, 164
Gastrin-releasing peptide receptor (GRPR) antagonist, 81
Gold nanoparticles, 196
Gross tumor volumes (GTV), 45, 119

H
Head and neck cancer
  epidemiology, 5
  rodent animal models, 208, 209
Hepatic artery infusion chemotherapy (HAIC), 91
Hepatic tumors
  ablation, 97–99
  HAIC, 91
  intra-arterial treatments for, 90, 91
  percutaneous thermal ablation, 96, 97
  TACE, 91–93
  TARE, 94–96
Hepatocellular carcinoma cells (HepG2), 206
High-dose-rate (HDR), 55, 56, 120–122
High-specific-activity (HSA), 64
Hodgkin's lymphoma, 5
Human epidermal growth factor 2 (HER2), 2
Human serum albumin (HSA), 163

I
^{131}I gelatin microspheres (^{131}I-GMSs), 206
Image-guided IMRT (IG-IMRT), 50
I MIBG (metaiodobenzylguanidine), 68
Institutional Review Board (IRB), 242–245
Intensity-modulated radiation therapy (IMRT), 22, 47, 49, 50
Internal Review Board (IRB), 240
Internal target volume (ITV), 45
Internal tumor volume (ITP), 119
Interpolated analytical photon distribution (APDI), 138
Investigational Device Exemption (IDE), 250
Investigational New Drug (IND), 230
  Application, 239, 240
  pathway, 250
^{131}I sodium iodide (NaI), 68

L
LDR, *see* Low-dose-rate (LDR)
Leukemia, epidemiology, 5, 6
Liver cancer
  epidemiology, 4
  rodent animal models, 206–208
Local consolidative therapy, 57
Locoregional radionuclide cancer therapy (LRCT), 13
  animal tumor models (*see* Animal tumor models)
  clinical trials, 260
  depth dosimetry
    biodistribution, 119, 120
    estimation, 117
    interpolation and extrapolation, 117
    micrometastases, 119
    nonspherical masses, 119
    peripheral distribution model, 116
    ranges, 116
    target tumor volumes, 119
    uniform distribution model, 114, 115
    variations, 117
  detection and monitoring, 259
  HDR and LDR, 120–122
  injectate volume, 120
  locoregional toxicity/efficacy, 258, 259
  Monte Carlo radiation transport simulation, 113, 114
  peripheral distribution model, 113
    dimensions, 113
  potential use, 259
  radiation science, 259
  sealed radionuclides, 251, 252
  target dosimetry
    biodistribution, 119, 120
    control of tumors, 119
    estimation, 117
    GIMA, 117, 118
    interpolation and extrapolation, 117
    nonspherical masses, 119
    peripheral distribution model, 116
    target tumor volumes, 119
    uniform distribution model, 114, 115
  treatment modalities, 259
  uniform distribution model, 112
  unsealed radiopharmaceuticals (*see* Unsealed radiopharmaceuticals)
  volume-normalized S-values, 129
Locoregional therapy
  hepatic tumors
    ablation, 97–99
    HAIC, 91
    intra-arterial treatments for, 90, 91
    percutaneous thermal ablation, 96, 97
    TACE, 91–93
    TARE, 94–96

Locoregional therapy (*cont.*)
  musculoskeletal tumor ablation, 101, 102
  pulmonary tumor ablation, 99–101
  renal tumor ablation, 99
Low-dose-rate (LDR), 55, 120–122
Lung cancer
  epidemiology, 3
  rodent animal models, 209, 210
Lymphoma, epidemiology, 5

M
Macroaggregated albumin (MAA), 94
Malignant neoplasms, 2
Maximum a posteriori (MAP), 137
Maximum likelihood expectation maximization (ML-EM), 137
Melanocortin-1 receptor (MC1R), 200
Melanoma, epidemiology, 4
Metastatic castration-resistant prostate cancer (mCRPC), 68
Microcarcinomas, 77
Microwave ablation (MWA), 96, 97
Modular nanotransporter (MNT), 200
Monte Carlo simulation (MCS), 137
  radiation transport simulation, 113, 114
Musculoskeletal tumor, ablation, 101, 102
Myeloma, epidemiology, 5

N
National Association of Boards of Pharmacy (NABP), 236
National Formulary (NF) monographs, 236
Neuroendocrine tumors (NETs), 70, 71, 245
New drug application (NDA) process, 230, 236
Non-Hodgkin's lymphoma, 5
Non-small-cell lung cancer (NSCLC), 3, 57, 209
Nuclear medicine technologists (NMT), 232
Nuclear Regulatory Commission (NRC), 227–229, 235
Nuclear Tumor Vaccine in situ (NuTuVIS), 180
Nude male mice (BALB/c), 207

O
Objective response rate (ORR), 28
Occupational Safety and Health Administration (OSHA), 230, 231
Office of Regulatory Affairs (ORA), 242
Oligometastatic disease, 56, 57
Ordered subset expectation maximization (OS-EM) reconstruction, 137, 138
Organs at risk (OAR), 45, 46
Overall survival (OS), 78

P
Pancreatic cancer
  epidemiology, 4
  rodent animal models, 204–206
Pathologic complete response (pCR), 20
^{32}P BioSilicon, 207
Penalized likelihood function employing CT side information (PL-CT), 138
Peptide receptor radionuclide therapy (PRRT), 63
Peptide receptor scintigraphy (PRS), 63
Peripheral distribution model, 113
  dimensions, 113
  fractional depth dose, 126–127
  ranges, 128–129
  target dose, 125–126
  TD and DD, 116
Perturbation-based geometric transfer matrix (pGTM), 137
Pheochromocytoma, 68
Physician-sponsored IND, 240
Planned tumor volumes, 119
Planning target volume (PTV), 45
Positron emission tomography (PET), 236
Post-treatment inflammation, 11
Precision Oncology, 27
Primary cancer hallmarks
  angiogenesis, 8, 9
  biology and vulnerability, 6
  cancer initiation and development, 6
  growth suppressors evasion, 6, 7
  invasion and metastasis, 8
  programmed cell death, 7
  proliferative signaling, 7, 8
  replicative immortality, 7
Prostate cancer
  epidemiology, 3
  rodent animal models, 201–204, 214, 215
Prostate-specific membrane antigen (PSMA), 82, 133, 201
Pulmonary tumor, ablation, 99–101

R
Radiation Control Program, 234
Radiation Safety Committee (RSC), 226
Radiation Safety (RS) group, 226

Radiation safety officer (RSO), 231
Radioactive Drug Research Committee (RDRC), 241, 242
Radioactive iodine (^{131}I)
  challenges, 79, 80
  clinical care of, 72
  dose administration, 73, 74
  dosimetry based *vs*. empiric prescribed activity, 78, 79
  hyperthyroidism, 75, 77
  incidence-based mortality, 77
  patient stimulation, 75, 76
  recurrence, 73
  screening, 77, 78
  sestamibi uptake, 79
  therapeutic use, 72
  types, 72, 73
Radioactive materials (RAM), 228
Radiobiology
  definition, 39
  DNA damage, 39
  fractionation
    cell cycle, 41, 42
    radiation, 41
    rationale for, 41
    reoxygenation, 41
    repair, 41
    repopulation, 42
  mitosis, 39
  survival curves, 39, 40
Radiofrequency ablation (RFA), 96
Radioimmunotherapy (RIT), 210
Radioisotopes, 191
Radiolabeled lipiodol employing rhenium-188 (^{188}Re-ECD/lipiodol), 207, 208
Radioligand therapy (RLT), 63
Radionuclide therapy
  alpha emitters, 65–67
    LET, 64
    TAT, 64, 68
  beta-emitters, 65–67
    ^{131} I-Bexxar (tositumomab), 70
    NETs, 71
    ^{153}Sm- lexidronam (Quadramet), 69
    ^{89}Sr chloride (Metastron), 69
    ^{90}Y- Zevalin, 69
    challenges, 79, 80
    clinical care of, 72
    dose administration, 73, 74
    dosimetry based *vs*. empiric prescribed activity, 78, 79
    DTC, 72, 73
    hyperthyroidism, 75, 77
    I MIBG, 68
    incidence-based mortality, 77
    Indium-111 (^{111}In), 70, 71
    Lutetium-177 (^{177}Lu-), 71, 72
    NaI, 68
    NETs, 70, 71
    patient stimulation, 75, 76
    phosphorus-32 (^{32}P), 70
    polycythemia vera, 70
    radioiodine, 72
    screening, 77, 78
    serum thyroglobulin, 73
    sestamibi uptake, 79
    TgAb, 73
  clinical trials, 81–83
  locoregional therapy
    ^{32}P- chromic phosphate, 80
    ^{90}Y-Theraspheres and ^{90}Y-SIRSpheres, 81
  theranostics, 61–64
Radiopharmaceuticals
  DOT, 231, 232
  EPA, 231
  FDA, 228–230, 238, 239
  IND, 239, 240
  IRB, 243–245
  NRC, 227–229, 235
  OSHA, 230, 231
  paradigm of, 226
  RDRC, 241, 242
  rules and regulations, 245
  state regulatory agencies
    civil and criminal enforcement, 233
    nuclear pharmacy, 234–237
    RAM inspections, 233, 234
    regulatory scrutiny, 232
    TJC, 238
Radiosurgery, 51
RAM inspections, 233, 234
Renal cell carcinoma (RCC), 99
  epidemiology, 5
Renal tumor ablation, 99

S

Scatter correction (SC), 137
Sealed radionuclides, 251, 252
Secondary cancer hallmarks
  biology and vulnerability, 6
  cellular energetics, 9, 10
  genomic instability and mutation, 10, 11
  immune destruction, 9
  tumor-promoting inflammation, 9

Serum thyroglobulin (Tg), 73
Small-cell lung carcinoma, 3
Sociodemographic index (SDI), 2
Solid tumors, 2
Staging, 11
State Boards of Pharmacy, 236, 237
State Radiation Inspector, 231
Stereotactic ablative radiotherapy (SARS), 22
Stereotactic body radiation therapy (SBRT), 22, 51–53
Stomach cancer, epidemiology, 4

T

Target dosimetry (TD)
- biodistribution, 119, 120
- control of tumors, 119
- estimation, 117
- GIMA, 117, 118
- interpolation and extrapolation, 117
- nonspherical masses, 119
- peripheral distribution model, 116
- target tumor volumes, 119
- uniform distribution model, 114, 115

Targeted alpha therapy (TAT), 64, 68, 198, 199
Targeted radionuclide therapies (TRTs), 63
- accuracy and precision, 136
- bremsstrahlung imaging, 139–141
- gamma camera, 136, 137
- image reconstruction methods, 137
- quantitative SPECT/CT, 137–139, 141–144
- radiopharmaceuticals, 135–136
- spatial distribution of, 133
- 2D absorbed dose information, 134
- 3D dosimetric methods
  - cumulative activity, 148
  - data analysis, 149, 150
  - dose calibration, 144
  - dose conversion, 148, 149
  - dosimetric software, 150, 151
  - image registration, 145–147
  - VOI delineation, 144–146
- uncertainty propagation, 150, 152
- workflow, 134

T cell receptor (TCR), 29
Texas Department of State Health Services (TXDSHS), 233, 234
The Joint Commission (TJC), 238
Thyroglobulin antibodies (TgAb), 73
Thyroid cancer
- radioactive iodine (^{131}I)
  - challenges, 79, 80
  - clinical care of, 72
  - dose administration, 73, 74
  - dosimetry based *vs.* empiric prescribed activity, 78, 79
  - hyperthyroidism, 75, 77
  - incidence-based mortality, 77
  - patient stimulation, 75, 76
  - recurrence, 73
  - screening, 77, 78
  - sestamibi uptake, 79
  - therapeutic use, 72
  - types, 72, 73

Time activity curves (TAC), 142
Transarterial chemoembolization (TACE), 91–93
Transarterial radioembolization (TARE), 94–96
Triple energy window (TEW), 139
Tumor suppressor gene (TSG), 7
Tyrosine kinase inhibitors (TKIs), 28

U

Uniform distribution model, 112
- depth dose fraction, 130–131
- fractional depth dose, 124–125
- ranges, 127–128
- target dose, 123–124
- TD and DD, 114, 115

United States Department of Transportation (USDOT/DOT), 231
United States Pharmacopeia (USP), 236
Unsealed radiopharmaceuticals
- locoregionally administered soluble radiopharmaceuticals, 254–256
- *vs.* sealed radiopharmaceuticals, 255–258
- with tumor affinity, 252, 253
- without tumor affinity, 253, 254

Uterine cancer, epidemiology, 5

V

Volume-of-interest (VOI) delineation, 144–146
Voxel S value (VSV), 148, 149

Y

Years of life lost (YLL), 2

MIX
Papier aus verantwortungsvollen Quellen
Paper from responsible sources
FSC® C105338

If you have any concerns about our products,
you can contact us on
ProductSafety@springernature.com

In case Publisher is established outside the EU,
the EU authorized representative is:
Springer Nature Customer Service Center GmbH
Europaplatz 3, 69115 Heidelberg, Germany

Printed by Libri Plureos GmbH
in Hamburg, Germany